Primary care in the driver's seat?

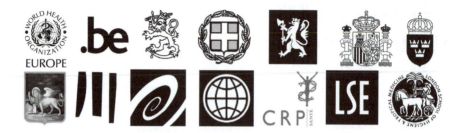

European Observatory on Health Systems and Policies Series
Edited by Josep Figueras, Martin McKee, Elias Mossialos and Richard B. Saltman

Primary care in the driver's seat?

Organizational reform in European primary care

Edited by

**Richard B. Saltman,
Ana Rico and
Wienke G. W. Boerma**

Open University Press

Open University Press
McGraw-Hill Education
McGraw-Hill House
Shoppenhangers Road
Maidenhead
Berkshire
England
SL6 2QL
email: enquiries@openup.co.uk
world wide web: www.openup.co.uk
and Two Penn Plaza, New York, NY 10121–2289, USA

First published 2006

A catalogue record of this book is available from the British Library
ISBN-10 0 335 21365 0 (pb)   0 335 21366 9 (hb)
ISBN-13 978 0 335 21365 8 (pb)   978 0 335 21366 5 (hb)

Library of Congress Cataloging-in-Publication Data
CIP data applied for

Typset by RefineCatch Limited, Bungay, Suffolk
Printed in the UK by Bell & Bain Ltd, Glasgow

European Observatory on Health Systems and Policies Series

The European Observatory on Health Systems and Policies is a unique project that builds on the commitment of all its partners to improving health care systems:

- World Health Organization Regional Office for Europe
- Government of Belgium
- Government of Finland
- Government of Greece
- Government of Norway
- Government of Spain
- Government of Sweden
- Veneto Region
- European Investment Bank
- Open Society Institute
- World Bank
- CRP-Santé Luxembourg
- London School of Economics and Political Science
- London School of Hygiene and Tropical Medicine

The series

The volumes in this series focus on key issues for health policy-making in Europe. Each study explores the conceptual background, outcomes and lessons learned about the development of more equitable, more efficient and more effective health systems in Europe. With this focus, the series seeks to contribute to the evolution of a more evidence-based approach to policy formulation in the health sector.

These studies will be important to all those involved in formulating or evaluating national health care policies and, in particular, will be of use to health policy-makers and advisers, who are under increasing pressure to rationalize the structure and funding of their health system. Academics and students in the field of health policy will also find this series valuable in seeking to understand better the complex choices that confront the health systems of Europe.

The Observatory supports and promotes evidence-based health policy-making through comprehensive and rigorous analysis of the dynamics of health care systems in Europe.

Series Editors

Josep Figueras is Head of the Secretariat and Research Director of the European Observatory on Health Systems and Policies, and Head of the European Centre for Health Policy, World Health Organization Regional Office for Europe.

Martin McKee is Research Director of the European Observatory on Health Systems and Policies and Professor of European Public Health at the London School of Hygiene and Tropical Medicine as well as a co-director of the School's European Centre on Health of Societies in Transition.

Elias Mossialos is Research Director of the European Observatory on Health Systems and Policies, and Brian Abel-Smith Reader in Health Policy, Department of Social Policy, London School of Economics and Political Science and co-director of LSE Health and Social Care.

Richard B. Saltman is Research Director of the European Observatory on Health Systems and Policies, and Professor of Health Policy and Management at the Rollins School of Public Health, Emory University in Atlanta, Georgia.

European Observatory on Health Systems and Policies Series

Series Editors: Josep Figueras, Martin McKee, Elias Mossialos and Richard B. Saltman

Published titles

Health policy and European Union enlargement
Martin McKee, Laura MacLehose and Ellen Nolte (eds)

Regulating entrepreneurial behaviour in European health care systems
Richard B. Saltman, Reinhard Busse and Elias Mossialos (eds)

Social health insurance systems in Western Europe
Richard B. Saltman, Reinhard Busse and Josep Figueras (eds)

Health care in Central Asia
Martin McKee, Judith Healy and Jane Falkingham (eds)

Hospitals in a changing Europe
Martin McKee and Judith Healy (eds)

Funding health care: options for Europe
Elias Mossialos, Anna Dixon, Josep Figueras and Joe Kutzin (eds)

Regulating pharmaceuticals in Europe: striving for efficiency, equity and quality
Elias Mossialos, Monique Mrazek and Tom Walley (eds)

Purchasing to improve health systems performance
Joseph Figueras, Ray Robinson and Elke Jakubowski (eds)

Forthcoming titles

Mental health policy and practice across Europe
Martin Knapp, David McDaid, Elias Mossialos and Graham Thornicroft (eds)

Human resources for health in Europe
Carl-Ardy Dubois, Martin McKee and Ellen Nolte (eds)

Contents

List of tables

List of boxes

List of plates & figures

Plates (these appear in the plate section)

Figures

List of contributors

Richard Baker is Professor and Head of the Department of Health Sciences at the University of Leicester in Leicester, United Kingdom.

Sven-Eric Bergman is Consultant in Health Policy and Management at Bergman and Dahlbäck AB in Stockholm, Sweden.

Wienke G. W. Boerma is Senior Researcher at NIVEL (The Netherlands Institute for Health Services Research) in Utrecht, Netherlands.

Mats Brommels is Professor of Health Services Management at the University of Helsinki, and Professor and Director of the Medical Management Centre at the Karolinska Institute in Stockholm, Sweden.

Michael Calnan is Professor of Medical Sociology at the Department of Social Medicine of the University of Bristol, United Kingdom.

Diana M. J. Delnoij is Senior Research Coordinator at NIVEL in Utrecht, Netherlands.

Anna Dixon is Lecturer in European Health Policy at the Department of Social Policy, London School of Economics and Political Science in London, United Kingdom.

Carl-Ardy Dubois is Assistant Professor at the University of Montreal (Canada) in the Faculty of Nursing Sciences.

Joan Gené-Badia is Family Doctor in the Castelldefels Primary Care Team at the Catalan Institute of Health in Barcelona, Spain.

Bernhard Gibis is Director of the Department of Quality Assurance at the National Association of Statutory Health Insurance Physicians (KBV) in Berlin, Germany.

Stefan Greß is Assistant Professor at the Institute of Health Care Management of the University of Duisburg-Essen in Essen, Germany.

Peter P. Groenewegen is Research Department Head at NIVEL and Professor of Social and Geographical Aspects of Health and Health Care at Utrecht University in Utrecht, Netherlands.

Jan Heyrman is Professor and Director of the Department of General Practice at the Catholic University Leuven (KULeuven) in Leuven, Belgium.

Jack Hutten was Research Coordinator at NIVEL in Utrecht, Netherlands. At present Senior Policy Advisor at the Curative Care Department of the Ministry of Health, Welfare and Sports in The Hague, Netherlands.

Michael Kidd is Professor and Head of the Discipline of General Practice at the University of Sydney, and President of The Royal Australian College of General Practitioners in Sydney, Australia.

Mårten Kvist is Director of the Laitila-Pyhäranta Health Centre in Laitila, Finland.

Miranda Laurant is Senior Researcher at the Centre for Quality of Care Research of the Universities of Nijmegen and Maastricht in Nijmegen, Netherlands.

Margus Lember is Professor and Head of the Department of Internal Medicine at the University of Tartu in Tartu, Estonia.

Martin Marshall is General Practitioner and Professor of General Practice at the National Primary Care Research and Development Centre of the University of Manchester in Manchester, United Kingdom.

Alison McCallum is Research Fellow, Outcomes and Equity Research, National Research and Development Centre for Welfare and Health (STAKES) in Helsinki, Finland, and Associate Professor at the Medical Management Centre of the Karolinska Institute in Stockholm, Sweden.

Toomas Palu is Senior Health Specialist at the Europe and Central Asia Development Department of the World Bank in Washington DC, USA.

Ana Rico is Associate Professor of Health Politics and Policy at the Department of Health Management and Economics of the University of Oslo, Norway.

Ray Robinson is Professor of Health Policy at the Health and Social Care Centre of the London School of Economics and Political Science in London, United Kingdom.

Valentin Rusovich is General Practitioner, Chairman of the Belarussian Associ-ation of General Practitioners and GP-teacher at the Department of General Practice of the Belarussian Medical Academy for Continuous Medical Education (BelMAPO), Department of General Practice in Minsk, Belarus.

Richard B. Saltman is Professor of Health Policy and Management at the Rollins School of Public Health, Emory University in Atlanta, USA, and Research Director of the European Observatory on Health Systems and Policies.

Anthony Scott is Reader in Health Economics at the Health Economics Research Unit of the University of Aberdeen in Aberdeen, United Kingdom.

Rod Sheaff is Senior Research Fellow at the National Primary Care Research and Development Centre of Manchester University in Manchester, United Kingdom.

Bonnie Sibbald is Professor of Health Services Research at the National Primary Care Research and Development Centre of the University of Manchester in Manchester, United Kingdom.

Igor Švab is Professor and Head of the Department of Family Medicine at the University of Ljubljana, Slovenia.

Hrvoje Tiljak is Senior Lecturer at the Andrija Štampar School of Public Health in Zagreb, Croatia.

Michel Wensing is Senior Lecturer at the Centre for Quality of Care Research of the Universities of Nijmegen and Maastricht in Nijmegen, Netherlands.

Series editors' introduction

European national policy makers broadly agree on the core objectives that their health care systems should pursue. The list is strikingly straightforward: universal access for all citizens, effective care for better health outcomes, efficient use of resources, high-quality services and responsiveness to patient concerns. It is a formula that resonates across the political spectrum and which, in various, sometimes inventive, configurations, has played a role in most recent European national election campaigns.

Yet this clear consensus can only be observed at the abstract policy level. Once decision makers seek to translate their objectives into the nuts and bolts of health system organization, common principles rapidly devolve into divergent, occasionally contradictory, approaches. This is, of course, not a new phenomenon in the health sector. Different nations, with different histories, cultures and political experiences, have long since constructed quite different institutional arrangements for funding and delivering health care services.

The diversity of health system configurations that has developed in response to broadly common objectives leads quite naturally to questions about the advantages and disadvantages inherent in different arrangements, and which approach is 'better' or even 'best' given a particular context and set of policy priorities. These concerns have intensified over the last decade as policy makers have sought to improve health system performance through what has become a Europe-wide wave of health system reforms. The search for comparative advantage has triggered – in health policy as in clinical medicine – increased attention to its knowledge base, and to the possibility of overcoming at least part of existing institutional divergence through more evidence-based health policy making.

The volumes published in the European Observatory on Health Systems and Policies series are intended to provide precisely this kind of cross-national health policy analysis. Drawing on an extensive network of experts and policy makers working in a variety of academic and administrative capacities, these studies seek to synthesize the available evidence on key health sector topics using a systematic methodology. Each volume explores the conceptual background, outcomes and lessons learned about the development of more equitable, more efficient and more effective health care systems in Europe. With this focus, the series seeks to contribute to the evolution of a more evidence-based approach to policy formulation in the health sector. While remaining sensitive to cultural, social and normative differences among countries, the studies explore a range of policy alternatives available for future decision making. By examining closely both the advantages and disadvantages of different policy approaches, these volumes fulfil central mandates of the Observatory: to serve as a bridge between pure academic research and the needs of policy makers, and to stimulate the development of strategic responses suited to the real political world in which health sector reform must be implemented.

The European Observatory on Health Systems and Policies is a partnership that brings together three international agencies, six national governments, a region of Italy, two research institutions and an international nongovernmental organization. The partners are as follows: the World Health Organization Regional Office for Europe, which provides the Observatory secretariat; the governments of Belgium, Finland, Greece, Norway, Spain and Sweden; the Veneto Region; the European Investment Bank; the Open Society Institute; the World Bank; the London School of Hygiene and Tropical Medicine and the London School of Economics and Political Science.

In addition to the analytical and cross-national comparative studies published in this Open University Press series, the Observatory produces Health Care Systems in Transition (HiTs) profiles for the countries of Europe, the journal *EuroHealth* and the newsletter *EuroObserver*. Further information about Observatory publications and activities can be found on its web site, www.observatory.dk.

Josep Figueras, Martin McKee, Elias Mossialos and Richard B. Saltman

Foreword

Primary care in Europe has grown dramatically in scope and respect over the past several decades. This reflects a concerted effort by academics, policy-makers, and national and international organizations to move primary care, as a core component of primary health care, into the centre of health system decision-making and responsibility. While the process has taken on different forms in different countries, the underlying goal has been broadly similar.

This process of organizational change has been a difficult and complicated exercise. In varying degrees, it has involved developing new and more balanced relationships between hospital and primary care, between specialist and general practitioner, between primary care and home care, and, in a number of environments, between inpatient and outpatient forms of care. These types of fundamental organizational adjustments are, by their very nature, long-term endeavours. Progress must be counted in years and requires focused and persistent efforts from key actors.

This study serves as a status report on this process of organizational change. Drawing on a broad range of information and perspectives, it charts primary care's progress to date in achieving what are important health policy objectives for all of Europe's health care systems. This progress is particularly notable in the recent rapid proliferation of innovative mechanisms such as care networks for the chronically ill and the elderly, and continuing experimentation with new funding instruments to support and extend these networks.

The assessment provided in this volume closely follows the view of many national policy-makers that Europe is in a period of extensive innovation in primary care. This intellectual and organizational ferment, if sustained, can help close the gap between the expectations of health policy-makers about the major role that primary care should play, on the one hand, and the day-to-day performance of real health systems, on the other hand.

There are, to be certain, additional dilemmas that still remain to be addressed. As the study rightly notes, some of the most important decisions about how primary care can best be institutionalized within modern health care systems – in particular the title's question as to whether primary care ought to be in the health system's 'driver's seat' – have yet to be determined. These decisions, and the associated issues that go with them, will continue to be a central focus of policy-making activity across Europe. Despite the undeniable reality that primary care has come a long way from where it began in the 1970s, there remains a great deal of work to be done if it is to achieve its full promise. In outlining the extent of the overall progress that primary care has accomplished to date, the reform innovations currently underway, and the complex issues yet to be resolved, this volume provides both policy-makers and scholars with a valuable perspective on this very important effort.

Marc Danzon
WHO Regional Director for Europe

Acknowledgements

The editors are grateful for generous contributions made to this project by numerous individuals and organizations. We are heavily indebted to our chapter authors, whose commitment of both time and knowledge made this study possible. We also thank John Wyn Owen and the Nuffield Trust for Research and Policy Studies in Health Services for their support, and for their superb hosting of the author's workshop on 21–22 May 2002 in London. Additional thanks are due to the external experts who joined us for that workshop: Martin Roland, Mikko Vienonen, Milagros Garcia-Barbero, Oliver Gröne, and Philippe Duprat. The final volume benefited greatly from the extensive comments on an early draft by four external reviewers: Allen Hutchinson, Chris van Weel, Leon Epstein, and Josep Goicoechea. Valuable suggestions for revision were made on the first three chapters by staff members at NIVEL.

Expert research and editorial support was provided by the Observatory team in Madrid – Hans Dubois, Marikay McCabe, and Wendy Wisbaum – with additional typing support from Charlotte Brandigi in Atlanta. Coordination with Open University Press/McGraw-Hill Education on the delivery and production process was provided by Francine Raveney and Nicole Satterley.

part one

Assessing the strategic landscape

chapter one

Coordination and integration in European primary care

Wienke G. W. Boerma

A book on stronger primary care

The title of this book appears to imply that the current driver of the health care system is not doing a satisfactory job and should be replaced by primary care. Indeed, it may be that in a number of European countries the provision of health care to patients is inadequately steered, but this is likely due to the fact that, too often, there seems to be nobody behind the wheel. This situation is not new. In the 1970s and 1980s, countries sought with varying degrees of success to make health services more efficient and more coherent (Abel-Smith and Mossialos, 1994; Maynard and Bloor, 1995; Saltman and Figueras, 1997). Several decades later, insufficient coherence and coordination in health care are still considered the main causes of lack of responsiveness to the needs of the population. Experience in several countries indicates that this problem can be tackled at the point where patients normally enter the health care system, where the scope of the patients' health problems is examined and where decisions are made about other possible providers to involve: that is, in primary care (WHO, 2002). Strengthening primary care by extending the skill mix or giving primary care control over other levels of care is often mentioned as key to the solution (Starfield and Shi, 2002). How feasible are these ambitions in the current health care context in Europe, which is extremely heterogeneous, particularly with regard to primary care? What are the conditions for strong primary care and what is known about effective measures and strategies? Although the organization and provision of health care are still largely a national affair, European integration has led to higher interest in foreign experiences in the field of health system development as the basis of policy-making (WHO, 2002).

The aim of this book is to consider the extent to which strengthening primary care can be a suitable strategy to improve the overall coherence in health care and to explore the conditions and instruments that fit into this strategy. The "driver's seat" in the book's title refers to the coordination and navigation function, for which primary care may have considerable potential. After completing our exploration we maintain the question mark in the title, however, because the answer is not unequivocal. The character and conditions of primary care in Europe are so diverse that a general judgement about the suitability of primary care for coordination and navigation is hard to make.

This volume explores the different approaches to primary care found across Europe and examines the success of different strategic alternatives in its design and operation. In this introductory chapter, we set the conceptual stage for the more detailed assessments that follow. We begin by examining the central issue of health system coherence and coordination, and assessing the role that primary care might play in resolving this dilemma. Drawing on this analysis, we then develop a working definition of primary care, which, in turn, serves as the basis for Chapter Two's subsequent mapping of primary care resources across the European region.

The problem

Despite constantly rising health expenditures in European countries, the health needs of growing subgroups of the population, such as the chronically ill, the elderly and those in need of hospice services in their homes, are not well met (McKee and Healy, 2001). Over the past years these needs have changed quantitatively and qualitatively and they will continue to do so, as a result of the epidemiological transition related to the ageing of populations and the general increase in wealth in most countries. Larger proportions of patients suffer from more than one disease and receive a mix of health (and social) care provided by several workers from different disciplines at the same time (Van den Akker *et al.*, 1998; Menotti *et al.*, 2001; Westert *et al.*, 2001). Such complex needs often are not adequately dealt with by a health care system which itself has also become much more complex. The inadequacy may result not only in unmet needs, but also in unnecessary treatments, medicalization and other threats to patients' safety. The increased system complexity is a side effect of specialization and sub-specialization in health care, by which professional "inward-directedness" has tended to grow at the expense of attention to integration with other disciplines. The implementation of new care arrangements, such as those based on shared care, substitution and teamwork, is hampered by this fragmentation. More coordination will be needed to offer users of complex care the guidance and navigation to find their way through the system. Problems of coordination are likely to arise at key interfaces: between primary and secondary care, between curative care and public health services, and between specialities within particular subsectors (Renders *et al.*, 2001; Faulkner *et al.*, 2003; Rat *et al.*, 2004).

Another development that underlines the need for more coherence and coordination is the growing importance of anticipatory medicine and prevention. These are expected to bring further population health gain in terms of quality of life and life expectancy. Health care may be increasingly asked to look actively and systematically for conditions in their early stages and to identify factors that are known to be health risks. Screening, monitoring and follow-up, which are still relatively new tasks in primary care, can only be carried out effectively by the coordinated the efforts of various professional groups on the basis of information concerning the population they serve (Isles *et al.*, 2000; Murchie *et al.*, 2003; Oakeshott *et al.*, 2003; Campbell, 2004). Where preventive interventions already go beyond the boundaries of standard health care, extended coordination will be needed to include other sectors such as social services or education.

The pressures for change originate not only from public dissatisfaction about poor responsiveness of health care and the need to find effective ways of promoting health and preventing disease. Policy-makers, financers and others responsible for health care expenditure have long worried about the growing costs of health care (Abel-Smith, 1992; OECD, 1995). They are looking for incentives and mechanisms to enhance accountability and the awareness among health care providers of the common goal of efficiency. Currently, there is demand for reform measures that can improve coordination across health systems as well as stimulate a more efficient use of resources. Thus, current pressures go beyond the more targeted cost-containment measures that were dominant in the 1990s (OECD, 1995; Paton, 2000).

Although analysts tend to view health care as an integrated system, existing arrangements do not always provide a well-organized response to the health problems occurring in a society. The relevant characteristics of a system are not evident: operational goals are not always shared, the division of labour is far from perfect and, due to lack of coordination, the various elements of health care lack coherence (Van der Zee *et al.*, 2004). Poor communication between primary care, hospitals, and medical specialists has been well documented in many health care systems for decades. Similarly, curative health care and public health services are usually worlds apart. Furthermore, status and domain problems may prevent good working relations between doctors and nurses, in particular if the latter are working in separate organizations, such as independent practice and home care organizations (Poulton and West, 1993; Mur-Veeman *et al.*, 2001). Removing these barriers, for instance by creating incentives for teamwork, may improve the quality of care at the individual and facility levels of health care, but may not be sufficient to bring about increased coordination among levels and sectors of care. Other specific measures will be needed to establish new forms of supply that guarantee seamless interfaces, such as chains of care or integrated care networks.

Primary care: features and disciplines

Definitions of primary care are numerous and either more descriptive or normative, depending on the purpose they serve. The normative approach has been closely connected with the WHO Alma Ata Declaration in 1978 on Primary Health Care, in which the focus was on solidarity and equitable access to care; on the protection and promotion of health rather than on curing illness; on more influence of the population on health care instead of professional dominance; and on broad intersectoral collaboration in dealing with community problems (WHO, 1978).

Although the concepts of "primary care" and "primary health care" are often used as synonyms, they represent different aspects of the development and articulation of first level care. The subject of this book is not the broad societal strategy of primary health care as laid out at Alma Ata, but rather the more limited area of primary care as a subset of functions or services delivered specifically within the context of health care systems. Of course, a well-designed primary care sector can also serve broader primary health care goals as well. In the current European context of health care, the concept of primary care can be understood in the following ways: as refering to a level of care between informal care and hospital care; or to a set of functions and activities; or to a means of performing those functions and activities; or to a set of characteristics for the organization of health services (Starfield, 1992, 1998). One consistent thread within these variations is that primary care consists of the professional response when patients make first contact with the health care system. This approach to primary care is considerably broader than the care delivered by a general practitioner or a family doctor, yet is considerably more restricted than the intersectoral concept of primary health care promulgated at Alma Ata. It is precisely this intermediate category, however, which is at the centre of ongoing primary care development in many European countries (see as examples the four boxes in this chapter and Chapter Two) and which is the focal point for efforts to improve coherence and coordination in health care service delivery. For the purposes of this book, we will refer to this intermediate category as 'extended primary care.' As an initial step in the formulation of a working definition, we will address the functions or attributes of extended primary care, since they help identify which patients need adequate help, once they have taken the step to seek professional health care services.

The primary care process

Although the manifestations of primary care in Europe are diverse and the disciplines involved differ, its functions can be identified in most health care systems, although to differing degrees (Boerma, 2003; Raad voor de Volksgezondheid en Zorg, 2004). The most evident primary care function is serving as the point patients receive *first contact* professional care. This point lies at the transition from lay care to professional care, where a general identification of the problem takes place. Information about the previous visits of this patient and his or her medical history is taken into account. It may be necessary then to *clarify the demand*: what does the patient (actually) expect from health care and what are the patient's own options for dealing with the problem? At this stage already, large proportions of demands appear not to need further intervention and it will suffice to give *information, reassurance or advice*, sometimes combined with a follow-up appointment. For other patients a *diagnostic procedure* may be required. Diagnostic examinations will focus particularly on the identification or exclusion of severe illness. The diagnostic phase may be followed by *treatment*. Decisions on treatment are taken together with the patients because their motivation and possibilities are determinants of success. Depending on the kind of treatment it may be necessary to *involve other disciplines*, either in primary care or in secondary care. Involvement may vary from asking for advice to complete referral. If more than one health professional or health care facility is involved in the treatment, *coordination* is needed to avoid duplication and safeguard the *continuity* of the treatment. Closely related to the functions mentioned so far, which mainly apply to curative care, is *prevention* in primary care, which may start from knowledge about patients and their living situation and observations (weight or blood pressure, for instance) made during curative contacts. The preventive function may also extend to groups in the community.

The attributes or functions of primary care have been concisely summarized in the definition of the American Institute of Medicine (Donaldson *et al.*, 1996) referring to "the provision of integrated, accessible health care services by clinicians who are accountable for addressing a large majority of personal health care needs, developing a sustained partnership with patients and practicing in the context of family and community". Needless to say, the functions attributed to primary care may also apply to varying degrees to other levels of care.

Other dimensions

As a *level of care*, primary care is often represented as the base of the pyramid of health care. The middle layer is secondary care while tertiary care is situated at the top of the pyramid. Informal care is an unspecified area below the pyramid. Primary care is the response to unspecified and common health problems accounting for the vast majority of the population's health needs. Problems that require more specialized medical expertise are dealt with in secondary care, in hospitals or the outpatient context, while rare and very complex cases are treated in tertiary care (Fry, 1972). By the *characteristics of their services*, primary care is the kind of care that is ambulatory and directly accessible to patients, with a generalist character, situated in the community that it serves and with a focus on the individual in his or her home situation and social context (Van der Zee, 1989; Gervas *et al.*, 1994). Starfield has defined primary care more in the *content and the range of care*, including its integrative function: those services addressing the most common problems by providing a mix of preventive, curative and rehabilitative services; integrating care when more than one health problem exists, dealing with the context of illness; organizing and rationalizing the deployment of basic and specialized resources (Starfield, 1991).

Primary care is not a discipline itself, but it is provided by professionals with specialized training. Examining health care systems, disciplines can be listed which are, to varying extents, involved in the provision of extended primary care.

Primary care and general practice

A core discipline in primary care is general practice or family medicine. Primary care started to develop in medical territory not occupied by (medical) specialists. As specialization expanded and the number of specialties grew in the second half of the twentieth century, these "residual activities" became labelled as primary care and further developed to become its own specialty. In the Netherlands, for example, primary care was officially identified as a separate echelon in 1974 with the publication of a white paper on the structure of health care. The paper concluded that health care was not coherent, the financing fragmented and that too much emphasis was placed on the inpatient sector. (Ministerie van Volksgezondheid en Milieuhygiëne, 1974). In 1980 another paper, exclusively devoted to primary care, described the features of this echelon, the health professions involved, and launched measures to strengthen primary care (Ministerie van Volksgezondheid en Milieuhygiëne, 1980).

In Europe, primary care is not easily conceptualized without general practice, but these two concepts are not equivalent. The concept of extended primary care, as already noted, encompasses considerably more than general practice alone. How much more varies from one country to another. In those countries where general practice is well developed, the functions and characteristics of primary care largely overlap with those of general practice, and general practice may have a preferred position in primary care. In other countries, directly accessible primary medical care is also provided by specialists, such as paediatricians, gynaecologists, specialists in internal medicine and cardiologists. A definition of the general practitioner (GP), set out more than 30 years ago by the British Royal College of General Practitioners, covers many of these elements. According to this definition, a GP is

> . . . a doctor who provides personal, primary and continuing medical care to individuals and families. He may attend his patients in their own homes, in his consulting room or sometimes in hospital. He accepts the responsibility for making an initial decision on every problem his patient may present to him, consulting with specialists when he thinks it appropriate to do so. He will usually work in a group with other general practitioners, from premises that are built or modified for the purpose, with the help of paramedical colleagues, adequate secretarial staff and all the equipment which is necessary. Even if he is in a single-handed practice, he will work in a team and delegate when necessary. His diagnosis will be composed in physical, psychological and social terms. He will intervene educationally, preventively and therapeutically to promote his patient's health.
>
> (RCGP, 1972)

From this and the many definitions that came after, the following key characteristics of general practice or family medicine can be synthesized. First, it is *generalistic care*, meaning that it deals with the full range of unselected health problems and with all categories of the population, without exclusion on the grounds of age or gender. Second, as the provider of *first contact care*, services are available at all times and at a close proximity, in patients' homes, if necessary. Third, the *orientation to the patients' context* implies that the individuality of a patient is taken into account in the treatment as well as social network and living circumstances. Fourth, the focus is on *continuity*: the interventions are not limited to one episode of care but cover patients' health needs longitudinally. Fifth, *comprehensiveness* refers to the fact that services comprise curative, rehabilitative and supportive care, as well as health promotion and disease prevention. Finally, coordination means that patients are referred to other health professionals if necessary and that health care resources are properly allocated (Leeuwenhorst Group, 1974; WONCA, 1991, 2002; Boerma and Fleming, 1998; Van Weel, 1999; Olesen, 2002; Boerma, 2003). From this characterization, it follows clearly that general practice requires teamwork and collaboration with other disciplines.

Other disciplines in primary care

As in other sectors, the professional division of tasks and specialization have resulted in an increasing number of disciplines working in or with primary care. Obviously, not all characteristics of primary care – for instance the direct accessibility or a general approach – apply equally to all disciplines in every health care system in Europe. Furthermore, disciplines may be involved in primary-care-style activities but in hospitals or nursing homes as well. The typical profile of involvement of various disciplines in primary care is a distinguishing feature of the health care system in a country. In addition to general practice, the health professions outlined below can be regarded as the major providers of primary care (Boerma *et al.*, 1993; Bower and Sibbald, 2004; Pringle and Irvine, 2004; Raad voor de Volksgezondheid en Zorg, 2004).

Nursing is a crucial profession, which currently appears in primary care in various forms (Kinnersley *et al.*, 2000; Temmink *et al.*, 2000; Pringle and Irvine, 2004). The longest tradition involves *community nurses* (or district nurses), who care for patients in the home situation, mostly the very young, the elderly and those with chronic conditions. Examples of this type of care include washing patients, caring for wounds, administering medicines, giving information and support, and technical interventions after hospitalization or in a terminal phase. Psychiatric patients living at home are the target population of *community psychiatric nurses*. Activities of *practice nurses* include health promotion, perinatal care, vaccinations and routine monitoring of the chronically ill in the context of general practice. There is a tendency to involve practice nurses more in patient management (Shum *et al.*, 2000). In addition to the activities of practice nurses, *nurse practitioners* do certain diagnostic procedures and treatments including administering some medication. In addition, other *nurse specialists* are working in primary care teams for particular categories of patients, such as those with diabetes, asthma and coronary heart diseases (Calnan *et al.*, 1994; Vrijhoef, 2002).

The core task of *pharmacists* is to prepare and distribute of medicines prescribed by physicians. The density of pharmacists (and so their competition) varies greatly among European countries. In a number of countries, especially those where patients are usually registered with a pharmacy, providing patients and general practitioners with information has become an important task for pharmacies. Potentially, pharmacies are in a good position to develop a drug-prescribing policy with GPs in their area and to keep a careful watch on the safety of prescriptions (Hughes and McCann, 2003; Muijrers *et al.*, 2004; Silcock *et al.*, 2004). In the Netherlands cooperation between GPs and pharmacists has been strongly promoted since the early 1990s. Nowadays 71% of Dutch GPs have an explicit agreement with a pharmacist concerning their prescription policy. On average, Dutch GPs have meetings with pharmacists for 19 minutes per week (Braspenning *et al.*, 2004).

Physiotherapy is a rapidly growing profession in some countries, particularly in north-western Europe. Physiotherapists treat patients with musculoskeletal problems and they may work in institutions or in the community. In some countries patients may need a referral from a physician to see a physiotherapist (Koster *et al.*, 1991).

Midwifery is usually practiced in a clinical setting, where midwives are involved in prenatal care and deliveries under the supervision of obstetricians. In some countries midwives also work in the community (Page, 2001). In the Netherlands they have a unique position: midwives are responsible for about 40% of all deliveries most of which are at home (Wiegers *et al.*, 1998).

Finally, there are some disciplines with primary care functions although these workers are not always classified as primary care. Most important are *home helpers*, who give personal and domestic assistance, often in situations where community nurses also are involved (Hutten and Kerkstra, 1996). The deployment of the necessary mix of professional knowledge and skills for the specific needs of patients requires cooperation between professionals to ensure that their efforts match recipients' needs. The demand for better coordination in health care refers not just to increased cooperation between sectors or levels of care but also to the situation within primary care, which is considered to be too fragmented.

Vignette 1.1   The Almere experiment[1]

In 1968, the first steps were taken on the newly reclaimed land of "Zuidelijk Flevoland". In a part of this vast new polder, not far from Amsterdam, a new town was planned. In 1978, the first inhabitants entered their houses. Now, Almere has 165,000 inhabitants, with an average annual increase of 6500.

In the time that Almere was on the drawing boards, white papers were published about the urgent need to strengthen the Dutch primary care system to meet changing patient demand and to reduce the need for secondary care. There was a lack of coherence and coordination between specializations that led to fragmentation in primary care. At that time, GPs were private entrepreneurs mainly working in solo practice. Although the concept of integrated multidisciplinary health centres had been implemented in new housing estates, large-scale systemic change appeared to be very difficult.

Almere became a challenge to design a well-developed coherent system of primary care with a minimum amount of secondary level facilities. Supported by the authorities, a group of young health care workers, in collaboration with groups of active citizens, took the initiative in 1979 to start the Almere health care experiment, with the objective of avoiding the problems and shortcomings of the existing Dutch arrangements. Instead of care provided by individual private practiotners, integrated health centres would have a variety of professionals working in collaboration for the benefit of the population within well-defined catchment areas. Since the traditional combination of entrepreneur and caregiver was seen to be potentially confusing, a foundation was created to employ all GPs, physiotherapists, pharmacists, dentists, midwives and auxilliary staff. Later, social workers and community nurses were also employed by this foundation. GPs provided comprehensive services including first aid, minor surgery, child health care and major parts of ophthalmology. The goal was to reduce referrals to medical specialists. The use of antibiotics, particularly by children, was to be reduced, as were tonsillectomies. Furthermore, it was mandated that there would be at least one female GP in every health centre, so that patients who so wished could choose a female doctor.

From 1983 until 1992, the experiment had the legal status of a formal project, with special funding and regulations intended to establish new types of health care workers. One result of the Almere philosophy was that a small hospital was not opened until 1991. In the course of those years the use of hospital services was indeed lower. GPs and hospital specialists developed an intensive collaboration in a structural working group. A similar working relationship was established with a psychiatric centre that opened in 1997. In 1999, the foundation for primary care in Almere (EVA) merged with the organization running the nursing home and homes for the elderly.

The experiment has been successful in many regards as it has created a strong local network of health centres. Evaluation has shown that referral rates were lower than the national average, particularly when the age structure of the population was taken into account. Citizens of Almere are satisfied with the services and more than elsewhere health centres are involved in public health.

On the other hand, there have also been some setbacks. Most inhabitants of Almere previously lived in the old quarters of Amsterdam. They brought with them a pattern of expectations and health care consumption that was not always in line with the ideals of their new GP. These ideals may have suffered in the negotiation of this new healthcare strategy. The experiment also evolved in other respects as time went by. Those who subsequently worked for the Almere experiment were less idealistic and more pragmatic. They achieved an umbrella organization in Almere with working conditions that were still hard to realize elsewhere in the country.

There were three priorities that were central to the Almere experiment: teamwork, working part-time and delegation of tasks. In the Netherlands most professionals are not well prepared for teamwork because each profession fears losing their independence. In Almere, teamwork is the core of primary care provision and for many health care workers this was a reason to choose to work there. Newly attracted staff need to be trained for the working arrangements in the health centres. There has been much resistance in general practice concerning working part-time because it was seen as a threat to the concepts of personal, integral and continuous care. However, with the expanding proportion of female GPs in the Netherlands, there was a growing need for part-time work. At an early stage, these conflicting needs were reconciled in Almere. The result is that now 50% of the GPs in Almere are female, whereas the national proportion is 28%. Task delegation has also been well developed in Almere. Substitution has been realized between secondary care and primary care, but also within primary care. Some traditional GP tasks, for instance in care for the chronically ill and elderly, are now being delegated to newly introduced nurse practitioners and other staff. In Almere these changes have been implemented without fear of losing status in the health care market.

Recently, there have been additional innovations. GP service during evenings, nights and weekends has been reorganized. There is a better-equipped and staffed central GP facility for out-of-hours services for the city. Physiotherapy is becoming increasingly involved in guidance and follow-up with patients at risk of heart disease, the overweight and those with chronic diseases. Most physiotherapists have specialized in manual therapy, child physiotherapy or sport injuries. The supply of social services work has been extended with the introduction of primary care psychologists.

Almere is no longer an experiment, nor is it mainstream primary care in the Netherlands. Due to its special structure and its special population of health care workers, it is easier to implement changes, such that it will continue to be a model within the Dutch health care system.

Continuity of care

Continuity is the degree to which a series of discrete health care events is experienced as coherent and connected, and is consistent with the patient's medical needs and personal context (Haggerty *et al.*, 2003). Essential in this definition is the personal perspective of the patient: continuity is what patients perceive. Coordination and teamwork is what providers do for the benefit of continuity. In primary care, continuity is usually seen as the continued relationship between a patient and a particular provider – rather than a team – beyond care episodes. This is also referred to as personal continuity (Hjortdahl and Borchgrevink, 1991; Hjortdahl, 2004). However, the sense of affiliation between patient and caregiver is stronger in general practice than in some other professions, such as nursing, where a consistent approach is emphasized by the transfer of information. In addition to the personal perspective of a single patient, the second key element of continuity is longitudinality (Schers, 2004). The time frame may be relatively short, for instance an episode of care, or much longer, such as a long-standing relationship between patient and GP. Depending on the type of provider and the context of care, Haggerty *et al.* (2003) distinguish three types of continuity: informational, managerial and relational.

Informational continuity is the use of information, either documented or in the memory of providers, on past events and personal circumstances, to make current care appropriate for the individual. Information links care from one provider to another and from one event of care to another. *Managerial* continuity is the consistent and coherent approach of several professions to the management of health conditions (especially if chronic or complex) that is responsive to a patient's changing needs. Continuity is achieved if services are delivered in a complementary and timely manner, for instance by means of protocols. *Relational* continuity is the ongoing therapeutic relationship between patient and provider(s). Continuity is a quality relevant to care at different levels: in the relationship between patient and provider; among providers of one discipline; between disciplines and between organizations, levels or sectors of care. In the context of this book, informational continuity and managerial continuity are most relevant.

Coordination, teamwork, integration

When more than one provider is involved in administering care to an individual patient, some form of coordination will be necessary to realize continuity. The degree of coordination needed in specific situations depends on the complexity of the case and the options open to the patient. The conceptual framework developed by Boon *et al.* (2004) has distinguished seven models of care provision on the continuum between strict solo provision on the one hand and full integration of disciplines for the provision of curative, rehabilitative and preventive services on the other. In the non-coordination model, called *parallel practice*, practitioners work independently and carry out a formally defined set of services. In *consultative practice*, information concerning particular patients is shared informally and on a case-by-case basis. In the *coordinated* model, the communication and exchange of patient records is related to particular diseases or therapies and is based on a formal administrative structure; a case coordinator monitors the transfer of information. More articulated, more formalized and usually more numerous is the *multidisciplinary team*, led by a team leader and possibly sub-teams and sub-team coordinators. When members of a team start making group decisions or developing shared care policy, facilitated by regular face-to-face meetings, the multidisciplinary team has become an *interdisciplinary team*. Finally, the model of *integrative team care* is reached if the interdisciplinary team, based on a shared vision, provides 'a seamless continuum of decision making and patient-centred care and support' (Boon *et al.*, 2004).

A major reason why health care and primary care are still neither very coherent, nor very cost-effective, and why curative and preventive services are still too separate, is that coordination and teamwork are difficult to achieve. The success of new arrangements – such as shared care or several forms of substitution within primary care or between primary and secondary care – depends on cooperation and teamwork. The extensive literature on multidisciplinary collaboration has described the obstacles that have to be overcome. In addition to basic problems, related to differences in social status, employment, education, power and gender (Mur-Veeman *et al.*, 2001), there is little evidence on what the optimum model of collaboration looks like and how effective teams should be led. And even if teams work effectively it should not be assumed that it is automatically cheaper (Wolters *et al.*, 2004). It may be concluded that improving the collaboration and teamwork in primary care requires a multifaceted approach from decision-makers, management and health care workers (Poulton and West, 1993; West and Slater, 1996; Winkler, 2000). Health care systems in Europe differ considerably as far as the degree to which this has been successful is concerned (Boerma and Fleming, 1998). Not surprisingly, in countries with strong primary care systems there has been relatively greater attention paid to the development of collaboration and teamwork in primary care and to the smoothening of the interface between primary care and secondary care (Van Weel, 1994; Busby *et al.*, 1999; Temmink *et al.*, 2000; Iliffe *et al.*, 2002; Brown *et al.*, 2003; Rummary and Colemen, 2003). These experiences may be useful to further developing primary care in other countries.

Working definition

In the previous sections, primary care has been considered from several points of view. This has clarified the type of care provided in extended primary care and the disciplines potentially involved. We have seen why continuity is an important requirement and how collaboration, teamwork and other methods of coordination can promote the continuity of care for different categories of patients. Our working definition summarizes the features of extended primary care that are important in the context of this book. Primary care:

- refers to directly accessible, first contact ambulatory care for unselected health (related) problems;
- offers diagnostic, curative, rehabilitative and palliative services in response to the bulk of these problems;
- offers prevention to individuals and groups at risk in the population served;
- takes into account the personal and social context of patients;
- is provided by a variety of disciplines, either within primary care, secondary care or related sectors;
- assures patients continuity of care over time as well as between providers.

This definition can serve as a yardstick in the examination of primary care systems across Europe. The wide diversity in primary care in European countries, as discussed below, points to different conditions for the provision of primary care. For instance, continuity of care is not readily achievable if the organization of primary care is small scale and fragmented, or if there is no single point of entry to the health care system. Structural characteristics of health care, such as the mode of financing, determine possibilities for the provision of primary care. Financing arrangements influence not only how and where patients enter health care, but also the opportunity to establish a longer term relationship between patient and primary care provider, for providers to keep patient records routinely, to maintain adequate professional education and quality of care, or to foster cooperation between providers at different levels. How such conditions emerge and what strategies are effective to support primary care in particular countries depends on the prevailing national governance and health care structure.

Potential of primary care

There is considerable agreement, especially among international organizations and academics, that a strong primary care system is the linchpin of effective health care delivery and that it can help resolve the lack of continuity and responsiveness in health care in general (Saltman and Figueras, 1997; WHO, 2002). There is indeed considerable logic in thinking that the entrance point to the system is the obvious place where improved coordination should take place. Although there are critics who question the evidence for these arguments (Maynard and Bloor, 1995; Sheaff, 1998), studies have suggested that strong primary care based systems are cheaper to operate than more "open" systems and that their health outcomes are better (Starfield, 1994; Doescher *et al.*, 1999; Shi *et al.*, 2002; Macinko *et al.*, 2003). One study conducted in OECD countries found that systems with gatekeeping GPs were better able to control the costs of ambulatory care (Delnoij *et al.*, 2000). It therefore could be concluded provisionally in the European context that primary care-based systems are more cost effective. At meso and micro level there have been many studies on the effectiveness of collaborative, team and "shared" approaches to care, either within primary care or involving various levels of care, showing that these can promote continuity of care and be effective in dealing with new tasks (although they are not necessarily cheaper) (Poulton and West, 1993; Vierhout *et al.*, 1995; Calnan *et al.*, 1996; Shum *et al.*, 2000; Temmink *et al.*, 2000; Renders *et al.*, 2001; Brown *et al.*, 2003; Faulkner *et al.*, 2003; Murchie *et al.*, 2003; Oakeshott *et al.*, 2003; Vlek *et al.*, 2003; Campbell, 2004; Rat *et al.*, 2004; Wolters *et al.*, 2004). There is no direct evidence available about continuity of care, although greater cost-effectiveness may have resulted from better cooperation and coordination mechanisms.

Reservations

The positive expectations among policy-makers for a more central coordinating role of the primary level of health care, however, are in contrast to the diversity of opinions about the organizational mechanisms best suited to achieve that aim. This is due to the fact that health care functions are similar in any country, but the organizational system and the providers involved are quite diverse. This reflects the European reality, with quite different situations of primary care, as explained below. At present some health care systems are already formally based on primary care, including a referral system to secondary care and gatekeeping general practitioners (GPs) with broad task profiles, while others are based more on specialist services with a less exclusive domain for GPs (Boerma and Fleming, 1998). Other differences that create incomparable conditions relate to the financing structure, the mode of governance and the role of professional organizations. A more centralized NHS system, like in the UK, offers quite different conditions for policy-making and coordination than a social security environment, for example in Germany or France, where more parties are involved in decision-making (Saltman *et al.*, 2004).

Another issue, however should, probably precede questions about whether primary care *could* be installed in the driver's seat, how that could be realized, and whether it is *desirable* to do so. The delegation of coordination powers to providers in primary care, for instance GPs, may entail a dual role as both coordinators and providers of care. This may create a conflict of purpose (also discussed in Chapter Four). The important question is whether primary care has the capacity to handle new, complex tasks without losing hold of its main responsibility as the provider of care. First and foremost, GPs are the agents of their patients with professional values that require investing as high a level of resources as possible in those patients. However, to become efficient coordinators, they must incorporate "higher level concerns", and may therefore find themselves divided between these different responsibilities. Vice versa, one may even wonder about the influence of "coordinating doctors" on their professional values. A good division of tasks within primary care teams could potentially offer a solution to this conflict.

And what about the decision-makers: are they in favour of strengthening primary care? In their analysis of reforms in primary care systems in OECD countries, Macinko *et al.* (2003) found that only a few countries have been able to improve essential features of primary care since 1970. Does that reflect the stubbornness of health care reform or the absence of reasons for profound changes? Policy-makers, professionals and the public in countries where primary care is not well developed may not feel strongly attracted to the idea. They may come to see primary care as useful for cost containment, yet generally consider it a lower grade service compared to specialist care. In Central and Eastern Europe, countries had little choice but to change fundamentally their health care systems. Their experiences have taught us about the impact of radical reforms and the time it takes before the reformed system finds stability again.

Different possibilities

For most countries in Europe, the conclusion that neither extended primary care nor general practice specifically serve as the firm basis of health care is justified. Instead, primary care and GPs offer a heterogeneous set of services, often in competition with specialist services (Boerma and Fleming, 1998). In countries where it is hard to identify clear boundaries between levels of care, coordination and continuity of care is difficult to achieve, and possibilities for a steering role of primary care are obviously limited. But even in countries where citizens are on the list of a gatekeeping GP, primary care is usually not the most powerful echelon of health care. This creates a paradoxical situation: the tension between the relative weakness and unattractiveness of this level of care versus the intention to assign critical strategic functions to it. This *primary care paradox* is a basic concern that runs throughout this volume. Available strategies need to be considered that could tip the balance of the health care system towards primary care.

The three chapters that follow in Part One seek to provide a range of perspectives on the context for this central paradox. Chapter Two maps out the existing distribution of key primary care resources across Europe and examines in close detail the type and form of activities in which primary care personnel engage. Chapter Three analyses the process of governance in primary care, detaching the ways in which it has evolved and providing a framework for thinking about how it might develop in the future. Lastly, Chapter Four draws together the central themes that tie the volume together, exploring in particular the major challenges that primary care currently faces.

In Part Two, the chapters utilize both conceptual theories as well as national experience to probe more deeply into a number of key aspects of primary care raised in Part One. Chapters Five, Six, and Seven explore the changing institutional arrangements in European primary care, assessing the issues of coordination, purchasing, and the public-private mix. Chapters Eight, Nine, and Ten review changing work arrangements, including task profiles, training, and financial incentives. Finally, Chapters Eleven and Twelve examine changing quality standards, assessing efforts to emprove quality of care as well as to introduce new information and communication technologies. Taken together, the eight chapters in Part two are intended to provide the detailed case-based depth that can help amplify and reinforce the conceptual perspective and analysis presented in the four chapters of Part One.

Note

1   This vignette was written by Bert Groot Roessink, GP and Director, Curative Care, Almere, the Netherlands.

References

Abel-Smith, B. (1992). Cost containment and the new priorities in the European Communities, *The Milbank Quarterly* **70**(3): 417–416.

Abel-Smith, B. and Mossialos, E. (1994). Cost containment and health care reform: a study of the European Union, *Health Policy* **28**(2): 89–132.

Boerma, W.G.W. (2003). *Profiles of general practice in Europe. An international study of variation in the tasks of general practitioners*. Utrecht: NIVEL (dissertation).

Boerma, W.G.W. and Fleming, D.M. (1998). *The role of general practice in primary health care*. Norwich: WHO Europe/The Stationery Office.

Boerma, W.G.W., De Jong, F. and Mulder, P. (1993). *Health care and general practice across Europe*. Utrecht: NIVEL.

Boerma, W.G.W., Groenewegen, P.P. and Van der Zee, J. (1998). General practice in urban and rural Europe; the range of curative services, *Social Science and Medicine* **47**: 445–453.

Boerma, W.G.W., Van der Zee, J. and Fleming, D.M. (1997). Service profiles of general practitioners in Europe, *British Journal of General Practice* **47**: 481–486.

Boon, H., Verhoef, M., O'Hara, D. and Findlay, B. (2004). From parallel practice to integrative health care: a conceptual framework, *BMC Health Services Research* **4**: 15.

Bower, P. and Sibbald, B. (2004). The health care team, in R. Jones, N. Britten, L. Culpepper *et al.* (eds). *Oxford Textbook of Primary Medical Care*. Volume 1. Oxford: Oxford University Press.

Braspenning, J.C.C., Schellevis, F.G. and Grol, R.P.T.M. (2004). *Tweede Nationale Studie naar ziekten en verrichtingen in de huisartspraktijk: kwaliteit huisartsenzorg belicht*. Utrecht/ Nijmegen: NIVEL/Centre for Quality of Care Research (WOK).

Brown, L., Tucker, C. and Domokos, T. (2003). Evaluating the impact of integrated health and social care teams on older people living in the community, *Health and Social Care in the Community* **11**(2): 85–94.

Busby, H., Elliott, H., Popay, J. and Williams, G. (1999). Public health and primary care: a necessary relationship, *Health and Social Care in the Community* **7**(4): 239–241.

Calnan, M., Canr, S., Williams, S. and Killoran, A. (1996). Involvement of the primary care team in coronary heart disease prevention, *British Journal of General Practice* **46**: 465–468.

Calnan, M., Cant, S., Williams, S. and Killoran, A. (1994). Involvement of the primary health care team in coronary heart disease prevention, *British Journal of General Practice* **44**(382): 224–228.

Campbell, N.C. (2004). Secondary prevention clinics: improving quality of life and outcome, *Heart* **90** (supplement 4): 29–32.

Delnoij, D.M.J., Van Merode, G., Paulus, A. and Groenewegen, P.P. (2000). Does general practitioner gatekeeping curb health care expenditure? *Journal of Health Services Research and Policy* **5**: 22–26.

Doescher, M.P., Franks, P. and Saver, B.G. (1999). Is family medicine associated with reduced health care expenditures? *Journal of Family Practice* **49**: 608–614.

Donaldson, J.S., Yordy, K.D., Lohr, K.N. and Vanselow, N.A. (eds) (1996). *Primary Care: America's Health in a New Era*. Institute of Medicine, Division of Health Care Services, Committee on the Future of Primary Care. Washington DC: National Academy Press.

Faulkner, A., Mills, N., Bainton, D. *et al.* (2003). A systematic review of the effect of primary care-based service innovations on quality and patterns of referral to specialist secondary care, *British Journal of General Practice* **53**: 496, 878–884.

Fry, J. (1972). Considerations of the present state and future trends of primary, personal, family, and general medical care, *International Journal of Health Services* **2**(2): 159–324.

Gervas, J., Perez Fernandez, M., and Starfield, B. (1994). Primary care, financing and gatekeeping in Western Europe, *Family Practice* **11**: 307–317.

Haggerty, J.L., Reid, R.J., Freeman, G.K., Starfield, B.H. and Adair, C.E. (2003). Continuity of care: a multidisciplinary review, *British Medical Journal* **327**: 1219–1221.

Hjortdahl, P. (2004). Continuity of care, In: R. Jones, N. Britten, L. Culpepper *et al.* (eds). *Oxford Textbook of Primary Medical Care*. Volume 1. Oxford: Oxford University Press.

Hjortdahl, P. and Borchgrevink, C.F. (1991). Continuity of care: influence of general practitioners' knowledge about their patients on use of resources in consultations, *British Medical Journal* **303**: 1181–1184.

Hughes, C.M. and McCann, S. (2003). Perceived interprofessional barriers between community pharmacists and general practitioners: a qualitative assessment, *British Journal of General Practice* **53**(493): 600–607.

Hutten, J.B.F. and Kerkstra, A. (1996). *Home Care in Europe. A Country Specific Guide to its Organisation and Financing*. Aldershot: Arena Ashgate Publishing Ltd.

Iliffe, S., Lenihan, P., Wallace, P., Drennan, V., Blanchard, M. and Harris, A. (2002). Applying community-oriented primary care methods in British general practice: a case study, *British Journal of General Practice* **52**: 646–651.

Isles, C.G., Ritchie, L.D., Murchie, P. and Norrie, J. (2000). Risk assessment in primary prevention of coronary heart disease: randomised comparison of three scoring methods, *British Medical Journal* **320**: 690–691.

Kinnersley, P., Andersen, E., Parry, K. *et al.* (2000). Randomised controlled trial of nurse practitioner versus general practitioners care for patients requesting "same day" consultations in primary care, *British Medical Journal* **320**(7241): 1043–1048.

Koster, M.K., Dekker, J. and Groenewegen, P.P. (1991). *The position and education of some paramedical professions in the United Kingdom, The Netherlands, The Federal Republic of Germany and Belgium.* Utrecht: NIVEL.

Leeuwenhorst Group (1974). *The General Practitioner in Europe. A Statement by the Working Party appointed by the Second European Conference on the Teaching of General Practice.* Dublin: Leeuwenhorst Group.

Macinko, J., Starfield, B. and Shi, L. (2003). The contribution of primary care systems to health outcomes within Organization for Economic Cooperation and Development (OECD) countries, 1970–1998, *Health Services Research* **38**(3): 831–865.

Maynard, A. and Bloor K. (1995). Help or hindrance? The role of economics in the rationing of health care, *British Medical Bulletin* **51**(4): 854–868.

McKee, M. and Healy, J. (eds) (1992). *Hospitals in a Changing Europe.* Buckingham: Open University Press.

Menotti, A., Mulder, I., Nissinen, A., Giampaoli, S., Feskens, E.J. and Kromhout, D. (2001). Prevalence of morbidity and multimorbidity in elderly male populations and their impact on 10-year all-cause mortality: The FINE study (Finland, Italy, Netherlands, Elderly), *Journal of Clinical Epidemiology* **54**(7): 680–686.

Ministerie van Volksgezondheid en Milieuhygiëne [Dutch Ministry of Health and Environmental Hygiene] (1974). *Structuurnota Gezondheidszorg [Policy note on health care].* Leidschendam: Ministerie van Volksgezondheid en Milieuhygiëne.

Ministerie van Volksgezondheid en Milieuhygiëne [Dutch Ministry of Health and Environmental Hygiene] (1980). *Schets van de Eerstelijnsgezondheidszorg [Primary care draft].* Leidschendam: Ministerie van Volksgezondheid en Milieuhygiëne.

Muijrers, P.E., Knottnerus, J.A., Sijbrandij, J., Janknegt, R. and Grol, R.P. (2004). Pharmacists in primary care. Determinants of the care-providing function of Dutch community pharmacists in primary care, *Pharmacy World and Science* **26**(5): 256–262.

Murchie, P., Campbell, N.C., Ritchie, L.D., Simpson, J.A. and Thain, J. (2003). Secondary prevention clinics for coronary heart disease: four year follow-up of a randomised controlled trial in primary care, *British Medical Journal* **326**: 84–90.

Mur-Veeman, I., Eijkelberg, I. and Spreeuwenberg, C. (2001). How to manage the implementation of shared care: a discussion of the role of power, culture and structure in the development of shared care arrangements, *Journal of Management in Medicine* **15**(2): 142–155.

Oakeshott, P., Kerry, S., Austin, A. and Cappuccio, F. (2003). Is there a role for nurse-led blood pressure management in primary care? *Family Practice* **20**(4): 469–473.

OECD (1995). *New Directions in Health Care Policy.* Paris: OECD.

Olesen, F. (2002). Do we need a definition of general practice/family medicine? *European Journal of General Practice* **8**: 138–139.

Page, L. (2001). Human resources for maternity care: the present system in Brazil, Japan, North America, Western Europe and New Zealand, *International Journal of Gynecology and Obstetrics* **75** (suppl.1): 81–88.

Paton, C. (2000). *Scientific Evaluation of the Effects of the Introduction of Market Forces into Health Systems. A Review of Evidence in the 15 European Union Member States.* Dublin: European Health Management Association.

Poulton, B.C. and West, M.A. (1993). Effective multidisciplinary teamwork in primary health care, *Journal of Advanced Nursing* **18**: 918–925.

Pringle, M. and Irvine, S. (2004). Practice structures, in R. Jones, N. Britten, L. Culpepper *et al.* (eds) *Oxford Textbook of Primary Medical Care.* Volume 1. Oxford: Oxford University Press.

Raad voor de Volksgezondheid en Zorg (2004). *European Primary Care*. The Hague: Raad voor de Volksgezondheid en Zorg.

Rat, A.C., Henegariu, V. and Boissier, M.C. (2004). Do primary care physicians have a place in the management of rheumatoid arthritis? *Joint Bone Spine* **71**(3): 190–197.

RCGP (1972). *The Future GP: Learning and Teaching*. London: Royal College of General Practitioners (RCGP)/BMJ Publications.

Renders, C.M., Valk, G.D., Griffin, S., Wagner, E.H., Eijk, J.T. and Assendelft, W.J. (2001). Interventions to improve the management of diabetes mellitus in primary care, outpatient and community settings, *Cochrane Database Systematic Review* 1, CD001481.

Rummery, K. and Coleman, A. (2003). Primary health and social care services in the UK: progress towards partnership? *Social Science and Medicine* **56**: 1773–1782.

Saltman, R.B. and Figueras, J. (1997). *European Health Care Reform: Analysis of Current Strategies*. Copenhagen: WHO Regional Office for Europe.

Saltman, R.B., Busse, R. and Figueras, J. (eds) (2004). *Social Health Insurance Systems in Western Europe*. Berkshire/New York: Open University Press/McGraw-Hill Education.

Schers, H.J. (2004). *Continuity of Care in General Practice. Exploring the Balance between Personal and Informational Continuity*. Nijmegen: Radboud University Nijmegen (dissertation).

Sheaff, R. (1998). What is "primary" about primary health care? *Health care Analysis* **6**: 330–340.

Shi, L., Starfield, B., Politzer, R. and Regan, J. (2002). Primary care, self-rated health, and reductions in social disparities in health, *Health Services Research* **37**(3): 529–550.

Shum, C., Humphreys, A., Wheeler, D., Cochrane, M.A., Skoda, S. and Clement, S. (2000). Nurse management of patients with minor illnesses in general practice: multicentre, randomised controlled trial, *British Medical Journal* **320**: 1038–1043.

Silcock, J., Rayner, D.K.T. and Petty, D. (2004). The organisation and development of primary care pharmacy in the United Kingdom, *Health Policy* **67**: 207–214.

Starfield, B. (1991). Primary care and health. A cross-national comparison, *Journal of the American Medical Association* **266**(16): 2268–2271.

Starfield, B. (1992). *Primary Care, Concept, Evaluation and Policy*. New York/Oxford: Oxford University Press.

Starfield, B. (1994). Is primary care essential? *The Lancet* **344**: 1129–1133.

Starfield, B. (1998). *Primary Care. Balancing Health Needs, Services, and Technology*. New York/Oxford: Oxford University Press.

Starfield, B. and Shi, L. (2002). Policy relevant determinants of health: an international perspective, *Health Policy* **60**(3): 201–18.

Temmink, D., Francke, A.L., Hutten, J.B., Van der Zee, J. and Huijer Abu-Saad, H. (2000). Innovations in the nursing care of the chronically ill: a literature review from an international perspective, *Journal of Advanced Nursing* **31**(6): 1449–1458.

Van den Akker, M., Buntinx, F., Metsemakers, J.F., Roos, S. and Knottnerus, J.A. (1998). Multimorbidity in general practice: prevalence, incidence and determinants of co-occurring chronic and recurrent diseases, *Journal of Clinical Epidemiology* **51**(5): 367–375.

Van der Zee, J. (1989). *Over de grenzen van de eerste lijn; vergelijkend onderzoek in een Europese regio [Over the borders of primary care. Comparative study in a European Region]*. Inaugural lecture. Utrecht/Maastricht: NIVEL/Rijksuniversiteit Limburg.

Van der Zee, J., Boerma, W.G.W. and Kroneman, M.W. (2004). Health care systems: understanding the stages of development, in R. Jones, N. Britten, L. Culpepper *et al.* (eds). *Oxford Textbook of Primary Medical Care*. Volume 1. Oxford: Oxford University Press.

Van Weel, C. (1994). Teamwork, *Lancet* **344**: 1276–1279.

Van Weel, C. (1999). International research and the discipline of family medicine, *European Journal of General Practice* **5**: 110–115.

Vierhout, W.P., Knottnerus, J.A., Van Ooij, A. *et al.* (1995). Effectiveness of joint consult-ation sessions of general practitioners and orthopaedic surgeons for locomotor system disorders, *Lancet* **346**(8981): 990–994.

Vlek, J.F., Vierhout, W.P., Knottnerus, J.A. *et al.* (2003). A randomised controlled trial of joint consultations with general practitioners and cardiologists in primary care, *British Journal of General Practice* **53**(487): 108–112.

Vrijhoef, H.J.M. (2002). *Is It Justifiable to Treat Chronic Patients by Nurse Specialists? Evaluation of Effects on Quality of Care.* Maastricht: Universitaire Pers Maastricht.

West, M. and Slater, J. (1996). *Teamworking in Primary Health Care: A Review of Its Effective-ness.* London: Health Education Authority.

Westert, G.P., Satariano, W.A., Schellevis, F.G. and Van den Bos, G.A. (2001). Patterns of comorbidity and the use of health services in the Dutch population, *European Journal of Public Health* **11**(4): 365–372.

WHO (1978). Declaration of Alma-Ata. International Conference on Primary Health Care: Alma-Ata, 6–12 September 1978 (http://www.who.int/hpr/NPH/docs/declaration_almaata.pdf, accessed 18 February 2005).

WHO (2002). *The European Health Report 2002.* Copenhagen: WHO Regional Office for Europe.

Wiegers, T.A., Van der Zee, J. and Keirse M.J. (1998). Maternity care in The Netherlands: the changing home birth rate, *Birth* **25**(3): 190–197.

Winkler, F. (2000). Multidisciplinary Collaboration in Primary Care. Paper presented at 4th meeting of St Petersburg Initiative. Minsk: World Health Organization.

Wolters, R., Wensing, M., Klomp, M. and Grol, R. (2004). Shared care and the manage-ment of lower urinary tract symptoms, *BJU International* **94**(9): 1287–1290.

WONCA (1991). *The role of the general practitioner/family physician in health care systems; A statement of the World Organization of National Colleges, Academies and Academic Associations of General Practitioners/Family Physicians.* Victoria: WONCA.

WONCA (2002). *The European Definition of General Practice/Family Medicine.* Singapore: World Organization of Family Doctors (WONCA).

chapter two

Mapping primary care across Europe

Wienke G. W. Boerma and Carl-Ardy Dubois

Although growing integration has reduced differences between European countries in a variety of economic sectors, the organization and provision of health care continues to be relatively diverse (Belien, 1996; Goicoechea, 1996; Helman, 1998). Reflecting this diversity as well as the practicality that health care is still mainly a national affair in the European Union, there is little comparable data available on organization and provision. The lack of information and evidence is particularly noticeable given the broad range of health care reforms that have occurred since the early 1990s, many of which have affected primary care. Examples of such reforms are the introduction of GP fundholding and the later Primary Care Groups and Trusts in the United Kingdom, family doctor systems in Sweden (later largely dropped) and Finland, and policies in Germany, France, Norway and Finland leading to voluntary patient list systems and a stronger coordinating role for GPs (Alban and Christiansen, 1995; Niemelä, 1996; Vehvilaeinen *et al.*, 1996; Le Grand *et al.*, 1998; Aguzzoli *et al.*, 1999; Bundesministerium für Frauen, Jugend und Gesundheit, 2000).

Vignette 2.1   Finnish primary health centre[1]

Janakkala is a middle-income town of 15,000 about 150 km north of Helsinki. Its main industry is a large forest products mill, thus it has a relatively large number of industrial workers as residents. In size, population distribution, and income, it is very close to the median for all Finnish municipalities. The primary health centre employs its full complement of 10 GPs, as well as a substantial number of nurses and aids. It also has on staff a social worker and several health education personnel. Facilities include clinic rooms and its own X-ray and laboratory facility. Like most primary health centres in Finland, it also has several wards of inpatient beds – referred to in Finland as a 'primary care hospital'. These 85 beds, in Janakkala's case, provide long-term skilled nursing care for elderly patients who are unable to remain at home but are not sick enough to warrant inpatient hospital treatment. The beds are oversubscribed, and the health centre recently added nine beds in order to reduce the number of elderly who had to be sent to the district hospital for care.

The health centre is owned and operated by Janakkala municipality. The elected municipal council makes general policy for all municipal services, while an appointed Health and Social Board, composed of several elected members of the council, the chief doctor in the primary care centre, and a municipal administrator responsible for health and social care, is responsible for supervising the municipality's health and social care activities. The board is also responsible for arranging inpatient hospital services for Janakkala's residents through a well-developed contracting process (see below).

Over the past 10 years, the municipality has gained considerable financial and managerial freedom in how it manages its health sector responsibilities. Previously, a wide variety of state controls over funding (the state provided a sliding subsidy to Finnish municipalities of 39–61 % of total health expenditures) and staff salary levels, a state-mandated municipal obligation to hold capital shares in the district and specialist hospital (and thus to send Janakkala's patients only to those institutions), and a near complete inability on the part of the municipality to influence either the hospital's overall budget or the portion to be paid by Janakkala, all had resulted in a sense within Finnish municipalities that, although they formally owned both their primary health centres and the hospitals, in practice they had little effective say in what they did or what it cost. By 2002, all of these restraints on municipal decision-making had been removed. For example, Janakkala decided in summer 2001 to solve its continuing problem of inadequate coverage for GPs. By decision of the municipal council, it raised the salary paid to GPs to well above the minimum required by the national union contract, enabling it to attract a full compliment of 10. Since it now had full control over how it spent its funds and also the salary range paid to staff, this solution became possible.

Janakkala municipality has signed four separate contracts for specific medical services to supplement those provided by its own primary health centre. They were for:

- specialist hospital services;
- visiting specialist clinics organized in Janakkala's primary health centre;
- endoscopic services in the primary health centre;
- out-of-hours emergency coverage.

While the second, third and fourth contracts are relatively straightforward efforts to supplement on-site clinical services with outside providers; the first contract is quite complex. It is a public contract, agreed between two publicly owned and operated entities (the municipality and the hospital district). There is no state supervision or approval in Finland of either the contract terms or the contract process – a legacy of the municipalities' 'Spring Revolt' in 1987 that resulted in the state granting nearly full operating control over health care to municipal governments.

The hospital contract is based on the past two and a half years' experience of inpatient use by Janakkala patients in the nearby public specialist hospital (of which Janakkala is still technically an owner and for which it sits on the Hospital District Board). For each fiscal year (same as the calendar year), the hospital makes a "proposal" to the municipality. The municipality then responds, and the two ultimately agree on a final amount. For fiscal year 2003, the agreed figure is 5.2% higher than for fiscal year 2002 (not inflation adjusted). It is a fixed price contract: the municipality will receive nothing back if volume or costs are lower than expected, while the hospital receives nothing more if volume or costs are higher than expected. The contract does contain a clause, however, that if during the contract period the current level of municipally provided services in primary or social care should materially change – for whatever reason, and whether to be more or less comprehensive or extensive – then the contract amount will be opened up for reconsideration. The only aspect of the current contract that concerns Janakkala's health and social care administration is that the contract has no quality of care specifications – although to date there has been no adverse consequences for Janakkala's patients, as the quality of care at the specialist hospital is considered to be quite good as compared with all Finnish hospitals.

Two additional aspects of the Janakkala primary care centre are worth noting. First, although Janakkala had considered sending their laboratory work to the specialist hospital and closing their own facility, they decided against it for both financial (few substantial savings) and patient convenience issues (patients would have to travel to the hospital for certain tests). Second, Janakkala had decided to terminate its own in-house pharmacy service, opting instead to have its drugs prepared by the (much bigger) specialist hospital pharmacy and then sent out to the primary care centre and hospital.

Both the chairwoman of Janakkala's health and social board as well as the municipal administrator for health and social care felt that the municipality's health services were working rather well. They were pleased with their progress in the last several years, including the fact that all 10 GPs saw patients for approximately 80% of their working time (a relatively high ratio for a publicly operated health centre). They were not content, however, with the fact that patients still had to wait for up to two weeks for a regular (non-urgent) appointment with their regular GP, since they could jump to the private sector and see a GP within one-two days. Janakkala's administrator also would like to have quality of care parameters included in the contract with the specialist hospital.

The context of funding and politics

Taxonomies of health care systems often take an approach based on the funding mechanism, with countries divided into tax-based and social insurance systems. Although the method of funding is an important factor in shaping the system, it alone is insufficient to explain the diversity in health care delivery. For this reason, we take an additional dimension into account, namely, the political context.

The *economic dimension* in health systems encompasses both funding (including the collection and pooling) and the purchasing and provision of services (Dixon *et al.*, 2004). Functions that relate to primary care include the process of mobilizing and distributing resources for primary care, the methods of remuneration of primary care providers, the methods of organizing provision of primary care services and the types of primary care services that are provided.

At the beginning of the 1990s, health care systems in Europe could be divided into three broad models: the social health insurance model ("Bismarck systems"), tax funded models ("Beveridge systems"), and the Soviet model ("Semashko system"). However, no European health care system is an exact replica of any specific model. Rather, each country has its own variation, in which the basic model is adjusted to national particularities (Marrée and Groenewegen, 1997). Furthermore, health care financing is not static. The institutional arrangements in the Beveridge and Bismarck countries have been subject to considerable experimentation intending to promote choice, encourage competition, increase resources for health care, enhance responsiveness to consumers' wishes, expand coverage or counteract high labour market costs (Saltman and Von Otter, 1992; Dixon and Mossialos, 2001). At the same time countries in central and eastern Europe as well as a number of former Soviet Republics are abandoning the Semashko model, most of them implementing insurance-based models and decentralized governance. Reforms include the creation of independent practitioners, new methods of funding, combining elements of capitation payment with incentives to undertake certain activities, programmes of training and professional development, and mechanisms to provide capital funding to upgrade facilities and equipment (Preker *et al.*, 2002).

The *political dimension* includes both the balance of power between actors involved in health care delivery and territorial administrative structures. Differences between health care systems do not lie in the types of actor, but in the way these relationships are configured. The categories include patients or consumers of services, providers of services (those directly contacted by patients and those available via first level providers), funders or insurers of health care, and central governments and regional authorities (Evans, 1981; OECD, 1992). The interaction between the actors relates to the provision of services to patients, referrals

Vignette 2.2 Family medicine in Romania[2]

Historical overview

During the communist period, health care in Romania was hospital centred. Family doctors existed, but they worked in dispensaries that reported to hospital directors and did not have an autonomous professional identity. This was the result of a medical education system which was exclusively hospital oriented, without any attention to the morbidity pattern that family doctors deal with. The fact that family doctors were subordinated to the hospitals resulted in lower quality premises and equipment that severely limited their diagnostic and therapeutic possibilities. All doctors were state employees and as such badly underpaid As a result patients often had to pay 'under the table'. Home care by nurses and home helpers was virtually unknown, therefore bedridden patients were forced to be hospitalized.

Until the mid–1990s, different family doctors treated different members of one family, since there were separate family doctors for children, for adults, for industrial workers, for soldiers and for railway personnel. This system changed in 1995, but still today former paediatricians may prefer to have children on their lists instead of adults. Often mothers are the patients of a former adult doctor, while the child is on the list of a former paediatrician.

There are also large differences in the content and workload of family practice in towns and in rural regions. Because the distance to hospitals in villages can be great, the rural population expects family doctors to provide a greater range of medical services than those living near hospitals. As a result, rural family doctors have more opportunities to develop adequate family medicine skills than their urban colleagues.

The current situation

After the 1989 revolution, a group of progressive family doctors established the *Societatea Nationala de Medicina Generala* (SNMG). They organized continuing education, produced two medical journals and they sought to represent family doctors at the national level. Three years of postgraduate training for family doctors was established, including one year in a kind of teaching practicum. A small minority of family doctors completed this programme.

State funding for the health care system was replaced in 1998 by a health insurance system, which meant that the Ministry of Health no longer dominated the health care system. This task was taken over by Health Insurance Offices established in each district and also a National Health Insurance Agency for the whole country. These new organizations became responsible for both the structuring and financing of regional health care. Paying premiums was a big change for the population.

Another change was the requirement that all inhabitants choose a family doctor.

The changed structure of health care has been beneficial to Romania as a pre-accession country of the EU, since a well-functioning primary care system is one of the conditions of membership. Recently however, the National Health Insurance Agency has come under the influence of the Ministry of Health again and there is a widespread belief that the government is diverting health care resources that have been paid by employees and employers to cover other debts.

Family doctors continued to be plagued by financial issues. On the one hand, earnings have improved and they now receive a fee, partly *per capita* and partly for service, which has created a better relationship between workload and income. However, the problem remains that fees are paid in "credit points", the value of which is variable, set retrospectively, and subject to devaluation.

Family doctors have also become responsible for their own offices, this too was formerly the responsibility of the hospital director. Family doctors now receive a budget for their premises, equipment, heating and electricity and nurses' salaries. This is a considerable step forward but the budget often does not cover the real costs. In addition, many offices are in poor condition and family doctors cannot invest in improvements because the offices are part of a 'commodity system', which means for five years the doctors cannot buy the premises. Overall, the income of family doctors has improved compared to the previous situation (now about $150 per month on an average), but most doctors still have financial problems. Negotiations with the Health Insurance offices are conducted by the College of Physicians, in which medical specialists are the great majority, and the Society of Family Doctors has only a consultative role.

Theoretically, the new health care structure constitutes a significant improvement and makes family medicine the gatekeeper for health services. In practice, however, this goal is not supported by the Ministry of Health, which is still strongly influenced by specialists who view family doctors as competitors.

from first level to second level providers, patients' payment of insurance premiums (or taxes), payments for services and regulation by government. In western Europe, a number of reforms have included initiatives aiming to bestow greater power on intermediate or local tiers of governance. In central and eastern Europe, health care policy-making is gradually shifting towards a less hierarchical and more decentralized organization of health services. Notwithstanding this trend, the political organization of health care at subnational levels in European countries follows diverse pathways and gives rise to a mosaic of institutions, many rooted in historical, cultural and religious traditions (Blanpain, 1994; Chinitz *et al.*, 2004).

Resources for primary care

A number of health sector reforms during the 1990s have sought to readjust the division of tasks between primary and secondary care. The role of primary care in managing the entrance to and exit from secondary care has tended to increase. In addition, inpatient care is required for a diminishing proportion of those who enter the health care system and stays in hospitals have become shorter (White *et al.*, 1961; McKee and Healy, 2001). Many more patients can be treated in the primary care setting, so that these services can account for up to 90% of all health care activity (Hobbs, 1995). This figure highlights the need to achieve an appropriate balance of resources between primary and secondary care, with adequate financial and human resources being directed towards the primary care sector, and in line with changes in the task division between primary and secondary care (Forrest and Starfield, 1996; Jepson, 2001).

Availability of data

Information on the allocation of resources in health care is not plentiful. More studies have focused on the hospital sector than on primary care, perhaps in part because definitional problems related to primary care make comparison difficult. As a consequence there is no source of comparable data on, for example, the financial resources allocated to the primary care sector in Europe. Neither the OECD database nor the Health-for-All database do not provide these data. Some national databases give information on resources allocated to primary care but differences in definitions, parameters, and data retrieval make comparison difficult (Lagasse *et al.*, 2001). With regard to human resources, data on primary care practitioners are also incomplete and not always adequate. Despite of the central role of human resources in the health sector, international attention to human resources for health has only recently emerged on the health policy agenda (Dubois *et al.*, 2005 forthcoming).

Financial resources

Existing data on expenditure in primary care suggest that less than a quarter of the health care budget generally goes to primary care in western Europe (Hobbs, 1995; Goicoechea, 1996; OHE, 2000). Overall, health care resources across Europe have increased in real terms over recent decades, reflected in increases in health expenditures. Indirect indicators, however, do not indicate that the proportion for primary care has increased drastically over time. In central and eastern Europe, where concerted attempts are being made to develop primary care, data from the European Health For All database indicate that to date only Latvia and Hungary have significantly reduced the proportion of the health budget devoted to inpatient care. In other countries such as the former Yugoslav Republic of Macedonia and Slovenia, the fraction of health resources allocated to inpatient care has continued to increase (WHO, 2004). Data from western European countries suggests a modest trend towards reducing or containing the share of inpatient expenditure in total health expenditure (WHO, 2004). This is consistent with significant decreases in hospital capacity and efforts to contain hospital costs. At the same time, however, changes in skill mix and technological developments have enabled substitution of primary care for secondary care. OECD Health Data do not suggest a shift of resources towards the primary care sector and outpatient care. In some countries (Finland, France, Iceland, Italy, Luxembourg, Netherlands, Spain, Switzerland, Belgium and Turkey), the proportion of total health care spending devoted to outpatient care throughout the 1990s has remained relatively stable or has decreased. Only two countries have significantly increased the proportion of resources channelled to outpatient care: Austria (+ 6 %), and Denmark (+ 3 %) (OECD, 2004).

GP density

Tracking the distribution of the workforce between levels of care is a way to obtain evidence on possible changes in the accent on primary and secondary care. Available data on the supply of physicians do not suggest growth in the proportion working in primary care. The density of GPs across Europe is shown on the map in Figure 2.1 (see plate section) and also in Table 2.1.

The map shows considerable variations across countries. Countries with most GPs per 1000 population in 2002 are Austria, Belgium, Finland and France. The lowest densities are found in Latvia, Poland, Slovakia and Switzerland. Details on the number of GPs per 1000 population both in 1990 and 2002 are given in Table 2.1.

Comparison of the figures from 1990 and 2002 shows that the numbers have remained relatively stable in most countries. In 10 out of 19 countries for which data were available for both years there has been an increase in GP density, with a relatively strong increase in Austria, Finland and Norway. In eight countries the density was the same in both years. Only in Portugal only was there a decrease in the number of GPs in relation to the population. Countries with a GP referral system have been indicated in the table, as this feature can be taken as an indicator for a well-developed primary care system. The table shows that GP referral systems are not related to a high or low GP density. Between countries with such a referral system there is also a considerable variation. Within this group, in Norway and Italy the number of GPs per 1000 population is about double the number in Netherlands, Portugal and Slovenia. Concerning nurses, no current data are available to estimate what proportion are involved in primary care.

Income

Recruitment for general practice is influenced by the income that medical students can expect to earn as a GP, compared to the income of medical specialists. Differences in income reflect differences in status between medical specialties. Existing data suggest that physicians' incomes, both generalists and specialists, are in general in the top 25% of the population, similar to senior civil servants (Anderson, 1998; OECD, 2000; Reinhardt *et al.*, 2002). However, there is enormous variation between countries. Physicians in western Europe receive higher compensation than their colleagues in central and eastern Europe. GPs'

Table 2.1 Number of GPs per 1000 population in European countries in 1990 and 2002

Countries	GPs per 1000 population		Difference 1990–2002
	1990[1]	*2002[1]*	
Austria	1.1	1.4	+0.3
Belgium	1.9	2.1	+0.2
Czech Republic	0.7	0.7	0
Denmark[g]	0.6	0.7	+0.1
Estonia	n.a.	0.7	n.a.
Finland	1.3	1.7	+0.4
France	1.6	1.6	0
Germany	1.1	1.1	0
Hungary	0.7	0.7	0
Iceland[g]	0.6	0.7	+0.1
Ireland[g]	0.5	0.6	+0.1
Italy[g]	0.9	0.9	0
Latvia	n.a.	0.4	n.a.
Lithuania	n.a.	0.7	n.a
Luxembourg	0.8	0.9	+0.1
Netherlands[g]	0.4	0.5	+0.1
Norway[g]	0.7	1.1	+0.4
Poland	n.a.	0.2	n.a.
Portugal[g]	0.7	0.5	−0.2
Slovakia	n.a.	0.4	n.a.
Slovenia	n.a.	0.5	n.a.
Sweden	0.5	0.5	0
Switzerland	0.4	0.4	0
Turkey	0.5	0.7	+0.2
United Kingdom[g]	0.6	0.6	0

Note: [g] Countries with referral system/patients registered with a GP
[1] Or nearest available year.
n.a. = not available / not applicable
Sources: OECD (2004), Arnoudova (2005).

incomes have been increasing in many countries over recent years, but data available for a few OECD countries show a gap between average physicians' income (specialists and generalists) and average GPs' income in most of these countries (OECD, 2000). In some countries such as Norway, systematic efforts have recently been made to narrow the income gap between generalists and medical specialists (Furuholmen and Magnussen, 2000).

In all countries, the average income among physicians was superior to the average income among nursing and midwifery professionals (OECD, 2000). In general, physicians' average wages go up to more than twice as high as wages for nursing and midwifery professionals (Gupta *et al.*, 2002). There are no specific data on primary care nurses.

Although more accurate and thorough information is clearly needed to tease out the issue of the distribution of resources between the different levels of care in Europe, the evidence to date suggests several conclusions:

- an absence of significant changes in the financial resources allocated to primary care;
- an unequal density of GPs across European countries;
- little or no change in most countries in GP density between 1990 and 2002;
- a financial situation that in most cases continues to be more favourable to medical specialists than GPs.

Mapping primary care practice in Europe

To what extent do primary care systems in Europe comply with our definition? Is there one single point in the health system where first contact care is provided with a generalist approach from a long-term perspective? To what extent have nursing disciplines developed and been integrated into the context of primary care? Are services available in patients' homes? Are providers collaborating and are their interventions coordinated? It will be difficult to answer all these questions, because, here again, the available information is not up to date and not sufficient to provide answers.

The first part of this section briefly reviews the general organization of home care activities in 15 European countries, and to a lesser extent their provision. The information reflects the situation in these countries in the mid-1990s and has been derived from an international study (Hutten and Kerkstra, 1996). The remaining part of this section describes the organization and provision of services in general practice in 32 countries in Europe, based on a 1994 study (Boerma *et al.*, 1997; Boerma and Fleming, 1998; Boerma, 2003).

Home care

Ageing populations and societal developments result in increasing demand for professional home care in Europe. The old and very old are a growing proportion of the population. As family size decreases and mobility increases the availability of relatives for informal care will continue to decline. Moreover, substitution policies in health care result in the transfer of tasks from hospitals to the home situation. Consequently, home care is increasing both quantitatively and qualitatively (Tjassing *et al.*, 1998). In the countries of central and eastern Europe, home care is a relatively new concept; however, it is now being developed in a number of these countries as part of primary care (Vladu, 1998; Fedullo *et al.*, 2004).

A variety of disciplines provide medical, nursing and domestic care in the home situation. GPs make home visits as do practice nurses in some countries. Social and geriatric services may also visit their clients at home, and churches may be involved as well. The European study of Hutten and Kerkstra (1996) focused on structurally embedded care provided at home by professional organizations. It was limited to two core disciplines: home nursing and home help services. Home nursing included rehabilitative, supportive, promotive or preventive and technical nursing and was mainly aimed at sick people at home. Preventive mother and child care, school health nursing and occupational nursing were not covered by this study. Home help services included house-work, such as cooking, cleaning, washing, shopping, personal care and adminis-trative paperwork. Organizations for the provision of only one item of service, such as "meals on wheels", were not included.

The *assessment of needs* with "patients" or "clients" is an important first con-tact function in home care, related to the mode of funding. In countries where home care is prescribed by a physician, such as in France, he or she may be the one to decide what care is needed. In many other countries needs assessment and the delivery of care are not separated and are carried out by an employee of the home care organization involved (Parry-Jones and Soulsby, 2001). In the Netherlands, where no referral is needed for home care, since 1998 broad needs assessment has been undertaken by independent assessment agencies. The Netherlands has also introduced uniform assessment instruments in order to make the intake procedure more objective (Algera *et al.*, 2003).

Home nursing

In the 15 countries of the pre-2004 EU, home nursing is usually part of the health care system, but it is organized, quite differently often reflecting histor-ical development. In Belgium, Denmark, Finland, Ireland Netherlands and the United Kingdom, home nursing has a long tradition, while it is still only devel-oping in Austria, Greece, Italy, Luxembourg, Portugal and Spain. Also, *organiza-tion* is not always uniform within countries. There may be two or more modes of organization or circuits, for instance parallel provision by municipalities, non-profit organizations, hospitals, charity associations, and initiatives affiliated with political parties, in addition to independently established nurses.

Organizations for home nursing are usually not-for-profit. However, with the introduction of market elements in health care for-profit organizations have also entered the sector. Basically, there are two *funding models*. In one, resources come from general taxation with fixed budgets for the organizations. The size of the budget is usually related to the number and composition of the inhabitants in the working area. In countries with this funding scheme, such as Denmark, Ireland, Italy, Portugal and Spain, patients do not need a referral for home nurs-ing. In the second model, where resources have been collected from social health insurance premiums, a fee-for-services scheme is used. In these cases (Austria, Belgium, France, Germany) patients need a referral from a physician. The assessment of need for home nursing differs in both funding schemes. If no referral is required, needs are assessed by the home nursing organization, while in the second model needs are usually assessed by the referring physician. Payments can be based on different mechanisms. In the case of fee-for-service payment, services have been specified in a nomenclature; a list of (technical) nursing activities. In a pay-per-home visit scheme, usually two types of visits (and tariffs) are distinguished: those for personal hygiene and those for tech-nical nursing. Another option is payment per patient for a fixed period of time, for instance one month. The level of payment is then determined by the assessed needs of the patient. Mixes of these modes of payment also occur, either with or without co-payment by the patient.

Concerning *human resources* in the provision of home care, usually two levels of expertise are distinguished: a lower level nurse more involved in personal hygiene and uncomplicated nursing tasks and a higher level nurse for more technical nursing and complex situations.

Home help services

In contrast to home nursing, home help services are not a part of health care but are considered as social services, except in Ireland, the Netherlands and to some degree in Germany. In Greece and Italy home help services started to develop only in the early 1980s, while in other countries it has had a longer tradition. In most countries home help services are organized by local authorities, such as municipalities and no referral is needed. Needs are assessed by an organizer or team leader of the home help organization who is usually a social worker. In cases where home nursing and home help services are integrated in one organization, as in the Denmark, Ireland and Netherlands, home nurses may also assess the patients' need for home help. Since the mid-1990s there has been a trend towards integrating home care nursing and home help services. There is increased collaboration and there have been mergers between these organizations.

The workforce in home help services is large, but the level of required education is relatively low. In most countries there is little formal training for home help-ers – they may have had a short course or have been trained on the job. There are enormous differences in the availability of home helpers, as Table 2.2 shows.

The supply of home helpers in countries like Belgium, Denmark, Finland, the Netherlands and Sweden is at least 10 times the supply in Italy, Luxembourg and Spain (referring only to the Genoa region, since in the south of the country home help services are even less developed). In countries with relatively few home helpers, informal care plays an important role in the provision of personal and domestic assistance to relatives, friends and neighbours.

Table 2.2 Number of full-time home helpers per 1000 population in European countries

Country	Population per home helps per 1000 population
Austria (Vienna area)	1.34
Belgium (Flanders)	2.23
Denmark	6.21
Finland	1.89
France	0.71
Ireland	0.86
Italy (Genoa area)	0.18
Luxembourg	0.16
Netherlands	2.01
Spain	0.20
Sweden	9.01
United Kingdom	0.91

Source: Hutten and Kerkstra (1996).

In many countries both home nursing organizations and home help services reported problems in efforts to collaborate with hospitals, GPs and other services in primary care, and with social services. The most frequently reported complaints were lack of information and poor communication with patients transferred from one level or service to another or concerning joint patients (Hutten and Kerkstra, 1996).

General practice

General practice has the potential to be the core of primary care, but this potential is utilized to different degrees in European health care systems. Arguably the strength of primary care very much relates to the strength and position of general practice in a country. Many elements of our working definition of primary care apply to services provided in general practice if it is well positioned in a health care system.

The position and strength of general practice in Europe will be discussed in light of our working definition. In particular, the focus will be on the following elements: the role of GPs as the doctor of first contact for a broad spectrum of health problems; the range of curative and preventive services offered to patients; the available medical equipment to allow diagnostic services and treatment; mono- and interdisciplinary cooperation; and conditions favouring continuity of care.

Information for this comparison is from the European study of GP Task Profiles, in which well over 8000 GPs in 32 countries answered detailed questions on the organization of their practice and the provision of services (Boerma et al., 1997; Boerma and Fleming, 1998; Boerma et al., 1998). Data were collected in 1994 and so changes may have taken place in a number of countries since then. This will be particularly true in countries in central and eastern Europe and should be taken into account when interpreting the results. However, the study was recently replicated in one of these countries and demonstrates that the effects of health reforms on the task provision of doctors in primary care should not be overestimated. Another indication of the relative stability of GP services over time are the results from the Second Dutch National Study in General Practice, which were recently updated 14 years after the first edition. The results indicate that GPs work more efficiently now, for example by delegating tasks to other providers of out-of-hours care, and a slight decrease in specialist referrals suggests a higher level of curative activities in primary care. In general, however, there are no indications of fundamental change. All groups in the population still find their way to the GP and the gatekeeping role of GPs is unchanged (Schellevis et al., 2004).

Results by country are presented by maps with colours representing the ranking of the country regarding aspects of GP task provision, as mentioned above. Tables with the rank positions per country are in the annex at the end of this chapter. In these tables, the countries have been listed according to three categories: those with a tax-funded health system, those with a social health insurance system and the countries in transition located in central and eastern Europe.

First contact care

The five columns on the left-hand side of Table 2.A in the annex show data on the role of general practice as the entry point of health care. This role was measured by means of 27 short case descriptions about which GPs could answer according to a four-point scale regarding the extent to which a problem would be presented first to the GP when it would occur in the practice population. Four dimensions could be identified according to the type of health problem: acute problems, problems specific to children, those specific to women, and psychosocial problems. The first column in Table 2.A shows the overall ranking with respect to the total list of problems. This has also been depicted in Figure 2.2 (see plate section). The second to the fifth columns give the countries' position as regards the subcategories.

Countries with GPs in a strong position as the entry point of health care appear to be the Denmark, Ireland, Netherlands, and the United Kingdom, followed at a short distance by Norway, Portugal and Spain. It is not surprising that these are countries with GPs in a gatekeeping position, since this role generally requires health problems to enter via the GP. The transitional countries have the lowest rankings, however, with the exception of Croatia and Slovenia, which are the only transitional countries with gatekeeping GPs.

The highest ranking countries also are strong in terms of the point of entry when subcategories of problems are considered (see Table 2.A). This appears to reflect a stronger position in terms of first contact with problems related to children and women. In the other countries, it seems that for these problems people bypass GPs. For first contact with acute health problems, for instance, the role of GPs is similar irrespective of their gatekeeping position. In most transitional countries, GPs have a much weaker entry position, but with respect to first contact with acute problems this gap is smallest. The differences between countries with tax-funded health services and those with social health insurance schemes seem to be evident, but can be attributed to the fact that tax-funded health systems more often have GPs in a position as gatekeeper. Ireland and the Netherlands are both social health insurance countries with gatekeeping GPs and interestingly, both countries are in the highest ranking group.

Generalism and comprehensiveness

General practice is not only the place where health problems are presented, but also diagnosed and treated. This is true for acute cases as well as for chronic diseases. Comprehensiveness and generalism refer to the range of curative services provided by GPs, as well as his or her role in the domain of prevention and health education (Calnan *et al.*, 1994). The following groups of activities by GPs were taken into account. First, involvement in the treatment of diseases. This was measured by means of 17 short case descriptions about which GPs could respond according to a four-point scale. Second, the involvement of GPs in the provision of medical technical procedures, including minor surgical treatments, was measured. This was gauged by means of 14 questions structured in a similar way to the questions pertaining to treatment of diseases.

Furthermore, the uptake of cervical smears and health education in clinics or groups concerning smoking cessation, healthy diet or problematic drinking was surveyed. Finally, the involvement of GPs in family planning was measured.

The relative positions of countries on the comprehensiveness of the GPs' curative and preventive services, as mentioned above, have been summarized in Figure 2.3 (see plate section). Positions on each of the services can be found in Table 2.A at the end of this chapter.

Considering all services together, Figure 2.3 shows that countries where GPs provide the most comprehensive mix of services are mostly situated in western and northwestern Europe. More specifically, these countries are: Austria, Denmark, France, Germany (western), Iceland, Ireland, Norway, Switzerland and the United Kingdom. Five of these countries have gatekeeping GPs, but these are only half of the countries with GPs in such a position. Two countries with gatekeeping GPs, Italy and Spain, are among the countries where GPs provide a relatively small set of services, as in transitional countries such as the Czech Republic, Poland and Romania.

Teamwork and cooperation

The provision of comprehensive services and coordination of care can be facilitated by teamwork and good working relations with other health care workers, both in primary care and in secondary care and hospitals. In small scale (solo) practices it may be difficult for GPs to provide a broad range of services around the clock and to coordinate with care provided by others. Larger practices can hire ancillary staff, purchase equipment more efficiently and have regular meetings for coordination and joint policy-making. Group practices can be seen as institutionalized forms of professional social control (De Jong et al., 2003).

In most countries, general practice used to be dominated by individual practices. In most social health insurance countries the majority of GPs still work in solo practices (see Table 2.B). Turkey is an exception in this group, and also, though less so, the two gatekeeping countries (the Ireland and Netherlands). Countries with few solo practices (less than 20%) are mostly found in the tax-funded health system group: Finland, Iceland, Portugal, Sweden and the United Kingdom. Italy, however, has a majority of solo practices and has gatekeeping GPs. In three transitional countries there are few solo GPs: Bulgaria, Latvia and Ukraine. In this group of countries Poland is the exception with many soloists.

Cooperation was further explored via questions about the prevalence of regular meetings (at least once per month) with colleague GPs, with ambulatory medical specialists, with medical specialists in hospitals, with primary care nurses and with social workers. Details have been reported in Table 2.B.

Taken together, the measures of collaboration with GPs, medical specialists and other professional groups, the map in Figure 2.4 (see plate section) shows the relative position of the countries.

Countries where GPs have relatively most intensive collaboration with other professional groups tend to be at the periphery of Europe (see Figure 2.4). These countries are: Bulgaria, Finland, Iceland, Latvia, Lithuania, Portugal, Sweden,

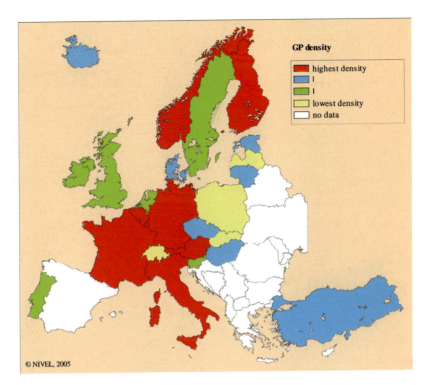

Figure 2.1   Density of GPs in Europe

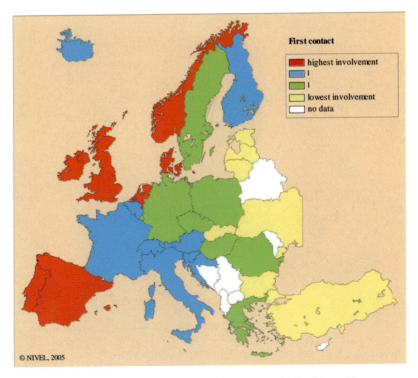

Figure 2.2   Role of GPs as the doctor of first contact with health problems

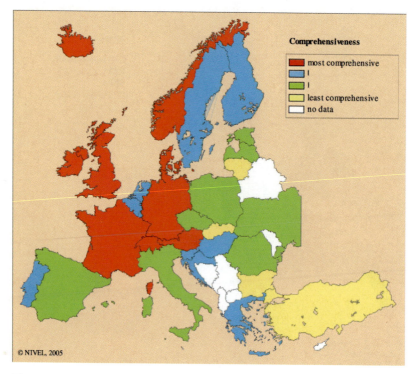

Figure 2.3 Comprehensiveness of curative and preventive services by GPs

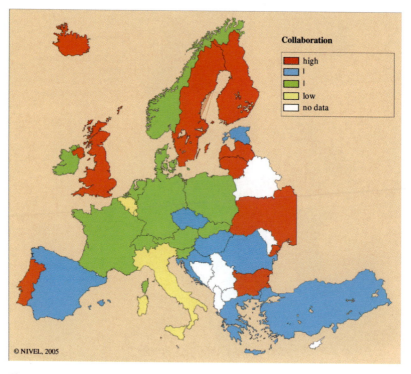

Figure 2.4 Collaboration of GPS with several disciplines

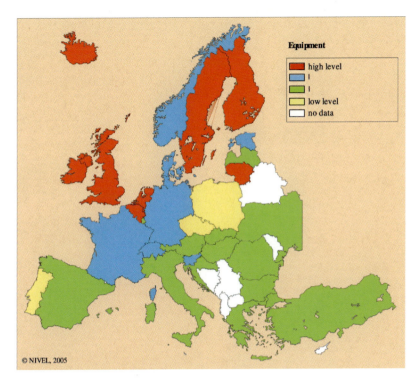

Figure 2.5   Medical equipment in general practice

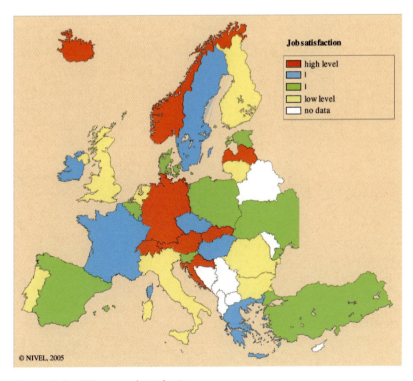

Figure 2.6   GP's sense of satisfaction

the United Kingdom and Ukraine. GPs in Belgium, Italy and Luxembourg have few collaborative relations compared to GPs elsewhere.

Vignette 2.3   Slovenian primary care[3]

In the 1950s, under the influence of Andrij Stampar, the then socialist government of Yugoslavia made large investments in primary health care. A range of preventive activities were implemented: well-baby clinics, well-mother clinics, clinics for women, clinics for people with tuberculosis, clinics for trachoma, clinics for workers, clinics for schoolchildren and students, etc. Many of the physicians working in these clinics pursued their professional careers in one of these specialist fields. Under these circumstances, there was a decline in holistic and generalist thinking and a polyclinic approach to health care, hence, general practice was on the verge of extinction. Only a few enthusiasts believed in family medicine as an important source of health care.

In the 1960s, family medicine (at that time known as general medicine) was declared a specialist field, although vocational training was not a pre-requisite for working in general practice. In November 1995, the Department of Family Medicine was established at Ljubljana University. It has an unique curriculum. Four days each week, students meet with specially trained tutors in a primary care practice to test their communication skills, medical record keeping and other ordinary skills. One day a week, students work with an assistant teacher in small groups presenting reports about their experiences.

In 1992 Slovenia's health care system was transformed from a state-run system to a decentralized model with one insurance company, the National Health Insurance Institute (NHII). Health care is provided by both public (hospitals and primary health care centres) and private providers. Inhabitants of Slovenia are insured through their employment status and local communities cover the unemployed. The compulsory health insurance covers over 80% of all health care costs. Additional coverage is available through voluntary insurance, which includes co-payments.

Patients must now choose their own 'personal' family physician. The personal family physician has the responsibility to provide primary care for their patients, which includes emergency care 24 hours a day provided by physicians working in rotation outside of regular office hours. Family physicians' gatekeeping role also makes them a focus for cost containment and quality assurance efforts. These goals could present a potential threat to the quality of the doctor-patient relationship.

Family physicians work as independent contractors to NHII or employees in non-for-profit Primary Health Care Centres (PHCCs) which are group contractors to NHII. PHCCs are very evenly distributed throughout the country and mainly located in the community centres. The PHCC in Radovljica is a typical example of such a centre. Radovljica lies in the north-west part of Slovenia, 50 km from the capital Ljubljana. It is one of the 60 Health Care Centres (HCCs) in Slovenia and is neither the biggest nor the smallest. PHCC Radovljica provides care for approximately 18,200 inhabitants.

Primary health in the Radovljica PHCC combines public and private physicians. Nearly half of all employees are private with public contracts and only one health care profession, acupuncture, is completely private. Private medical staff receives money directly from the National Insurance Company (ZZZS). The PHCC in Radovljica performs the following activities and employs the following staff:

General practice	7 GPs, 6 of them specialists
Paediatric and school medicine	1 paediatrician, 1 specialist for school med.
Occupational medicine	1 specialist
Dental care for adults	4 dentists
Dental care for children	2 dentists
Orthodontics	1 specialist
Physiotherapy	3 physiotherapists
Neurophysiotherapy	1 neurophysiotherapist
Gynaecology	1 gynaecologist
Otorinolaringology	1X/week otorinolaringologist
Ophthalmology	3X/week ophthalmologist
Acupuncture	every day; medical doctor
Medical care for imprisoned people	2X/week GP

This includes a certain number of nurses.

PHCCs provide on call, emergency and out of hours services. PHCCs also provide medical care for the elderly in a home with 206 beds. Approximately half of these beds are for elderly people needing specialized medical care but not hospital care. There is also a home for youth with disabilities which has with 75 beds.

The owner of the PHCC's premises is the municipality, except for two family practice offices, which are a part of a new wing that private doctors bought this year. The municipality has some influence on policy in the PHCC, but is not very important. The PHCC is integrated with Primary Care of Gorenjska (Gorenjska is a region, where Radovljica lies). The PHCC of Radovljica has premises in several locations: the main building and majority of offices are situated in Radovljica, there is a branch office in Kropa (a village approximately 20 km from Radovljica); there are homes for the elderly and people with disabilities, and two dental surgeries located in primary schools.

An appointment system was introduced to make the services more accessible to patients. However, primary health care services are already very accessible, perhaps even too accessible since patients often walk in without appointment. The visiting rates in the Radovljica PHCC are more than eight times per year per person. Due to heavy workload and expansion of the cardiovascular programme, an additional family physician had to be employed.

A few years ago a nationwide cardiovascular prevention programme was introduced for 35–65-year-old men and for 45–70-year-old women. Workshops to teach healthier lifestyle habits (smoking cessation, weight control, healthy eating, physical activity, etc.) are offered for people with more than a 20% risk of having a cardiovascular problem. Patients also receive anticoagulant treatment and diabetics are seen in the PHCC.

In conclusion, following a long history of investing in primary care the health care system in Slovenia has had a relatively smooth transition to a decentralized model that recognizes the importance of primary care to continuity and the coordination of patient services.

Continuity of GP care

The following indicators are available for continuity of care: the percentage of GPs in a country who visit their hospitalized patients, GPs actively involved in evening, night and weekend services and GPs routinely keeping medical records for (almost) all attending patients (see Table 2.B). Making home visits has not been taken into account, because in all countries, except Turkey and Finland, it was reported as a task by a large majority of GPs. Hospitalized patients are visited by about three quarters of GPs in the Netherlands and Belgium and by 40% to well over 50% in France, Italy, Portugal, Romania and Ukraine. Such visits are rarely made by GPs in Denmark, Latvia, Norway, Slovenia and Sweden.

Countries where at least 80% of GPs are actively involved in out-of-hours primary care (for instance, in a rota group) are the Austria, Belgium, Finland, Iceland, Ireland, Luxembourg, the Netherlands, Sweden, Switzerland and the United Kingdom (see Table 2.B). In contrast, only small minorities of GPs are involved in these services in Croatia, Estonia, Italy, Lithuania and Poland. GPs in countries with a social health insurance system appear to be more involved in out-of-hours services than those in the tax-funded systems.

Keeping comprehensive medical records on a routine basis are indispensable for maintaining continuity of care. In Finland, Germany, Luxembourg and Switzerland records are kept routinely by more than 90% of the GPs. This is also true for most countries where GPs hold a gatekeeping position, with the exception of Italy and Spain, where it is reported by only 70% of GPs (see Table 2.B). Bulgaria, Greece and Romania rank lowest in this respect (around 40% or less).

Practice equipment

The use of medical equipment was measured with a list of 25 items; GPs were asked to indicate if it was available and used in the practice. The list included, among other items: haemoglobinometer, blood glucose test, cholesterol meter, ophthalmoscope, gastroscope, ultrasound, audiometer, peakflow meter, electrocardiograph, set for minor surgery and defibrillator. Equipment assumed to be used everywhere, for example the sphygmomanometer, was not included. As Figure 2.5 (see plate section) and Table 2.C show, GPs in Germany, Lithuania, the Netherlands, Nordic countries and Switzerland have the most items of equipment, 12 or more from the list. Relatively low levels of equipment (four to six) are in general practice in the Czech Republic, Hungary, Italy, Poland, Portugal and Romania. Thus, it can be surmized that although GPs in Italy and Portugal are gatekeepers, they do not have much equipment in their practices.

Indicators of the availability of X-ray and diagnostic laboratory facilities were the presence of appropriate equipment in the GP practice or externally, with results available within 48 hours (see Table 2.C). Five of the countries having most of the items from the list of 25 are here again in the group with the highest scores (availability among at least 90% of GPs). These countries are Finland, Iceland, Lithuania, the Netherlands and Sweden. In Belgium and the United Kingdom more than 75% of GPs have X-ray and laboratory facilities at their disposal with quick reporting of results. Countries with high levels of practice equipment but limited X-ray and laboratory facilities for GPs are Austria, Denmark, Germany, Norway and Switzerland. GPs, particularly in the Czech Republic and Poland, but also in Croatia, Hungary, Portugal and Turkey are worst off in term of X-ray and laboratory facilities and practice equipment.

Job satisfaction

The European Task Profile Study of general practice contained questions on different aspects of job satisfaction. Most GPs indicated interest and enjoyment in their work; only 14% would prefer other work. Seventy per cent of GPs reported an administrative overload. Satisfaction about the balance between effort and reward was not high overall, but quite low in the countries of central and eastern Europe and in Portugal and Turkey (Boerma and Fleming, 1998). About half of the GPs felt that some parts of their work did not make sense (this is shown in Figure 2.6 (see plate section) and in Table 2.C).

The largest proportion of GPs who believe that parts of their work do not make sense are in Bulgaria, Finland, Italy, Lithuania, the Netherlands, Portugal, Romania and the United Kingdom. It seems that in countries where GPs are gatekeepers, they are somewhat less satisfied on this respect than GPs in other countries. The reason for this may be that gatekeeping GPs, as the regular point of entry, cannot easily make a selection in their case mix to exclude tasks regarded as less reasonable.

The state of primary care in Europe: conclusions

Probably more important than the evident great differences in general practice across Europe is how these differences are related to the way health care and primary care are organized in different countries. A number of conclusions can be drawn from a European study (Boerma, 2003). The organization of a health care system is an important determinant of the way primary care services are provided. In countries with a *referral* or *gatekeeping* system, GPs generally provide a more comprehensive range of services, although they work fewer hours than GPs in countries with parallel access to medical specialists. In countries with *self-employed* GPs paid on a fee-for-service basis, the GPs are more involved in the treatment and follow-up of diseases and they spend more of their working hours on direct patient care than GPs in other countries. *Salaried GPs provide fewer treatment services than self-employed GPs.* The prevailing payment system also influences how GPs respond to varying workloads. Furthermore, there is a consistent contrast between the post-communist countries and the western European countries. In the western European countries, GPs have more comprehensive service profiles than in central and Eastern Europe, particularly regarding point of entry into the health system and the provision of medicotechnical procedures. Among post-communist countries distinctions are also found between the countries of the "former Yugoslavia" and countries previously belonging to the Soviet Union.

On the basis of these results, a number of implications can be drawn. The chapters that follow will expand on these themes.

- Gatekeeping GPs are well positioned in the patient flow at the entrance to health care systems to respond to a wide range of ordinary conditions. This position favours a coordinating role. Many countries are currently examining flexible forms of GP gatekeeping. In countries with gatekeeping GPs, this system is sometimes felt to be too rigid (for instance, in care for the chronically ill), whereas some countries without a gatekeeping system are trying to introduce one, initially on a voluntary basis.
- With respect to coordination and continuity of care, a system in which patients are registered with a GP appears favourable in that it offers a greater likelihood that medical information will be stored in one place, than do systems without patient lists. A patient list system is not sufficient, however. Individual GPs need to keep comprehensive medical records and maintain good working relations with other health professionals in primary and secondary care.
- The mode of employment and payment of GPs should strive for a balance between meeting patients' needs and avoiding overtreatment. Self-employed GPs appear to be more active than salaried GPs, both in terms of services offered and working hours. Services like preventive screening, which are not demand-driven, are unlikely to be provided under simple capitation payment systems, which means that additional target payments are needed.
- There is a trend of expanding responsibilities in primary care, resulting from task transfer from secondary care, as well as the stronger involvement of primary care in screening, prevention and health promotion. If financial obstacles for these services are removed, practices need to be prepared for these increased activities. It has been demonstrated that practices with more staff and equipment provide a wider range of services. Moreover, GPs working in groups may be more efficient because they work fewer hours with similar workloads.
- Computerized medical records are not just helpful for coordination and in providing continuous care to individual patients. A good practice database is also indispensable for the systematic screening and follow-up of chronic patients. Routinely kept medical records become a major source of information for epidemiological and health services research, and can help develop the currently inadequate body of knowledge on primary care in Europe (Rosser and Van Weel, 2004).

Table 2.A General practice: point of first contact care; generalist approach and comprehensiveness

Country	GPs' role as first contact with health problems					Generalism/Comprehensiveness				
	all health probl.[1]	acute probl.[2]	childr. probl.[3]	women's probl.[4]	ps./soc.-probl.[5]	treatm.of disease[6]	technic. proc.[7]	cervical screen.[8]	health educ.[9]	family plann.[10]
Tax-funded health systems										
Denmark[G]	1	2	1	1	1	1	1	1	4	1
Finland	2	2	2	2	3	3	1	2	2	2
Greece	3	3	3	3	3	3	2	3	2	3
Iceland[G]	2	2	1	2	2	2	1	2	1	1
Italy[G]	2	3	1	2	2	3	4	2	3	3
Norway[G]	1	2	1	1	2	1	1	2	1	1
Portugal[G]	1	3	1	1	1	2	3	1	1	1
Spain[G]	1	1	2	1	2	3	3	3	3	3
Sweden	3	3	2	2	2	2	1	3	2	3
United Kingdom[G]	1	2	1	1	1	1	1	1	1	1
Social insurance systems										
Austria	2	2	2	2	2	1	2	3	2	2
Belgium	2	2	2	2	1	2	2	2	4	1
France	2	2	2	2	1	1	2	2	3	2
Germany	3	2	2	3	2	1	2	3	1	2
Ireland[G]	1	1	1	1	1	1	2	2	4	1
Luxembourg	3	3	3	3	3	2	2	3	4	2
Netherlands[G]	1	1	1	1	1	3	1	1	4	1
Switzerland	2	2	3	3	2	1	1	2	3	1
Turkey	4	4	3	4	4	4	3	4	4	3

Transitional countries

	1	2	3	4	5	6	7	8	9	10
Bulgaria	4	4	4	4	4	4	4	3	1	4
Croatia[G]	2	1	2	2	1	2	3	4	2	2
Czech Republic	3	2	4	4	3	3	3	4	4	4
Estonia	4	4	3	4	4	3	4	3	1	4
Hungary	3	1	4	3	2	2	3	4	1	1
Latvia	4	4	4	4	4	3	4	2	4	3
Lithuania	4	4	4	4	3	3	4	–	3	4
Poland	3	3	3	4	3	3	4	3	2	4
Romania	3	3	3	3	4	4	3	3	1	3
Slovakia	4	3	4	4	4	4	4	4	3	4
Slovenia[G]	2	1	3	3	2	3	2	4	2	3
Ukraine	4	4	4	3	3	3	3	2	2	3

Note:
Ranking of European countries (1 = countries with highest average involvement scores; 4 = countries with lowest average involvement scores; 2 and 3 = countries with intermediate scores)

[G] Countries with GPs holding a gatekeeping position

[1] All health problems (27 short case descriptions; answered on 4-point scale)

[2] Acute problems (subscale on 5 cases, e.g. burnt hand, first symptoms of paralysis, sprained ankle, first convulsion)

[3] Problems related to children (subscale on 5 cases, e.g. rash, enuresis, hearing problem, physical abuse)

[4] Problems related to women (subscale on 5 cases, e.g. oral contraception, irregular menstruation, lump in breast)

[5] Psycho-social problems (subscale on 5 cases, e.g. relationship problems, suicidal inclinations, work-related stress)

[6] Treatment/follow-up of disease (4-point scale on 17 short case descriptions, e.g. hyperthyroidism, acute CVA, ulcerative colitis, myocardial infarction)

[7] Medical technical procedures (4-point scale on 14 specified procedures, e.g. removal of wart, insertion of IUD, removal of rusty spot from cornea, joint injection)

[8] Involvement in taking cervical smears systematically (e.g in a community programme)

[9] Involvement in groupwise health education or life style clinic on smoking, diet or alcohol intake

[10] Involvement in family planning and contraception

Sources: Boerma *et al*. (1997), Boerma *et al*. (1998).

Table 2.B General practice: cooperation and continuity of care

Country	Teamwork and cooperation						Continuity of care		
	2 or more GPs in practice	regularly meetings with other GPs[1]	regular meetings with ambulatory specialist[1]	regular meetings with hospital specialist[1]	regular meetings with PC nurse[1]	regular meetings with social worker[1]	% GPs making hospital visits[2]	% GPs active in out-of-hours care[3]	% GPs keeping comprehens. medical records[4]
Tax funded health systems									
Denmark[G]	2	4	4	4	4	4	4	3	1
Finland	1	1	2	3	1	1	2	1	1
Greece	3	3	1	1	4	1	2	3	4
Iceland[G]	1	1	3	3	1	3	2	1	1
Italy[G]	4	3	3	1	4	3	1	4	3
Norway[G]	2	4	4	4	3	3	4	2	1
Portugal[G]	1	1	3	2	1	2	1	4	1
Spain[G]	2	3	4	4	4	1	4	3	3
Sweden	1	1	4	4	1	4	4	1	2
United Kingdom[G]	1	2	3	3	1	2	2	2	1
Social insurance systems									
Austria	4	2	1	1	3	3	3	1	2
Belgium	4	4	2	1	4	3	1	1	2
France	4	2	2	2	2	3	1	2	2
Germany	4	1	1	1	2	2	3	3	1
Ireland[G]	3	3	4	4	3	4	3	1	1
Luxembourg	4	4	2	2	3	1	2	1	1
Netherlands[G]	3	1	4	3	3	2	1	1	1

Country								
Switzerland	4	1	1	2	2	3	2	1
Turkey	1	4	4	4	3	2	3	3
Transitional countries								
Bulgaria	1	1	2	3	4	4	4	4
Croatia[G]	2	2	4	1	2	3	4	1
Czech Republic	3	2	3	3	2	3	2	1
Estonia	4	2	3	3	2	3	4	1
Hungary	2	3	2	2	1	2	2	2
Latvia	1	1	2	3	4	4	3	1
Lithuania	2	3	2	1	3	3	4	2
Poland	3	3	1	1	1	2	4	2
Romania	3	3	3	2	1	1	3	4
Slovakia	3	2	3	3	3	2	2	1
Slovenia[G]	4	4	4	2	4	4	2	2
Ukraine	2	1	1	2	3	1	3	3

Note: Ranking of European countries (1 = countries with highest average involvement; 4 = countries with lowest average involvement scores; 2 and 3 = countries with intermediate scores)

[G] Countries with GPs holding a gatekeeping position

[1] Regular meetings at least once per month

[2] GPs who visit their hospitalized patients

[3] GPs involved in evening, night and weekend services

[4] GPs routinely keeping medical records for (almost) all attending patients

Sources: Boerma *et al.* (1997), Boerma *et al.* (1998).

Table 2.C General practice: medical equipment and diagnostic facilities; job satisfaction

Country	Medical equipment and diagnostic facilities			Job satisfaction
	Medical equipment[1]	X-ray[2]	Labo[2]	Work makes sense[3]
Tax funded health systems				
Denmark[G]	1	3	3	3
Finland	1	1	1	4
Greece	3	2	2	2
Iceland[G]	1	1	1	1
Italy[G]	4	2	2	4
Norway[G]	1	4	4	1
Portugal[G]	3	4	4	4
Spain[G]	3	2	3	3
Sweden	1	1	1	2
United Kingdom[G]	2	1	1	4
Social insurance systems				
Austria	2	4	4	1
Belgium	2	1	1	3
France	2	2	2	2
Germany	1	4	3	1
Ireland[G]	2	1	1	2
Luxembourg	2	3	3	2
Netherlands[G]	1	1	1	4
Switzerland	1	4	4	1
Turkey	3	3	3	3
Transitional countries				
Bulgaria	2	3	3	4
Croatia[G]	3	4	3	1
Czech Republic	4	4	4	2
Estonia	2	3	2	3
Hungary	3	3	3	2
Latvia	2	3	3	1
Lithuania	1	1	1	4
Poland	4	4	4	3
Romania	4	2	2	4
Slovakia	3	2	3	1
Slovenia[G]	2	3	1	3
Ukraine	4	2	2	3

Note: Ranking of European countries (1 = countries with highest average scores; 4 = countries with lowest average scores; 2 and 3 countries with intermediate scores)
Sources: Boerma et al. (1997), Boerma et al. (1998).
[1] Medical equipment being used from a list of 25 items
[2] X-ray/laboratory facilities within the practice or external with results within 48 hours
[3] % GPs disagreeing with: "Some parts of my work do not really make sense".
[G] Countries with GPs holding a gatekeeping position.

Notes

1   This vignette was written by Richard B. Saltman.
2   This vignette was writen by Elvira Chirila, GP, Romanian coordinator of the Dutch-funded Matra programme and Jan C. van Es, MD, PhD, general coordinator Matra programme.
3   This vignette was written by Marjana Grm, GP and Janko Kersnik, GP, Radovljica, Slovenia.

References

Aguzzoli, F., Aligon, A., Com-Ruelle, L. and Frerot, L. (1999). *Choisir d'avoir un médecin référent. Une analyse réalisée à partir du premier dispositif mis en place début 1998 [Choosing to have a gatekeeper. An analysis, starting from the first mechanism established in 1998].* Paris: CREDES.
Alban, A. and Christiansen, T. (1995). *The Nordic Lights; New Initiatives in Health Care Systems.* Odense: Odense University Press.
Algera, M., Francke, A.L., Kerkstra, A. and Van der Zee, J. (2003). An evaluation of the new home care needs assessment policy in the Netherlands, *Health and Social Care in the Community* **11**(3): 232–241.
Anderson, G.F. (1998). *Multinational Comparisons of Health Care. Expenditures, Coverage and Outcomes.* Baltimore: Johns Hopkins University, Center for Hospital Finance and Management (http://www.cmwf.org/usr_doc/Anderson_multinational.pdf, accessed 18 February 2005).
Arnoudova, A. (2005). *10 Health Questions about the 10.* Copenhagen: World Health Organization (http://www.euro.who.int/eprise/main/WHO/InformationSources/Publications/Catalogue/20040607_1, accessed 18 February 2005).
Belien, P. (1996). Health care reform in Europe, *Pharmacoeconomics* 10 (Supplement 2): 1994–1999.
Blanpain, J.E. (1994). Health care reform: the European experience, in Institute of Medicine (ed.) *Changing the Health Care System: Models from Here and Abroad.* Washington, DC: Institute of Medicine.
Boerma, W.G.W. (2003). *Profiles of General Practice in Europe. An international study of variation in the tasks of general practitioners.* Utrecht: NIVEL (dissertation).
Boerma, W.G.W. and Fleming, D.M. (1998). *The Role of General Practice in Primary Health Care.* Norwich: WHO Europe/The Stationary Office.
Boerma, W.G.W., Groenewegen, P.P. and Van der Zee, J. (1998). General practice in urban and rural Europe; the range of curative services, *Social Science and Medicine* **47**: 445–453.
Boerma, W.G.W., Van der Zee, J. and Fleming, D.M. (1997). Service profiles of general practitioners in Europe, *British Journal of General Practice* **47**: 481–486.
Bundesministerium für Frauen, Jugend und Gesundheit (2000). *Gesundheitsreform 2000 [Health Care Reform].* Berlin: Bundesministerium für Frauen, Jugend und Gesundheit.
Chinitz, D., Wismar, M. and Le Pen, C. (2004). Governance and (self-)regulation in social health insurance systems, in R.B. Saltman, R. Busse, and J. Figueras (eds) *Social Health Insurance Systems in Western Europe.* Berkshire: Open University Press/McGraw-Hill Education.
De Jong, J.D., Groenewegen, P.P. and Westert, G.P. (2003). Mutual influences of general practitioners in partnerships, *Social Science and Medicine* **57**(8): 1515–1524.

Dixon, A. and Mossialos, E. (2001). Funding health care in Europe: recent experiences, in T. Harrison and J. Appleby, *Health Care UK*. London: King's Fund.

Dixon, A., Langenbrunner, L. and Mossialos, E. (2004). Facing the challenges of health care financing, in J. Figueras, M. McKee, J. Cain and S. Lessof (eds) *Health Systems in Transition: Learning from Experience*. Copenhagen: World Health Organization/ European Observatory on Health Systems and Policies.

Dubois, C-A., McKee, M., and Nolte, E. (2005, forthcoming). *Human Resources for Health in Europe*. Berkshire/New York: Open University Press/McGraw-Hill Education.

Evans, R.G. (1981). Incomplete vertical integration: the distinctive structure of the health-care industry, in J. Van der Gaag and M. Perlman (eds) *Health, Economics and Health Economics*. Amsterdam: North Holland Publishing Company.

Fedullo, E., Jansone, A. and Ignatenko, E. (2004). Innovative home care and hospice. Cross partnerships in Russia and Latvia, *Caring* **23**(1): 22–25.

Forrest, C.B. and Starfield, B. (1996). The effect of first-contact care with primary care clinicians on ambulatory health care expenditures, *Journal of Family Practice* **43**: 40–48.

Furuholmen, C. and Magnussen, J. (2000). *Health Care Systems in Transition: Norway*. Copenhagen: WHO/European Observatory on Health Systems and Policies.

Goicoechea, J. (1996). *Primary Health Care Reforms*. Copenhagen: WHO Regional Office for Europe.

Gupta, N., Diallo, K., Zurn, P. and Dal Poz, M. (2002). Human resources for health: an international comparison of health occupations from labour force survey data. Syracuse, NY: Syracuse University [Luxembourg Income Study Working Paper Series, No. 331].

Helman, C.G. (1998). *Culture, Health and Illness*. Oxford: Reed Educational and Professional Publishing.

Hobbs, R.H. (1995). Emerging challenges for European general practice, *European Journal of General Practice* **1**: 172–175.

Hutten, J.B.F. and Kerkstra, A. (1996). *Home Care in Europe. A Country Specific Guide to its Organisation and Financing*. Aldershot: Arena Ashgate Publishing Ltd.

Jepson, G.M.H. (2001). How do primary health care systems compare across Western Europe? *Pharmaceutic Journal* **267**: 269–273.

Lagasse, R., Desmet, M., Jamoulle, M. *et al.* (2001). *European Situation of the Routine Medical Data Collection and their Utilisation for Health Monitoring*. Brussels: Université Libre de Bruxelles.

Le Grand, J., Mays, N. and Mulligan, J.A. (eds) (1998). *Learning from the NHS Internal Market: A Review of the Evidence*. London: King's Fund.

Marrée, J. and Groenewegen, P.P. (1997). *Back to Bismarck: Eastern European Health Care Systems in Transition*. Aldershot: Avebury.

McKee, M. and Healy, J. (2001). The changing role of hospitals in Europe: causes and consequences, *Clinical Medicine* **1**(4): 299–304.

Niemelä, J. (1996). *Health Care Systems in Transition: Finland*. Copenhagen: WHO Regional Office for Europe.

OECD (1992). *The Reform of Health Care: A Comparative Analysis of Seven OECD Countries*. Paris: OECD.

OECD (1995). *New Directions in Health Care Policy*. Paris: OECD.

OECD (2000). *OECD Health Data 2000*. Paris: OECD.

OECD (2004). *OECD Health Data 2004: A Comparative Analysis of 30 Countries*. Paris: OECD (first edition).

OHE (2000). *12th Compendium of Health Statistics*. London: Office of Health Economics (OHE).

Parry-Jones, B. and Soulsby, J. (2001). Needs-led assessment: the challenges and the reality, *Health and Social Care in the Community* **9**(6): 414–428.

Preker, A.S., Jakab, M. and Schneider, M. (2002). Health financing reforms in central and eastern Europe and the former Soviet Union, in E. Mossialos, A. Dixon, J. Figueras and J. Kutzin (eds) *Funding Health Care: Options for Europe*. Buckingham: Open University Press.

Reinhardt, U., Hussey, P. and Anderson, G.F. (2002). Cross-national comparisons of health systems using OECD data, *Health Affairs* **21**(3): 169–181.

Rosser, W.W. and Van Weel, C. (2004). Research in family/general practice is essential for improving health globally, *Annals of Family Medicine* 2 (s2–s4) (http://www.annfammed.org/cgi/content/full/2/suppl_2/s2, accessed 16 March 2005).

Saltman, R.B. and Von Otter, C. (1992). *Planned Markets and Public Competition: Strategic Reform in Northern European Health Systems*. Philadelphia: Open University Press.

Schellevis, F.G., Westert, G.P., De Bakker, D.H. *et al.* (2004). Nog altijd poortwachter. Rol en positie van huisartsen opnieuw in kaart gebracht [Still being a gatekeeper. Role and position of GPs mapped again], *Medisch Contact* **59**(16): 622–625.

Tjassing, H., Kling, T., Janssens, P., Van Gorp, J., Bramall, J. and Bowman, A. (1998). Home care business opportunities in Europe, *Caring* **17**(9): 53–57.

Vehvilaeinen, A.T., Kumpusalo, E.A. and Takala J.K. (1996). A list system can help to reduce the proportion of out of hours referrals for male patients, *Scandinavian Journal of Primary Health Care* **14**: 148–151.

Vladu, V. (1998). Home care in Romania: a whole new concept, *Caring* **17**(R): 36–37.

White, K., Williams, T.F. and Greenberg, B.G. (1961). The ecology of medical care, *New England Medical Journal* **265**: 885–892.

WHO (2004). *WHO European Health for All Database*. Copenhagen: WHO Regional Office for Europe, June.

chapter three

Changing conditions for structural reform in primary care

Wienke G. W. Boerma and Ana Rico

Introduction

The 1970s and 1980s have witnessed many attempts in European countries to enhance integration among primary care services and to improve coordination with the specialist and hospital sector and with social services. These initiatives have demonstrated that there is room for experimentation and initiative, producing extensive experience on possible policy options to solve well-known problems of poor coherence among services in primary care. However, implementation has not gone beyond the activities of motivated idealists. In the meantime, since the 1990s, a new division of roles and new governance mechanisms have combined to change the organizational character of health care. New approaches to strengthening primary care need to take these changes into account as part of the increased complexity and diversity in health care.

Regulating health care and making reforms work is complex, not least because it depends so much on the motivation of diverse professionals within the health care system. The context of health governance is not only highly typical per country but it is also changing. Increasingly, governments tend to refrain from direct involvement in financing and provision of health care. In the domain of regulation, governments are leaving the details to lower level authorities or to other parties in health care. But governments can only make this shift from "rowing to steering" to the extent that the other actors are capable of taking up compensating roles.

Probably more than in other health care sectors, changes in primary care are difficult to achieve. As we have seen, the units of provision are usually numerous and small. Also many disciplines are involved, each with their professional backgrounds and employment status. Improving coordination and continuity in this complex situation requires a mix of policy instruments and the involvement of authorities, financers and organizations of professionals at different levels. This chapter reviews the kind of reform tools available, which in turn influence recent developments in health sector governance. It also discusses what it means for primary care to be accountable and what requirements are necessary for stronger primary care to be realized.

Reform tools for primary care

At the level of health care organizations, governance is shared by managers and health professionals to different degrees across countries, sectors and time periods. As in the case of health system governance, the trend over the last decades has been less towards "command-and-control", management-centred approaches, and towards more "steer-and-channel", clinical governance approaches. Organizational governance is heavily influenced by the regulatory and financial environment, and by the actors operating within it: central, regional and local authorities, funding bodies, organizations of professionals and patients and individual health care workers. Regulation for effective primary care, including potentials for coordination and continuity, deserves special attention. Such primary care systems do not emerge spontaneously in a laissez-faire environment. Rather, the system must be financed, planned and regulated, at different levels, in such a way that primary care providers are willing and able to take responsibility for the health of the population assigned to them (Groenewegen *et al.*, 2002). Experiences in several countries have shown that such approaches are not incompatible with current trends of more contractual freedom between providers and purchasers, more budgetary power for primary care professionals (for instance for particular services in secondary care) or the privatization of primary care practice.

Governance of health care organizations

In organizational terms, governance can be defined as the combination of two tasks: (a) decision-making (also called coordination); and (b) guaranteeing compliance (motivation and control). Organizational decision-making consists of dividing tasks across units, and reintegrating them through coordination. Governance is operating successfully when personal and organizational goals are reconciled, and actors are effectively performing the agreed tasks. Individual compliance can be achieved either through *motivation* (when actors perceive tasks as beneficial or useful) or through *control* (where the execution of tasks can be imposed on the actors) or a combination of both.

Organizational governance can be realized by means of three possible mechanisms: markets, hierarchies and networks (Williamson, 1985). In *market situations*, the central mechanism of coordination is prices, with the assumption that there is a spontaneous diffusion of information on costs, products and innovations. Motivation in markets is mainly achieved via financial incentives.

In *hierarchies*, coordination is mainly achieved through plans and routines, often designed at the top of the hierarchy, by managers. In hierarchies, means of guaranteeing compliance is through the hierarchical power held by managers, and ultimately, the threat of dismissal. In *networks* (also called *cooperation*), coordination is accomplished by interaction between interdependent actors; for example, negotiation or collective decision-making on the distribution and content of tasks. The means for realizing compliance in networks are less straightforward than in markets and hierarchies, since networks rely heavily on voluntary adherence to social norms (trust, reciprocity). Informal social control plays an important part too: fear of loss of reputation on the one hand, and threats of exclusion from the network, on the other.

When the applicability of these notions to primary care is examined, it should be noted that features of the demand side as well as of the supply side make it an atypical industry in which not all models of governance and coordination are equally suitable (Webb, 1991; Scharpf, 1994). Market-based coordination is adequate for certain purposes and under strict conditions, but price mechanisms are not effective, as a result of imperfect competition and asymmetry of information. Such market failures need to be compensated for by complementary state regulation. Furthermore, competition in a market strategy should not inhibit necessary joint working among competitors. An obstacle for hierarchical coordination is the flow of information. The top levels in hierachies have difficulties in getting access to information from the lower levels. Furthermore, the division of labour in hierarchies tends to be strict and rather rigid, creating relatively independent organizational units among which interaction is difficult. Whenever coordination across hierarchical organizational units and boundaries occurs, it is usually the result of network interactions. The public sector is a favourable environment for network-like structures, because of its relative stability and shared social norms (Webb, 1991; Scharpf, 1994).

Multi-level approach

For the achievement of network mechanisms of governance, which is an indispensable strategy in strengthening primary care, regulation (and particularly self-regulation) is required at different levels. At system (national) level, the scope of services provided in primary care is set by means of governmental rules, incentives and standards. Professional bodies, regional authorities and health insurers play, each according to their possibilities, a steering role at the intermediate level. At micro level, the behaviour of professionals can be influenced by budgetary and social control mechanisms, for instance within group practices (Groenewegen *et al.*, 2002).

Governance in primary care, or at least within disciplines, is usually firmly based on forms of self regulation and mechanisms of network interaction. Organization of (medical) professionals at different levels plays a role in developing norms and maintaining adherence. At practice level, peer groups serve as the last link in the chain of social control. Peer control, for instance in partnerships, has traditionally been the predominant mode of coordination, even within health care systems with formally hierarchical governance structures, such as the National Health Service-type (Goddard *et al.*, 2000). Indeed, GPs within partnerships are more similar in their behaviour, and to a lesser extent in their attitudes, than GPs not working in such groups. This convergence appears to be related to partner selection in groups and to the practice circumstances (for instance, the availabilty of specialist inpatient care). So, medical practice variation is patterned by social processes in partnerships and group practices and by local circumstances (De Jong *et al.*, 2003).

Using social interaction in peer groups appears to be a more effective quality improvement strategy than just giving feed back without such an educational context (Verstappen *et al.*, 2004). Although social processes among peers may also have less positive influences on the quality of services, partnerships and group practices must be appreciated for the opportunities they offer to realize types of network coordination. Since general practice in many countries is mainly provided from single-handed practice, incentives for the merging of practices would be a good step towards better conditions for primary care coordination. The next step would be to facilitate effective peer review among practitioners, supported by national and regional structures.

The role of professions

Medical professions are suited to making cooperative coordination mechanisms work, given their common process of socialization (through medical education), the high salience of reputation, and their shared value system. After graduation, professional colleges and associations are valuable for maintaining this process by setting internal norms and defending the interests of the profession vis-à-vis other professions, the government, health insurers or other actors in health care.

In many countries supervision of the quality of services has, to some extent, been delegated to medical professional bodies. Examples are the maintenance of medical discipline and regular procedures of accreditation and reaccreditation. Self-regulation, which fits well in decentralization, may be more comprehensive and extend to initiatives for quality assurance. The Netherlands, with its "Polder model", is a country with a relatively strong self-regulatory role of professional organizations. Accreditation of continuing medical education and the five year relicensing of GPs have been delegated to the profession. The Dutch College of GPs has been active in practice-based research and has undertaken many quality assurance initiatives. For instance, a tool for mutual practice visitation has been developed and implemented. Feedback from these – voluntary – practice visits resulted in marked changes in practice management of the visited GP (Van den Hombergh *et al.*, 1999). The development of professional standards or guidelines is another example. In some countries national bodies produce these, such the National Institute for Clinical Excellence (NICE) in the United Kingdom. In the Dutch environment of shared power, guideline development has been a successful activity of the Dutch College of GPs. Enabled by government subsidies since the early 1990s the College has produced a large set of evidence-based guidelines, each developed by GPs and for the benefit of GPs; centrally developed, tested on applicability with GPs and locally implemented.

Implementation of the guidelines has received much attention; evaluation has shown that multi-level approaches with extensive support and feedback are most effective for the acceptance and adoption of the guidelines (Grol, 1993; Grol and Grimshaw, 2003). The dissemination and implementation strategy of professional organizations usually differs from the approach used by independent bodies. Professional organizations, such as GP Colleges emphasize the implementation and the acceptance of the guidelines more than national agencies do (Burgers *et al.*, 2003; Hutchinson *et al.*, 2003).

Against the merits of quality improvement through self-regulated cooperative arrangements, a number of limitations and weaknesses should be mentioned. First, its scope is limited to the borders of each discipline; interdisciplinary coordination may be a subject for improvement, for instance with "transmural" medical guidelines, but will probably remain exceptional, particularly between medical and non-medical disciplines. Cooperation based on self-regulation may even increase the inward directedness and not necessarily result in efficient larger scale system coordination (Scharpf, 1994). Some of the barriers to efficient coordination within network-type arrangements are especially prominent in health care, namely, disregard of aspects perceived as less relevant (for instance costs); distrust of actors outside one's own network (for instance, other professions, including health care managers); and higher coordination power of members with higher prestige (e.g. specialists versus general practitioners) (Grundmeijer, 1996; Vehviläinen *et al.*, 1996; Somerset *et al.*, 1999). Another limitation is the informal character of these arrangements, which creates poor conditions for accountability and does not improve coordination in a structural way. However, if supplemented by external incentives and stronger management, cooperation becomes less informal and may gain in effectiveness.

Professional bodies also have an important role to play in health politics. Many of the disadvantages of network governance can be attenuated or counterbalanced by appropriate regulation and financing mechanisms. Cooperation between the state and primary care professional associations is critical to guarantee that adequate mechanisms are in play. For primary care professionals to gain leverage over hospital colleagues, powerful, politically mobilized primary care professional associations are essential. In countries in which primary care associations are strong, their participation in policy-making is more active, contributing to policies which further strengthen primary care (Rico *et al.*, 2003).

The reform context

During the 1990s, the field of primary care in Europe witnessed a wealth of experiments and a variety of different organizational changes. To some extent the diversity of reform strategies reflected the specific features of the primary care field, such as the functional and structural diversity observed in Chapters One and Two. However, the approaches were also related to the changing policy paradigms within the health care sector. Considered from the perspective of strengthening primary care, both internally and in relation to other levels of care, reform initiatives can be categorized in three broad groups of strategies (Rico *et al.*, 2003):

(1) reforms that increase the power of primary care (as purchaser or coordinator) over other care levels;
(2) reforms directed at broadening the service portfolio of primary care (as provider); often these services are transferred from other levels of care;
(3) reforms dealing with supporting conditions (resources and control systems), which are necessary to promote a stronger role for primary care.

The first two strategies affect the division of tasks in health care. The first implies an extension of coordination power across the interface; secondary care services become subordinate to primary care. The redistribution of tasks in the second strategy may result in better coordination between existing and the newly transferred services within the primary care level. Supporting conditions, such as measures to enhance collaboration and teamwork in primary care and other organizational resources, are essential, but are particularly effective if combined with measures from the two other groups.

Mixes of governance

The role of the state in health care differs from country to country and ranges on a continuum from strong ("command-and-control") to relatively weak (forms of "steer-and-channel" regulation) (Saltman and Busse, 2002; Van der Zee *et al.*, 2004). In the 1980s and 1990s state dominance in health care decreased in favour of the various options of steering and channelling. The extreme of *command and control*, where the central government has full power over regulation, financing and provision of health care, has become increasingly unusual. Where state authority in health care is shared, for instance with regional or local authorities, it is termed *decentralization*. Through decentralization, regional and local circumstances can better be taken into account. Power can also be shared with NGOs or semi-state bodies, such as health insurance funds or organizations of professionals. This type of delegation of power is called *self-regulation*. Advantages of self-regulation include a strong commitment to one's own rules as well as low administrative costs. *Privatization* applies to situations in which certain tasks, usually the provision of services, are transferred from the public to the private sector. In social health insurance systems, primary care is usually provided privately. Private provision typically requires stronger external supervision of quality. This inspection of privatized provision is not necessarily in the hands of the state. The task of regular external review of quality of services on the basis of fixed standards, which is *accreditation* or *licensing*, can also be fulfilled by independent agencies (Saltman and Busse, 2002).

Relatively strong state involvement was traditionally found in those systems funded through taxation and largely providing in-kind services to the population. However, private practice can also co-exist, for instance through GPs who work under contract within the system, or parallel to the system in private practice. In social health insurance systems, originally, the state had a more facilitating role, for instance by harmonizing existing arrangements in health care; health care provision being primarily left to private institutions and providers (usually not-for-profit), contracted by "sickness funds". At present, it is increasingly difficult to position particular health care systems on the basis of this simple dichotomy, in that the nature and extent of relations between actors have changed so much. Countries with tax-funded systems have experimented with changes that promote consumer choice and responsiveness, encourage competition among providers and increase resources for health care. The British NHS is no longer the pure public delivery model that it used to be, and the introduction of competing sickness funds has changed the character of the social health insurance systems. In many countries during the past decades, managerial control and market mechanisms have reduced the traditional power of the professions, however, accountable professional organizations have received new roles in the context of self-regulation. In central and eastern Europe, reforms included the introduction of independent practitioners, new modes of financing and payment with incentives to stimulate the provision of specific services as well as engagement in continuing medical education (Dixon and Mossialos, 2001).

Health system governance

Although there is some similarity among the general themes of reform pro-grammes in different countries, this may not necessarily result in more similar health care systems and structures of governance. The reform agendas have common influences from international organizations such as the World Bank, the OECD and the European Union, but details of implementation reflect differ-ent national structures. Convergence is challenged by an opposite trend of increased power at the regional level (Defever, 1995).

The question is whether certain types of health care systems offer better con-ditions for change towards stronger primary care than others. As we have seen, primary care is well developed in both the United Kingdom and the Nether-lands, but health care governance in these countries is not easily comparable. In the centralized British NHS the government holds a relatively strong position, while decision-making in the Dutch context is determined by negotiation, con-sensus and compromise among actors. Yet, decisiveness seems to be stronger in the centralized model, given, for instance, the greater success in the United Kingdom in restructuring general practice into groups and later, in the 1990s, the implementation of pro-primary care reforms that we have grouped under category 1: the introduction of fund-holding schemes, later to be replaced by the less market-oriented Primary Care Groups/Trusts. In contrast, the Dutch policy on promoting integrated health centres in primary care has not been very successful, the fundamental Dekker reform plans have never been implemented and at present it is difficult to reinforce the agency role of the health insurance funds in the Netherlands (Boerma, 1989; Schut and Doorslaer, 1999). Sweden, with a tax-based system and largely public control and provision of services, has implemented important reforms in the early 1990s. The Patient Choice and Care Guarantee scheme laid grounds for competition between hospitals and resulted in a reduction of the large waiting lists in those days. The Family Doctor reform allowed GPs to start a private practice and patients could choose their family doctor, either in private practice or in the polyclinic. This reform, as well as other pro-competitive reform measures, were discontinued in 1994, when the Social Democrats returned to power (Harrison and Calltorp, 2000; Quaye, 2001).

The German system, part of the Social Health Insurance group, is a federation with powers shared between central government, the *Länder* and non-governmental corporate bodies (for instance the physicians associations and the umbrella of the – hundreds of – sickness funds). Decision-making is quite separate among different parts of the health care system, with corporate institutions particularly powerful in ambulatory and primary care. The German Government has not improved the position of family doctors in primary care, which is still dominated by ambulatory medical specialists, and it has been difficult to introduce a gatekeeping role for GPs (Busse, 1999; Wendt *et al.*, 2004). In France, ambulatory care is provided by privately established GPs and medical specialists, inpatient care is a public domain and funding is provided through social health insurance. Policies on the rationing of access to care and the consumption of medicines have been hard to implement. During the 1990s, there were initial attempts to control demand and improve quality of care, for instance, by the introduction of voluntary patient health records (*carnet de santé*) and voluntary referring physicians, a kind of gatekeeping system (*médecins référents*) (Lancry and Sandier, 1999). In 2005, however, a mandatory national gatekeeping system was introduced (Saltman and Dubois, 2005).

It is plausible that centralized systems could push through structural reforms more easily while reform processes in countries with "shared power" may proceed more incrementally (Saltman and Figueras, 1997), but these examples do not provide strong support to this supposition. Using dichotomies such as central versus decentralised schemes or state versus market orientation may be oversimplistic. Overall, the introduction of market elements has changed the role of governments in all health care systems. Boundaries between the public and the private sector are blurring; however, the introduction of private sector approaches is only compatible with sufficient government regulation to safeguard principles of equity and solidarity. The role of the state has changed, though it has not been reduced. A suitable mix of governance requires a balance between regulation and entrepreneurship (Defever, 1995; Saltman and Busse, 2002). Another reason why the traditional classification of health systems as conditions for health reform is losing ground is the use of foreign best practice models for health policy (Wendt *et al.*, 2004). In financing there is a general shift from public to private financing; in both tax-based and social insurance systems the ongoing growth of health care expenditures will be realized in the private sector. In regulation, health care systems tend to rely more on "uncommon" coordination mechanisms. Social health insurance countries, for instance, continue to implement gatekeeping arrangements, which used to be associated with tax-based systems. By introducing an internal market in the NHS, the British government reduced direct regulation and increased the role of competition.

Changing priorities

In the 1990s the focus of health policy has been on cost-containment, by means of budget caps, expenditure ceilings and, in a number of countries, the introduction of market mechanisms (Saltman and Busse, 2002). It was expected that coordination and coherence between services and levels of care would also benefit from these measures. By the late 1990s these expectations turned out to be too optimistic (Goddard *et al.*, 2000; Rico *et al.*, 2003). However, an interesting phenomenon could be observed in some countries where pro-competition policies prevailed. Cooperative behaviour developed among health care organizations, rather than competitive behaviour, in order to face the problems related to poor coordination (Goddard and Mannion, 1998; Harrison and Calltorp, 2000). More generally, among health professionals and citizens, the belief in the potential of market mechanisms has been reduced and countries previously endorsing market-based reforms have started to be more open to pro-cooperation policies (Busse, 2000; Harrison and Calltorp, 2000; Robinson and Dixon, 2000; Donatini *et al.*, 2001).

Towards new care arrangements

Attempting to formalize informal networks seems to be contradictory. A reduction of the informal character by transferring coordination power and resources to a steering entity may arouse distrust and thus negatively affect the motivation of members. Yet interest in new forms of "managed cooperation", with a possible coordinating role of primary care, is growing. However, past experience has taught that voluntary informal schemes are insufficient to this end. The challenge is to design and implement policy instruments to promote co-operation and integration within primary care and across levels of care, based on a mix of innovative market-like principles and more traditional hierarchical measures, while leaving sufficient freedom to health care providers.

Culture of accountability

Developing a set of technical policy instruments may not be enough. There may also be a need for a change of culture. This can be done with "implicit notions of quality, building on the philosophy that the provision of well-trained staff, good facilities and equipment [is] synonymous with high standards". New forms of leadership could empower teamwork, create an open and questioning culture, and ensure that clinical governance remains an integral part of every clinical service (Halligan and Donaldson, 2001). Indeed, the launch of clinical governance, the British NHS programme of work to join up initiatives to improve quality, has elicited high expectations. Clinical governance came in 1998 as a reaction to a number of medical scandals in the United Kingdom, but also as a reaction to the situation in primary care, where some practices were able to secure a wider range of services or faster access for their patients than other practices. Clinical governance was not merely intended to improve quality, but also to ensure it (Baker, 2000). Clinical governance is connected to activities such as audit, evidence-based practice, continuing professional development, risk assessment procedures, critical incident reporting, and systems to identify and help poorly performing professionals. The scheme was launched as an organizational innovation requiring a cultural change in the health sector, and senior managers of Primary Care Groups and Trusts seem to agree with this view. They regarded a need for greater accountability as one of the most important aspects (Marshall *et al.*, 2002).

Clinical governance is not an isolated development. There are more signs, also in other countries, indicating that requirements concerning the quality of primary care, including cooperation and continuity, are increasing. Participation in quality assurance activities, or in collaboration with colleagues, local hospitals or home care services is no longer at the discretion of individual GPs. Increasingly it will be a contractual obligation for practices and institutions to account for their activities and the quality of their services to various stakeholders. Allen (2000) distinguishes between downwards accountability, upwards accountability and horizontal accountability. "Downwards" refers to the local community where the practice is situated. It can be realized by means of patient participation. Upwards accountability is directed to the health care hierarchy, for instance in Britain, the local health authorities; in social health insurance countries, the health insurers with whom contracts are held. Horizontal accountability is towards other providers in the practice or health centre or to local providers of other disciplines (Allen, 2000). Major subjects of accountability are the *process*, which concerns the proper use of sound procedures, such as records of patient care; the *programme*, which concerns the activities undertaken as well as their quality, for instance as proven by audits; *priorities*, referring to the relevance and appropriateness of the activities chosen; and a *financial* explanation, for instance the clarification of expenditure (Allen, 2000).

Tendencies towards growing accountability can be observed in a number of countries. Current schemes for continuing medical education and procedures for periodical re-accreditation of GPs are becoming more performance orientated, instead of input orientated (hours spent on CME activities). The term "continuing medical education" is being replaced by "continuing professional development" (see Chapter Nine, Heyrman *et al.*). In the Netherlands the government and medical professions are jointly developing schemes for measuring performance in general practice. After these schemes have been established, they can be used to allow patients to compare practices and thus make an informed choice of their GP. Health insurers, who have the option of selective contracting, can use the information to decide about contracts.

Not surprisingly there is a general need for performance indicators at all levels of health care. Most indicators have been developed for clinical work; but indicators on practice management can also enable patients and insurers to compare services and providers (see Van den Hombergh *et al.*, 1999). European unification may demand indicators that can be used for international comparison (Engels *et al.*, 2005).

The growth of rational approaches, such as evidence based medicine and the use of systematic evaluations (i.e. for the purpose of accountability) has resulted in a need for increased research capacity. In the United Kingdom, for instance, a national network of primary care organizations will be established to host shared research management structures (Shaw *et al.*, 2004).

In the past decade entrepreneurship and competition have increased in most European countries, not least those in central and eastern Europe. This has not been favourable for the development of strong primary care systems, which are easier to develop in a less competitive and more regulated environment (Starfield, 1996; Delnoij *et al.*, 2000). Development of pro-primary care conditions, such as comprehensiveness, continuity and integration with other services fits, better in an environment with accountable GP entrepreneurs who take responsibility for care and coordination to a defined patient population (Groenewegen *et al.*, 2002).

Diversity or uniformity?

Current primary care arrangements in most European countries will have to go a long way to be able to cope with the expanding range of services at primary level, including continuity and coordination for complex care, and become more accountable to their environment as well. Tasks and activities of individual practitioners and sectors need to be reconsidered and tuned. Many experiments, supported by stimulating policies, have produced a wealth of experience about possible future models of provision. Fifteen years ago a so-called scenario study on primary care and home care, commisioned by the Dutch Government, formulated new patterns of primary care provision to solve the problem of fragmented supply in the light of increasing demand for complex care (Steering Committee on Future Health Scenarios, 1993). Given the pluriformity of Dutch primary care provision, the scenario team designed several possible models of organizational integration for complex care, based on two dimensions: central versus decentralized control; and either observing or not observing the traditional division of tasks between sectors and levels. Two scenarios, the "extramural network" (with cooperation and coordination among independent providers through agreements and protocols) and the "extramural centre" (with stronger integration of providers and disciplines, usually in shared premises) are purely primary care scenarios. Interestingly, the extramural centre can either be built around an extended GP group practice, or around other organization in primary care, for instance a home care association. In the "transmural network" scenario, intramural organizations are more closely involved, for instance nursing homes or hospitals (Steering Committee on Future Health Scenarios, 1993).

This study suggests that there is no single best solution for a country; depending on local circumstances, different solutions can exist alongside each other. If, despite incentives, a merger between primary care services is not feasible, a federation may be an option. Furthermore, it is not necessarily general practice that should take the lead; if home care is well organized it can be a better place for coordination than small and fragmented general practice. In some countries pharmacies are in a good position for a coordinating role, in particular in systems where patients are registered with a pharmacy and where these are well (electronically) connected to GP practices. The above mentioned "transmural network" has good possibilities for coordination across levels of care. But primary care needs to be able to manage this type of coordination. If not, the scenario proposes to put the "intramural" partner, the hospital or the nursing home, in the driver's seat. This points to the fact that pro-coordination innovations are not dependent on the availability of strong primary care. This is in line with an international study on cross-level integration in nursing care that found that such innovations took place both in primary care-oriented systems and in secondary care-oriented systems. The approaches, however, were different (Temmink *et al.*, 2000).

Requirements for primary care coordination

Central regulation is necessary to create preconditions and positive incentives for primary care, but in itself it is not sufficient to achieve goals like better coordination and continuity of care. Similarly, efforts from within the professions alone are not likely to be sufficient. As we have seen, a multi-level and multi-actor approach is more promising. Thus, a first requirement for successful primary care reform is that relevant actors at different levels, including governmental, non-governmental and professional, agree on policy aims and modes of implementation. Furthermore, the aims and scope of reforms in a country are obviously limited by the level of sophistication and development of actors and their organizations and by current features of primary care. For instance, attempts to implement fundholding schemes in the 1990s in central and eastern Europe were doomed to fail, above because recently introduced general practice was unable to fulfil the related role. Similarly, it is useless to try to expand the range of services in primary care if providers lack the competence for it. In addition to requirements related to the health care system and the professions, there are conditions related to the practical working environment. These three groups of requirements are elaborated below.

Conditions at system level

In addition to the general requirement of sufficient political and professional support for changes, the central level is extremely important in setting general conditions for primary care. An example of a notorious obstacle to coherence and coordination are the different funding schemes prevailing in primary care. Home care may be partly funded from the health care budget and partly from the budget for social services. Cooperation between primary medical care and social work is not only hampered because of different sources of funding, but also because social services may have been delegated to lower level authorities (for instance, municipalities) than other primary care services. Furthermore, there may be poor grounds for cooperation if catchments – or working areas – are not similar. This may be the case if the practice population of GPs is not geographically defined, because patients are free to choose their GP, and community nurses are working in strictly defined areas. Many of these obstacles can be taken away at central level. Another responsibility that should also be dealt with is the education of professionals. Policy on curricula and volumes should result in the production of sufficient numbers of providers – and no more than that – who are prepared for their tasks in primary care (including cooperation and coordination). Education for health care may be the joint responsibility of the ministry of health and the ministry of education, a situation that may cause conflicts. Planning the medical and nursing workforce is an important function in order to avoid shortages or oversupply.

The position of general practice in the health care system is also a subject of central regulation. If general practice is to play an important role in both patients' first contact and the coordination of care, its position needs to be approved. A strong position for general practice is not readily compatible with directly accessible medical specialists who compete with GPs to provide first contact care (this can be solved by introducing a referral system). Similarly, continuity of care requires that patients have appropriate incentives to see the same GP for each new episode of care (this is usually realized with a patient list system; patients register with a GP of their choice). As far as these arrangements spoil market forces, appropriate incentives should be in place to eliminate the potential disadvantages of this monopoly. If funding mechanisms are used for regulation, health insurers have a role in addition to the government. The payment system may serve as an important vehicle for the incentives that can help realize the objectives for primary care and general practice. Most powerful are so-called mixed schemes, including a mix of basic payments (salary or capitation) with separate payments for certain additional tasks. Combined with a gatekeeping role for GPs (and registered patients) this creates incentives for delivering primary contact according to the principles formulated in Chapter One. Since payment systems may interact with other incentive structures, such as performance monitoring, peer review and audit, fine-tuning may be needed.

The professions

Self regulation by professional bodies has become an increasingly important instrument in realizing health policy goals. It can only become important, however, to the extent that these bodies are able to take up this role. This differs between countries as well as between professions. The stronger the autonomy of a profession (and the higher its status and recognition) the more significant the instrument of self regulation may be (at the expense of hierarchical control). The degree of recognition of general practice by other medical specialties in a country is usually well reflected in its position in academia and education. Where GPs have a weak position, their professional identity and professional organization is weak, and their education relatively poor. Recognition follows the following steps: firstly, its specific field of knowledge is accepted; secondly, an academic body is established to develop this field of knowledge; thirdly, those who practice produce literature that describes that knowledge; finally, there is external recognition by the other medical disciplines, as well as by the state and society as a whole (Pereira Gray, 1989). A strong role of general practice in health care is related to advanced stages of recognition. Thus, professional development, not only in general practice, but also in other professions, is a requirement for strong primary care. The process of professional recognition of general practice developed differently in Europe, with successes in the Netherlands, Scandinavia and the United Kingdom and still marginal positions in countries like Austria, France, Greece and Italy. In several transitional countries, active groups of GPs are catching up with western Europe (Lember, 1998; Švab, 1998; Švab *et al.*, 2004).

In addition to academic efforts, professional recognition requires an organization for matters like registration, accreditation, quality assurance and professional discipline, and for external representation in negotiations and for defending the material interests of the discipline. These activities, which are important elements of self-regulation, are usually accommodated in the professional colleges and associations (Boerma and Fleming, 1998). Furthermore, institutional coordination powers should be transferred to primary care through state regulation. Last, but not least, the financial resources of primary care professionals and associations are critical to guarantee their autonomy as well as their market and political power (Rico *et al.*, 2003).

Other primary care disciplines may not have reached the same level of autonomy, but the professional development pathway shows similarities. In various countries nursing has developed from being an ancillary discipline to an independent profession with several specialties and related education and training, including academic chairs in nursing science. In primary care the following specialties have emerged: community nurses (sometimes called district nurses), practice nurses and nurse practitioners. These nursing specialties have been important in the expansion of tasks in primary care. Primary care nursing has not developed well in all countries. In transitional countries, many nurses are still "writing nurses" rather than "nursing nurses".

The professional development of pharmacists, in some countries, has been interesting for strengthening primary care. Especially in countries with well-developed primary care systems pharmacies have evolved from shops for the delivery of medicines and related articles to points of information and coordination of pharmaceutical care. In systems where patients are registered with a pharmacy, pharmacists are in a good position to give information and to enhance compliance among patients. In the Netherlands, regular meetings of pharmacists and GPs in the working area of drug prescribing policy have been institutionalized. In this way pharmacies have become an active link in the chain of primary care.

The practice environment

Proper housing is an important condition. The concentration of various primary care services in shared premises may be efficient, create better cooperative and working conditions for staff and improve access for patients as well. Although housing in most health systems is a local responsibility, there may be supporting incentives at central level. Each primary care centre or practice needs to safeguard physical access and availability of services to the patients; to contract allied staff and to purchase the necessary equipment; to organize cooperation with other providers in primary and secondary care; and to make arrangements for continuity of care. Here also, incentives at central level are indispensable in bringing about the desired working environment. The remuneration system for GPs, for instance, may include targeted payments for staff and equipment. Furthermore, there may be norms for the design of the offices and organization of services; contracts may include obligations concerning opening hours and availability during evenings, nights and weekends. Eventually it may be decided at operational level how primary care services are provided to patients. Alternatively how accessible services are, which resources are available, to what extent professionals cooperate; and whether or not continuity of care is being observed. These aspects will be dealt with shortly.

Patients' access should be available on a continuous basis and patients need to be informed as to how to obtain care. Practice premises should be located within a reasonable distance from patients' homes. Access also includes provision for out of hours and holiday services. The availability of necessary home visits is an essential aspect of access. Effective home visiting requires ready access to patient notes. If it is not the GP making the home visit, other professionals in the primary care team can fulfil this role (e.g. the practice nurse). Patients must have the option of consultation by telephone.

Teamwork and cooperation. Common working areas or boundaries of responsibility are prerequisites for cooperation. Training for effective teamwork can help team members to surmount problems which are related to different status and employment of team members; when some operate as independent contractors and others are employed externally, for instance in associations for home care. Cooperation between GPs and medical specialists deserves special attention. In a gatekeeping system, GPs have a much stronger position in secondary care than in systems where ambulatory specialists also provide primary care. Remuneration systems for GPs and specialists should be fine-tuned in order to avoid perverse incentives.

Responsibilities for *practice resources* differ from system to system. Where GPs are salaried the provision of practice premises and equipment is normally the responsibility of the health authorities or municipalities. In contrast, where GPs are independent entrepreneurs they are responsible for acquiring and developing adequate premises and equipment. Ancillary staff facilitates administrative operations within the practice. Nurses are involved in medical technical procedures and routine assessment of chronic patients and health education. In larger units managers may be in place.

Computer facilities are particularly important. Computer files are increasingly replacing paper records in many countries. However, the computer has more to offer than records. It may provide an integrated information system for the team and for secondary care. In this way it is an instrument for the continuity and coordination of care. It also serves prevention, for instance the identification and monitoring of groups at risk.

Continuity of care should avoid duplication of services and minimize the chance of patients receiving contradictory opinions. Long-standing relationships between providers and patients are good conditions for giving health education and enhancing patient compliance with therapies. Medical records are essential for an integrated provision of services. They allow immediate treatment of disease, serve as a reminder, define the risk status of the patient, and can be used for practice monitoring, audit, research and teaching.

Competence is a major necessity for each professional. Competence is enhanced by training and (continuing) education. The completion of specific training followed by accreditation needs to be a condition for entry into general practice. Procedures for periodic reaccreditation are a means of quality assurance. Evidence-based medicine has become an important approach for high quality and cost-effective care. Research feeds the body of knowledge. Research achievements should be disseminated not only among professionals to improve their competence, but also among policy-makers, insurers and health authorities to make them aware of best practice and its conditions (Van Weel and Rosser, 2004).

Conditions for primary care that has potential for a coordinative role in health care are numerous. Yet some specific elements stand out as key issues to be addressed. Whatever the model of governance, countries resort to the same set of policy instruments for restructuring primary care services: enhancing gatekeeping, developing teamwork, changing methods of remuneration of providers, increasing or reducing freedom of choice for providers and patients, shifting the balance of centralization and decentralization, and changing the balance between primary and secondary care. However, the options for reforming primary care in a particular country are not unlimited; there is only limited room for a wholesale restructuring. As Mariott and Mable (2000) suggest in their international review of primary care reforms, the evolution of the established primary care systems in western Europe reflects a process of refinement of pre-existing arrangements and continues to be consistent with their historical and institutional development. Only the alarming situations in central and eastern Europe have resulted in more rapid and substantial changes. For the rest, innovations are neither dramatic nor radical. Where important conditions for change, such as the recognition of professions, are the result of a long process, no quick structural changes can be expected.

References

Allen, P. (2000). Accountability for clinical governance: developing collective responsibility for quality in primary care, *British Medical Journal* **321**: 608–611.

Baker, R. (2000). Reforming primary care in England – again. Plans for improving the quality of care, *Scandinavian Journal of Primary Health Care* **18**: 72–74.

Boerma, W.G.W. (1989). Local housing scheme and political preference as conditions for the results of a health centre-stimulating policy in The Netherlands, *Health Policy*, **13**(3): 225–237.

Boerma, W.G.W. and Fleming, D.M. (1998). *The Role of General Practice in Primary Health Care*. Norwich: The Stationery Office.

Burgers, J.S., Grol, R., Klazinga, N.S., Mäkelä, M. and Zaat, J. (2003). Towards evidence-based clinical practice: an international survey of 18 clinical guidelines programs, *International Journal for Quality in Health Care* **15**(1): 31–45.

Busse, R. (1999). Priority setting and rationing in German health care, *Health Policy* **50**: 71–90.

Busse, R. (2000). *Health Care Systems in Transition*: Germany, Copenhagen: European Observatory on Health Care Systems.

De Jong, J.D., Groenewegen, P.P. and Westert, G.P. (2003). Mutual influences of general practitioners in partnerships, *Social Science and Medicine* **57**: 1515–1524.

Defever, M. (1995). Health care reforms: the unfinished agenda, *Health Policy* **34**: 1–7.

Delnoij, D.M.J., Van Merode, G., Paulus, A. and Groenewegen, P.P. (2000). Does general practitioner gatekeeping curb health care expenditure? *Journal of Health Services Research and Policy* **5**: 22–26.

Dixon, A. and Mossialos, E. (2001). Funding health care in Europe: recent experiences, in T. Harrison and J. Appleby (eds), *Health Care UK*. London: King's Fund.

Donatini, A., Rico, A., Lo Scalzo, A. *et al.* (2001). *Health Care in Transition Profiles: Italy*. Copenhagen: European Observatory on Health Care Systems.

Engels, Y., Campbell, S., Dautzenberg, M. *et al.* (2005). Developing a framework of, and quality indicators for, general practice management in Europe, *Family Practice* **22**: 1–8.

Goddard, M. and Mannion, R. (1998). From competition to cooperation: new economic relationships in the National Health Service, *Health Economics* **7**: 105–119.

Goddard, M., Mannion, R. and Smith, P. (2000). Enhancing performance in health care: a theoretical perspective on agency and the role of information, *Health Economics* **9**: 95–107.

Groenewegen, P.P., Dixon, J., and Boerma, W.G.W. (2002). The regulatory environment of general practice: an international perspective, in R.B. Saltman, R. Busse and E. Mossialos (2002) *Regulating Entrepreneurial Behaviour in European Health Care Systems*. Buckingham/Philadelphia: Open University Press.

Grol, R.P. (1993). Development of guidelines for general practice care, *British Journal of General Practice* **43**(369): 146–151.

Grol, R.P. and Grimshaw, J. (2003). From best evidence to best practice: effective implementation of change in patients' care, *Lancet* **362**(9391): 1225–1230.

Grundmeijer, H. (1996). GP and specialist: why do they communicate so badly? *European Journal of General Practice* **2**: 53–55.

Halligan, A. and Donaldson, L. (2001). Implementing clinical governance: Turning vision into reality, *British Medical Journal* **322**: 1413–1417.

Harrison, M.I. and Calltorp, J. (2000). The reorientation of market-oriented reforms in Swedish health-care, *Health Policy* **50**: 219–240.

Hutchinson, A., McIntosh, A., Anderson, J., Gilbert, C., and Field, R. (2003). Developing primary care review criteria from evidence-based guidelines: coronary heart disease as a model, *British Journal of General Practice* **53**: 691–696.

Lancry, P.J. and Sandier, S. (1999). Rationing health care in France, *Health Policy* **50**: 23–38.

Lember, M. (1998). *Implementing Modern General Practice in Estonia*. Tampere: University of Tampere, Acta Universitatis Tamperensis 603 (dissertation).

Mariott, J. and Mable, A.L. (2000). Integrated health organizations in Canada: developing the ideal model, *HealthcarePaper* **1**(2): 76–87.

Marshall, M., Sheaff, R., Rogers, A. *et al.* (2002) A qualitative study of the cultural changes in primary care organisations needed to implement clinical governance, *British Journal of General Practice* **52**: 641–645.

Pereira Gray, D.J. (1989). The emergence of the discipline of general practice, its literature, and the contribution of the College Journal, *Journal of the Royal College of General Practitioners* **39**: 228–233.

Quaye, R.K. (2001). Internal market systems in Sweden. Seven years after the Stockholm model, *European Journal of Public Health* **11**: 380–385.

Rico, A., Saltman, R.B. and Boerma, W.G.W. (2003). Organizational restructuring in European health systems: the role of primary care, *Social Policy and Administration* **37**(6): 592–608.

Robinson, R., and Dixon, A. (2000). *Health Care Systems in Transition: United Kingdom*. Copenhagen: European Observatory on Health Care Systems.

Saltman, R.B. and Busse, R. (2002). Balancing regulation and entrepreneurialism in Europe's health sector: theory and practice, in Saltman, R.B., Busse, R. and Mossialos, E. (2002) *Regulating Entrepreneurial Behaviour in European Health Care Systems*. Buckingham/Philadelphia: Open University Press.

Saltman, R.B. and Dubois, H.F.W. (2005). Current reform proposals in social health insurance countries, *Eurohealth* **11**(1): 10–14.

Saltman, R.B. and Figueras, J. (1997). *European Health Care Reform: Analysis of Current Strategies*. Copenhagen: WHO Regional Office for Europe.

Scharpf, F. (1994). Coordination in hierarchies and networks, in F. Scharpf (ed.) *Games in Hierarchies and Networks*. Frankfurt: Campus Verlag.

Schut, F.T. and Van Doorslaer, E.K.A. (1999). Towards a reinforced agency role of health insurers in Belgium and the Netherlands, *Health Policy* **48**: 47–67.

Shaw, S., Macfarlane, F., Greaves, C. and Carter, Y.H. (2004). Developing research management and governance capacity in primary care organizations: transferable learning from a qualitative evaluation of UK pilot sites, *Family Practice* **21**: 92–98.

Somerset, M., Faulkner, A., Shaw, A., Dunn, L. and Sharp, D.J. (1999). Obstacles on the path to a primary-care led National Health Service: complexities of outpatient care, *Social Science and Medicine* **48**: 213–225.

Starfield, B. (1996). A framework for Primary Care Research, *Journal of Family Practice* **42**(2): 181–185.

Steering Committee on Future Health Scenarios (1993). *Primary Care and Home Care Scenarios 1990–2005*. Dordrecht: Kluwer Academic Publishers.

Švab, I. (1998). General practice in the curriculum in Slovenia, *Medical Education* **32**(1): 85–88.

Švab, I., Pavlic, D.R., Radic, S. and Vainiomaki, P. (2004). General practice east of Eden: an overview of general practice in Eastern Europe, *Croatian Medical Journal* **45**(5): 537–542.

Temmink, D., Francke, A.L., Hutten, J.B.F., Van der Zee, J. and Huijer Abu-Saad, H. (2000). Innovations in the nursing care of the chronically ill: a literature review from an international perspective, *Journal of Advanced Nursing* **31**(6): 1449–1458.

Van den Hombergh, P., Grol, R.P., Van den Hoogen, H.J.M. and Van den Bosch, W.J.H.M. (1999). Practice visits as a tool in quality improvement: acceptance and feasibility, *Quality in Health Care* **8**: 167–171.

Van der Zee, J., Boerma, W.G.W. and Kroneman, M. (2004). Health care systems: understanding their stages of development, in R. Jones, N. Britten, L. Culpepper *et al.* (eds) *Oxford Textbook of Primary Medical Care. Volume 1*. Oxford: Oxford University Press.

Van Weel, C. and Rosser, W.W. (2004). Improving health care globally: a critical review of the necessity of family medicine research and recommmendations to build research capacity, *Annals of Family Medicine* **2** (suppl.2): s5–s16.

Vehviläinen, A.T., Kumpusalo, A. and Takala, J.K. (1996). Feed back information from specialists to general practitioners in Finland, *European Journal of General Practice* **2**: 55–57.

Verstappen, W.H.J.M., Van der Weijden, T., Dubois, W.I. *et al.* (2004). Improving test ordering in primary care: the added value of a small-group quality improvement strategy compared with classic feedback only, *Annals of Family Medicine* **2**(6): 569–575.

Webb, A. (1991). Coordination: a problem in public sector management, *Policy and Politics* **19**: 229–241.

Wendt, C., Grimmeisen, S., Helmert, U., Rothgang, H., and Cacace, M. (2004). Convergence or divergence of OECD health care systems? TranState Working Paper No. 9. Bremen: University of Bremen/Sfb 597 "Staatlichkeit im Wandel".

Williamson, O.E. (1985). *The Economic Institutions of Capitalism*. New York: Free Press.

chapter four

Drawing the strands together: primary care in perspective[1]

Richard B. Saltman

Primary care is one of the most complicated areas of European health care systems to assess and analyse (Boerma and Fleming, 1998; Boerma, 2003). Historically it has encompassed different activities in different countries, and has been performed by different types of medical professionals with different types of training: general practitioners, family doctors, community nurses, nurse practitioners, physician assistants, physiotherapists, polyclinic specialists, paediatricians and gynaecologists. Different primary care physicians have different levels or even types of professional training: some are board-certified specialists, others are not; some go through hospital rotations, others do not, and recently, with the advent of primary care training programmes in central European countries, some primary care doctors were not trained as general practitioners, but instead are rather hospital specialists with six months' additional training. Nursing and other disciplines in extended primary care also have been developed to quite different degrees across Europe.

Organizationally, primary care has been structured in a host of different arrangements. These cover the full spectrum, from being configured in some countries as a for-profit business in the private sector to being structured in other countries as a public service delivered by salaried civil servants. General practice, as a core element in primary care, can be delivered in a wide range of organizational settings: solo practice, group practice, primary health centres, occupational health centres, and specialist polyclinics. Depending upon the system and the country, its medical responsibilities range from first line curative care focused on individual patients to both individual and population-level prevention (Kark, 1981; Boerma *et al.*, 1997; Starfield, 1998). In some health systems, primary care sits at the centre of a complex primary health care system, coordinating a wide range of nursing home and home care services; in other systems, primary care has little formal connection to any other primary health care activity (Goicoechea, 1996).

All this diversity has made it difficult to settle on a universal definition to describe primary care. As explained in Chapter One, this volume relies upon Starfield's functionally rather than organizationally defined framework, which emphasizes what primary care does rather than who does it or in what part of the health care system it is carried out (Starfield, 1998). This functionally-oriented definition fits well with one of this volume's central characteristics, which is its pan-European approach to primary care. This broader comparative approach is one key factor that differentiates the preceding chapters from several other recently published, United Kingdom-focused studies of primary care (Dowling and Glendinning, 2003; Peckham and Exworthy, 2003).

A second dimension on which this volume has taken a different direction is visible in the pragmatic organizational focus of the issues discussed. The two United Kingdom volumes noted above focus on the politics and/or ideology of primary care and also primary health care reform, while two additional United Kingdom studies, moving to the other end of the spectrum, examine quality-related, performance issues inside individual primary care practices (Van Zwanenberg and Harrison, 2000; Marshall *et al.*, 2002). In contrast, the authors of this volume highlight the specific structural, personnel, and managerial configurations which exist and/or are possible within different organizational arrangements, as well as the supporting conditions necessary to operate primary care services efficiently and effectively. This emphasis fits well with the volume's broader cross-national approach. It also reflects this volume's central focus on key primary care policy-making issues currently under debate in a number of European health systems.

This study's cross-national and organizational perspectives serve to bring into view the long-term development that primary care has undergone across Europe over the past several decades. This perspective makes it possible to examine both the substantial organizational accomplishments of primary care to date, as well as the policy challenges – old and new – that still remain to be addressed. These two assessments, in turn, can then facilitate a more informative discussion of the central policy question raised by this volume's title, namely, whether primary care can be in the 'driver's seat' in European health care systems. Each of these three topics – organizational accomplishments, policy challenges, and the driver's seat question – will be considered in turn in this chapter.

As a prelude to this discussion, it may be useful to review briefly the central points raised in Chapter Five through to Chapter Twelve.

Drawing together the chapter contributions[2]

The evolving organizational arrangements in primary care across Europe can be approached from a number of different perspectives. Changes have been under way during the 1990s and first half of the 2000s in the institutional arrangements by which primary care is structured, in the work-life arrangements by which primary care personnel deliver services, and in the quality standards that influence the clinical and social appropriateness of the care delivered. Each of these topics is developed in the volume's expert, co-authored chapters. While each category contributes to the overall assessment of organizational reform in primary care, each also reflects sufficiently different components of the central topic as to deserve separate consideration.

Changing institutional arrangements

The three chapters in this section (Chapters Five, Six and Seven) probe aspects of the shifting interface between primary care and other sectors of the health service delivery system. All three lend support to an overarching perception that internal organizational arrangements for primary care across Europe are at present very much in flux.

This theme is clearly visible in Calnan et al. (Chapter Five) "The challenge of coordinating," which emphasizes three major points. The authors contend, first, that gatekeeping had been useful in the past in encouraging integration of services across the health system, and in particular for coordinating packages of care. However, second, they argue that the basic concept of gatekeeping no longer fits easily into a diversifying primary care world with large group practices, part-time GPs, specialist GPs, PC teams, and PC nurse triage. The chapter lists five challenges that are likely to reduce the overall role of gatekeeping in the medium term: 1) increased points of entry for patients to primary care; 2) single electronic patient records difficult to implement across the entire health system; 3) patients may no longer know the treating GP (larger practices, part-time GPs); 4) emerging specialist GPs (e.g. dermatology); and 5) use of nurse triage for first point of contact. All of these factors can be expected to dilute not only the authority of gatekeeping, but that of the traditional GP as well. Indeed, this profusion of non-GP-based points of entry into primary care suggests that the traditional notion of GPs as the appropriate coordinators of primary care, as well as of primary health care and hospital care more broadly, may be "outmoded". Following this line of logic to the next step, it may be that there will be increasing need for "new forms of coordination of care at the organization level, rather than at doctor-patient level" (Calnan, 2002).

Following along from this view, the authors' third observation is that a variety of additional and/or alternative policies will probably be necessary to improve the coordination role of primary care in the future. These new measures may include: 1) specifying patient populations; 2) establishing a common package of care for particular patient groups; 3) defining shared and separate responsibilities for primary care partners; 4) establishing clear financial arrangements in advance; and 5) introducing training in information and communication technologies in medical education.

Although they approach the shifting framework of primary care from a financial rather than an organizational perspective, McCallum et al. (Chapter Six) in "The impact of primary care purchasing" develop along a parallel logical line. The chapter focuses on the ability of different types of primary care led purchasing to influence both overall health system effectiveness and also the overall system-level influence of primary care. They contend that, conceptually, primary care purchasing can streamline decision-making as well as improve flexibility, timeliness and appropriate use of diagnostic services. They also deduce that purchasing works best when primary care practitioners have the clear ability to make choices about their financial liability and to control its size. Although they argue that effective primary care purchasing needs to combine clinical and financial decision-making so that spending reflects best clinical practice, they note that neither the organizational nor the professional conditions necessary to achieving this goal are currently met in most countries. Thus, just as Calnan *et al.* (Chapter Five) believe that gatekeeping is a good idea that can no longer coordinate care adequately, McCallum *et al.* (Chapter Six) find that primary care purchasing is a good idea but that most countries don't currently meet the necessary conditions to implement it effectively.

The third chapter in this set looking at institutional arrangements is Sheaff *et al.*, "The evolving public-private mix" (Chapter Seven). These authors describe a profusion of new variants in the delivery of primary care services, characterizing this development as a major break with past patterns and traditions:

"New European forms of primary care provision have included medical cooperatives; voluntary provision, including informal and self-care; 'public firms'; new forms of commercial primary care provision; non-medicalised primary care (including 'alternative' and 'traditional' methods); and networked provision (four types: virtual primary care organizations around a care pathway; professional networks promoting evidence-based medicine; policy implementation networks; and 'new public health' networks under WHO Healthy Cities)."

They trace the ongoing process of diversification in institutional arrangements to the impact of competition and privatization, on the one hand, and to state-promoted implementation of networks as a way to enhance accountability within primary care, on the other. The authors reinforce their first basic point by suggesting that the introduction of benchmarking, contestability and other instruments of competition have encouraged public forms of primary care to experiment with new organizational models, which have the potential to improve clinical quality and to better satisfy patients. Once again, although Sheaff *et al.* (Chapter Seven) trace the source of increasing diversity of organizational forms and function to a different source – here, governmental policies encouraging competitiveness and/or privatization – they support the broad conclusion that primary care is metastasizing into a variety of new organizational formats, without clear indication of a future dominant model.

Changing working arrangements

The second set of chapters (Chapters Eight, Nine and Ten) focuses on shifts under way in the range and scope of the workload that GPs perform. The central observation in all three is that the parameters of that workload vary considerably in response to a number of external needs and requirements, suggesting that GP job profiles are at least as much the product of the broader society and health system within which primary care sits as they are intrinsically generated by clinical and/or preventive criteria.

Sibbald *et al.* (Chapter Eight) in "Changing task profiles" argue that shifting work patterns for GPs can be attributed largely to forces in the broader society and health care system. They identify five key factors which drive these changes: 1) the broader organizational environment in the health care system; 2) policy preferences for multi-dimensional professional teams, assuming that these teams are more cost-effective; 3) payment systems that reward GPs for adopting the desired changes; 4) training requirements from governmental and/or professional bodies; and 5) attitudes of health professionals in renegotiating practice boundaries. The authors also examine specific organizational measures by which changes in skill mix occur: enhancement, substitution, delegation, and innovation. Further, the chapter notes that boundaries between general practice and other patient services can be altered by processes of transfer, relocation, and liaison. Ultimately, however, the authors conclude that, since there is little convincing evidence about the superior cost effectiveness of one approach as against another, the particular configuration that GP task profiles take appears to be contingent upon the specific circumstances within a given country and its health care system. Thus, the shape of the job GPs perform is likely to continue to vary over time and from country to country.

These observations are reinforced in Heyrman *et al.*'s chapter on "Changing professional roles in primary care" (Chapter Nine). The authors detail the wide range of responsibility among government, universities, and professionals for GP training and Continuing Medical Education, and the diverse criteria that different countries set for the content and objectives of these educational activities. They also review the role of international organizations such as WHO and WONCA in seeking consensus positions for training standards among these diverse national actors. The authors observe that one particularly important element for the future will be greater inclusion of a broader community orientation into professionally sponsored training activities. They conclude that if professional self-regulation is to be maintained, it will require increased flexibility and adaptability to the new GP roles that are now emerging.

The third chapter in this set, on using payment systems to manage GP behaviour, again suggests the fungibility of current thinking and tools regarding primary care. Greß *et al.* (Chapter Ten) review traditional economic thinking about behavioural responses to differing payment arrangements. Among other important points, they note that the additional transaction costs associated with close governmental regulation of integrated capitation systems should be included in assessments of the relative overall efficiency of capitation as against fee-schedule based approaches. Consistent with the two previous chapters, the authors caution that payment systems work within – and in interaction with – a broader institutional framework, making it difficult to transfer mechanisms successfully from one country context to another.

Changing quality standards

The two final chapters (Chapters Eleven and Twelve) focus on continuous quality improvement in primary care. Both chapters underscore the importance of encouraging ongoing processes of quality enhancement while recognizing that, particularly with new technology, new challenges also will need to be addressed.

Baker *et al.* in their chapter "Improving the quality and performance of primary care" detail the large number of ongoing quality improvement programmes in primary care across Europe (Chapter Eleven). Looking forward, they emphasize the importance of moving quality improvement programmes to a second stage that incorporates patients. This is not easy to achieve and as yet there is insufficient evidence to indicate that this second, shared stage is more effective. The authors also suggest that national programmes should promote a culture that emphasizes GPs' sense of self-esteem as a way to help make quality improvement a normal part of GPs' daily work routine.

Kvist and Kidd (Chapter Twelve) take a similarly hortatory perspective in their chapter on new information and communication technologies. They emphasize that primary care practitioners will need to keep up with patient expectations regarding the Internet and e-mail. Further, GPs will find that integrating these new information technologies can help improve quality in such areas as antibiotic prescriptions, drug dosing, and preventive care. However, the authors caution that GPs will have to be alert to new challenges reflecting problems relating to quality control of information (particularly on the Internet) as well as liability issues.

In sum

Taken overall, the eight co-authored expert chapters paint a picture of substantial innovation and change in primary care systems. The portrait that emerges from these chapters is one of growing complexity – in the content of primary care services, in its organizational structure, in its relationships (both formal and informal) with other sectors of the health care system, in its range of personnel and in the responsibilities that it assumes. This new level of complexity requires a substantially different level of managerial coordination than did the earlier, traditional model of primary care based on single-GP offices. A second observation is that, with regard to primary care as elsewhere in the health sector, context matters. In this case the importance of context can be seen in the varying scope of work that primary care personnel are expected to perform, in primary care relationships both upward with specialist hospital care and downward with other components of primary health care, and, lastly, in the impact of a diverse set of broader societal trends ranging from consumer involvement to electronic recordkeeping. A third observation is that the ongoing process of change in primary care does not point toward any single dominant organizational and/or behavioural framework.

Given the degree of change in primary care seen to date, it may be useful to provide a brief review of the organizational distance it has already come, and of the policy challenges that remain to be addressed. These two assessments then lead directly into a discussion about the specific role that primary care might appropriately play in the future leadership of the health care system – e.g. whether and/or to what degree primary care ought to be in the "driver's seat".

Primary care's accomplishments thus far

From an organizational perspective, primary care has undergone dramatic development over the past 30 years. At the beginning of the 1970s, most primary care in Europe was delivered in one of two geographically defined but broadly consistent manners. In western Europe, it was provided overwhelmingly in single-GP private practices and was almost exclusively curative in focus. In central and eastern Europe, the transition to the Semashko model had been largely completed with first contact care – also curative in focus – provided predominantly by specialist physicians in ambulatory polyclinics. In this traditional picture, primary care clearly sat at the periphery of the overall health care system, with specialist hospital care and the issues associated with secondary and tertiary level curative care dominating the centre of both health policy-making and health service delivery.

The first broadly systematic change in this picture came in Finland with the passing of the 1972 Primary Health Care Act. This required municipal authorities to provide preventive as well as curative primary care services to their inhabitants, and folded these services into broader primary health care centres, which combined primary care physicians, nurses, social workers, and health educators into a comprehensive team (Järvelin, 2002). Sweden adopted a similar primary health centre based strategy with its 1973 Primary Health Care Act (Hjortsberg and Ghatnekar, 2001). This Nordic initiative was soon followed by the global approach taken by the Alma Ata Declaration of 1978, which emphasized the centrality of primary health care to the operation of effective, efficient and equitable health services, particularly in developing country contexts (World Health Organization, 1978). Thus by the end of the 1970s, one could see the first cracks in the traditional GP-based model: the organizational framework for the delivery of primary care, the exclusive focus on curative medical treatment, and the role of general practitioners as solo practitioners had all for the first time come under principled conceptual and practical challenge, not just concerning developing countries but within the Nordic region in Europe as well.

The 1980s brought a wide range of initiatives that built upon the concept of primary health care, and the role of primary care as delivered within primary health centres. By the mid-1980s Sweden had articulated its primary health centre based system, and Finland was doing so as well. Countries like Greece, Netherlands, Spain, and also the United Kingdom, were developing a number of similar publicly operated, comprehensive centres. Symbolizing both the shift in policy-making emphasis and the growing hegemonic aspirations of the primary health care movement, WHO's Regional Office for Europe sponsored an "action research" project across a half-dozen countries that sought, as its name suggests, to "Tip the Balance Toward Primary Health Care". This project subsequently published a volume of research in 1995 (Rathwell *et al.*, 1995).

During this period there was arguably less change in the delivery of primary care services in the Social Health Insurance (SHI) countries of western Europe. Despite experiments with better coordination between GPs and hospital and/or other primary health care providers, as well as the emergence of some group-like responses to cover problem areas such as providing out-of-hours coverage, the vast majority of primary care continued to be delivered by solo practitioners (Boerma and Fleming, 1998).

The 1990s generated a dramatic upsurge in organizational change in primary care in both western and central Europe. As several chapters in this volume document, the solo GP in countries like the Netherlands and, to a lesser extent, Belgium became increasingly caught up in various voluntary network-like arrangements, coordinating services both with other primary health care providers and with some hospital clinics. In the United Kingdom's tax-based system, April 1991 brought the first wave of GP fundholders, transforming GPs into budget holders for a portion of their patients' elective hospital procedures (Glendinning and Dowling, 2003). Despite concerns about the "state agent" aspect of this new financial role, fundholding spread into a variety of more extensive models, including "total fundholding," which, in turn, became a model for the Primary Care Groups that were introduced in April 1999.

In central Europe, the 1990s were a period of major transformation in health care generally, and in primary care in particular (McKee *et al.*, 2004). Abandoning the Semashko model, state-run polyclinics were dismantled and replaced by private GPs. In the former East Germany, the West German model of independent solo and/or group practice was replicated. Countries like Estonia and Latvia established training programmes in primary care in their medical schools, providing specialists with six months retraining before they began new practices as GPs. Thus, after starting the decade with an almost entirely state-employed polyclinic approach to first contact medical care, many of the central European countries ended the 1990s with a largely private cadre of general practitioners (see Chapter Seven, Sheaff *et al.*).

The 1990s generated substantially less change in primary care in the SHI countries of western Europe, perhaps due to that system's highly articulated status (in Germany and the Netherlands) or the controlling role of *le médécin liberal* (in France). However, various experiments with networks of GPs were organized in the Germany, Netherlands, and in Switzerland, and, as detailed above by Sheaff *et al.* (Chapter Seven), a wide range of new activities appeared in such areas as coordinated care for the chronically ill and the elderly. While the rate and scope of change was considerably less than in tax-funded western Europe and dramatically less than in central European countries, nonetheless measurable change appeared to be under way.

When one steps back and reviews the overall process of change over the 30-year period since the Finnish Primary Health Care Act, one cannot help but be impressed with the remarkable growth and development that has taken place in the organizational structure, the capacities and range of personnel, the budgetary impact, and, perhaps most importantly, the policy legitimacy of primary care. It is a sector of European health care systems which began this period very much at the periphery, but which is now struggling to be taken seriously at the very centre of these systems. One of the most important aspects of this shift has been that in a number of countries primary care is now no longer viewed as completely overshadowed by and subordinate to hospital level care. Rather, it has begun the long and complex process of establishing itself as an equally legitimate partner of the secondary and tertiary care sectors. The wide range of experimentation currently under way, the broad diversity of new models and approaches – clinical, managerial, and financial – all speak to the accomplishments achieved by primary care to date, and bode well for its future.

Continuing challenges

Notwithstanding the recent accomplishments of primary care across Europe, there still remains a wide variety of organizational challenges that have yet to be adequately addressed. Based on the assessment presented in the preceeding chapters, it would appear that some of these challenges represent the fruits of primary care's considerable development to date, while others are long-standing dilemmas that have yet to be resolved. Viewed from a comparative European perspective, these challenges can usefully be grouped into three general topics. The first can be termed 'managing the network', a challenge which has both clinical and financial dimensions to it. The second challenge can be termed the 'credibility question', which involves the ability of primary care in general and GPs in particular to maintain and/or obtain the necessary respect and status to support further progress and development inside the health care system. The third challenge involves integrating information technology and electronic recordkeeping into GPs' offices and daily routines, especially patient consultations. Each of these three main challenges will be discussed in turn.

Managing the network

Perhaps the central development in the organization of primary care in western Europe over the past 10 to 15 years has been the growing role of networks. As discussed at length in Calnan *et al.* (Chapter Five), Sheaff *et al.* (Chapter Seven), and Heyrman *et al.* (Chapter Nine), a broad and diverse range of networks has emerged to help manage clinical services. In response to increases in the number of chronic care patients, as well as the improved technical capabilities of telecommunications and electronic technologies, GPs are finding themselves involved in three levels of patient care generated networks: upward to secondary and tertiary level hospital care (for care of specific conditions, for example diabetes or asthma); laterally with other elements of primary care (for example for community nursing and out-of-hours coverage); and downward with public health and basic health care services (for example school health care and occupational health services). As Calnan *et al.* noted (Chapter Five), the new GP coordinating role no longer looks like gatekeeping, with its single port of entry and its mandatory control over patient referral to specialist care. Rather, a form of "differentiated gatekeeping" appears to be emerging, in which chronically ill patients can elect to have a specialist as their main caregiver, while other patients can rely on the GP more as an advisor when they need to cross sectoral borders within the health care system, possibly in a voluntary rather than a mandatory gatekeeping arrangement. Although the type of physicians acting as gatekeepers would be expanded, in this new approach the list system remains in place, given its essential role in coordinating care and keeping patient information in a single location. This model may be more suited to those SHI countries which have previously had open access to specialist care, as highlighted by the differentiated structure of the new 2005 universal gatekeeping programme in France (although the new French arrangement is mandatory not voluntary in design). A more flexible approach may become more appropriate in the future in countries like the Netherlands, however, where the growth of networks is substantial as is a vocal patient empowerment movement (Wildner *et al.*, 2004). More generally, it may well be that gatekeeping will evolve differently in different national settings, with varying mixes of characteristics.

The issue of financial responsibility inside these new networks – or indeed for care delivered elsewhere in the health care system – raises a host of additional challenges for GPs. Beyond responsibility for managing patients' clinical pathways – in networks as previously in gatekeeping arrangements – the financial dimension requires GPs and/or primary care to take on further managerial roles vis-à-vis other providers in the health care system. McCallum *et al.* (Chapter Three) present a variety of arrangements in which GPs and/or primary care are budget-holders for some combination of services beyond just clinical primary care in their offices. However, if GPs individually (or general practice as a discipline) increasingly take on financial management responsibilities for care delivered elsewhere, particularly in hospitals, they are confronted with what can be termed the "state agent" problem (Saltman, 2005). Since most of the funds being managed are either publicly raised or publicly supervised, GPs either directly (themselves) or indirectly (through the decisions of other managers in their practice or in primary care) may find they are placed under growing pressure to contain costs even if such reductions would require trimming back necessary patient care (Ham and Honigsbaum, 1998). Here, the concern is the potential risk to the GPs' fundamental role as the representative of the best interest of the patient. A corollary aspect of this state-agent dilemma is the potential reduction in patient trust in his/her GP to make clinically appropriate decisions (Calnan and Sanford, 2003) – a situation which turned out to have serious long-term consequences when it was created by the admittedly different managed care arrangements found in the 1990s in the United States (Robinson, 2000).

As primary care looks forward, the twin challenges presented by both clinical and financial management of emerging network arrangements will become increasingly important. There are likely to be a variety of different solutions pursued, reflecting different arrangements for primary care across different countries (as highlighted in Chapter Two) as well as the range of different national cultures and social values that will necessarily come into play here as with restructuring in any health sector institution (Saltman and Bergman, 2005).

The credibility question

As suggested by the discussion about the state-agent issue just above, patient trust is an essential dimension of effective primary care practice. While recent research indicates that GPs in well-developed western European health systems such as Netherlands and Sweden receive high ratings from patients (Socialsty-relsen, 2002; Van der Schee *et al.*, 2003), they appear to lack the same levels of status and credibility of most of their specialist counterparts (Saltman, 2005). While some primary care experts do not see this as a serious problem, it would seem clear that GPs require adequate credibility with both medical specialists and with patients if they are to successfully manage the types of complex cross-border networks that are now emerging in a number of health care systems. The question of trust, respect, and status – summarized in the notion of credibility – is likely to require considerable attention in the future from advocates of increased primary care responsibility in the wider health system (Saltman, 2005).

Information technology

This would appear to be the least daunting of the likely future challenges, in that it appears to be 'only' a technical issue. In reality, as both Kvist and Kidd (Chapter Nine) and also Baker *et al.* (Chapter Eight) indicate, the process of integrating electronic technologies into primary care practice will involve a wide range of organizational and procedural challenges, including the ability to maintain patient privacy and confidentiality. It carries a range of implications for present and future professional behaviour as well. The introduction of full electronic records involves nearly every aspect of primary care and has the potential to improve and/or systematize a large number of GP decisions and activities. It also introduces the possibility of considerably more thorough external monitoring and evaluation of primary care services – a controversial issue for many GPs.

The driver's seat question

In previous sections, this chapter has sought to construct a broader organiza-tional and comparative context in which to place the ongoing changes in pri-mary care across Europe. Taken together, the preceding sections of this chapter serve to frame the main question contained in the volume's title, which has been a central question in the health policy debate for some 20 years. Namely, is primary care capable of taking a dominant role in running the whole health care system, and, second, if it is sufficiently capable, would it be wise to do so? An adequate consideration of these questions involves a number of related elements, many of which are raised either directly or indirectly in the Part Two chapters. One major issue involves the direction that primary care itself is taking in its own development – away from solo practice toward networks and other forms of coordination – as well as the pressing need mentioned by

Calnan *et al.* (Chapter Five) to consider alternative strategies to re-develop the concept of gatekeeping. Can primary care successfully pursue these next stages in its own evolution while at the same time taking on not just the clinical coordinating responsibilities for the evolving system of primary care and cross-border networks (as is evolving in the Netherlands) but also planning and financial responsibility for other health care providers as well (a model currently under construction as Primary Care Trusts in England)?

A wide range of questions and concerns arise in response to this potential new role for primary care generally and for GPs and general practice in particular. One wonders, for example, how giving general practice a greater 'state-agent' role across the entire health care system will affect the time GPs have to treat patients, and the trust with which they (and their medical advice) is viewed by patients. If a mix of general practitioner and/or general practice does take the driver's seat, clearly more time will need to be spent on coordination and state-agent functions. Who within general practice – or primary care more broadly – fulfils these administrative and managerial responsibilities then becomes a central question. If GPs specifically are expected to spend their time meeting these organizational needs, it is likely to decrease the time available to be providers of patient care. On the one hand, in terms of their overall credibility, this new financial and administrative role would clearly increase GPs power *vis-à-vis* hospital specialists and other primary care providers. Yet if GP power increases, there can be little certainty that it will increase their status, respect, or authority – which requires the legitimating assent of patients, specialists, and policy-makers (Weber, 1947; Pfeffer, 1981). It is equally difficult to be certain how it will affect the trust they are granted from patients (Saltman, 2005).

Coupled to these perspectives regarding power and credibility are the realities of what GPs themselves prefer. GPs often mention that they are trained to take care of patients, not to administer health care budgets. Some commentators have suggested that while a small group of GPs might be interested in an enhanced managerial role, the majority would prefer to simply treat patients.

One potential alternative to putting GPs and/or general practice in the driver's seat would be to put primary care as an organization in the driver's seat, with the GP in the back seat, so to speak. This would entail developing manager-ial capacity inside primary care, with the GP serving as an advisor to its exercise, but without tangling up GPs directly in financial contracts concerning providers elsewhere in the health care system. Examples already exist of giving this responsibility to public representatives of elected bodies in Sweden, where subcounty-level political boards (e.g. at district level inside Stockholm County) administer much of the hospital budget (Hjortsberg and Ghatnekar, 2001), and in Finland, where municipal health and social boards play much the same role (Järvelin, 2002). A third variant is the Primary Care Trusts (PCTs), which are taking on the contracting responsibilities once held either by fundholding GPs or by the now-defunct District Health Authorities (Bindman *et al.*, 2001).

One should note that all three of these variants have developed in tax-funded health systems – thus far an example of a similar managerial role for primary care has yet to emerge within social health insurance systems (Saltman *et al.*, 2004). A 1993 Dutch futures study suggested three possible alternative ways to provide coordinated primary care in an SHI system, based on, respectively, larger primary care units (such as primary health care centres), hospitals providing primary care, or an integrated home care organization providing primary care (Steering Committee on Future Health Scenarios, 1993). More than 10 years after this study, the future organizational structure for delivering primary care in the Netherlands or other SHI countries remains quite diverse and rather unsuited to taking up a driver's position. One possibility is that sickness funds may establish stricter requirements in their contracts with primary care providers concerning, for example, quality, coordination, and range of services, and thereby help to push primary care towards a broader organizational role.

How various primary care led models might develop in the future is contingent on a number of imponderables. Perhaps the most fundamental issue is whether emerging primary care approaches can develop a good working balance between the managerial needs of the health system and the practical service delivery concerns of providers. If growing coordination and state-agent functions are to be transferred to these primary care organizations, it will be essential to ensure that they develop methods of working that harmonize with – rather than disrupt – GPs' ability to provide appropriate clinical care to their patients. It may well be that these GP/Primary Care Manager balances will develop differently within different countries (or even within different parts of the same country, as the Dutch scenario study foresaw), dependent on a range of institutional and cultural considerations. How these new balances evolve is likely to be essential in determining their longevity. In the long run, it is possible that new GP/Primary Care Manager arrangements could form the basis for an as yet undefined new paradigm which might eventually emerge in primary care in Europe.

Notes

1   Prior versions of this chapter were presented in the John Fry Lecture of the Nuffield Trust, London; and at seminars in Lisbon, Almaty, CREDES, and at the London School of Economics. The current version benefits considerably from comments made by participants at these previous presentations and by Wienke Boerma.
2   Support for this section was provided by Hans Dubois.

References

Bindman, A.B., Weiner, J.P. and Majeed, A. (2001). Primary care groups in the UK: quality and accountability, *Health Affairs*, **20**(3): 132–145.
Boerma, W.G.W. (2003). *Profiles of General Practice in Europe*. Utrecht: NIVEL.
Boerma, W.G.W. and Fleming, D.M. (1998). *The Role of General Practice in Primary Health Care*. Copenhagen: WHO Regional Office for Europe.
Boerma, W.G.W., Van der Zee, J. and Fleming, D.M. (1997). Service profiles of general practitioners in Europe, *British Journal of General Practice* **47**: 481–486.
Calnan, M. (2002). Comment at author's workshop, 22 May, London.
Calnan, M. and Sanford, E. (2003). *Public Trust in Health Care in England and Wales. The System or the Doctor?* Bristol: University of Bristol.

Dowling, B. and Glendinning, C. (eds) (2003). *The New Primary Care: Modern, Dependable, Successful?* London: Open University Press/McGraw-Hill.

Glendinning, C. and Dowling, B. (2003). Introduction: "Modernizing" the NHS, in Dowling, B. and Glendinning, C. (eds) *The New Primary Care. Modern, Dependable, Successful?* Maidenhead: Open University Press.

Goicoechea, J. (ed.) (1996). *Primary Health Care Reforms.* Copenhagen: World Health Organization.

Ham, C. and Honigsbaum, F. (1998). Priority setting and rationing health services, in Saltman, R.B., Figueras, J. and Sakellarides, C. (eds) *Critical Challenges for Health Care Reform in Europe.* London: Open University Press.

Hjortsberg, C. and Ghatnekar, O. (2001). *Health Care Systems in Transition: Sweden.* Brussels: European Observatory on Health Systems and Policies.

Järvelin, J. (2002). *Health Care Systems in Transition: Finland.* Brussels: European Observatory on Health Systems and Policies.

Kark, S.L. (1981). *The Practice of Community-Oriented Primary Health Care.* New York: Appleton-Century-Crofts.

Marshall, M., Campbell, S., Hacker, J. and Roland, M. (2002). *Quality Indicators for General Practice: A Practical Guide for Health Professionals and Managers.* London: Royal Society of Medicine Press.

McKee, M., MacLehose, L., and Nolte, E. (eds) (2004). *Health Policy and European Union Enlargement.* Berkshire: Open University Press/McGraw-Hill.

Peckham, S. and Exworthy, M. (2003). *Primary Care in the UK.* Basingstoke: Palgrave Macmillan.

Pfeffer, J. (1981). *Power in Organizations.* Marshfield: Pitman Publishing.

Rathwell, T., Godinho, J. and Gott, M. (eds) (1995). *Tipping the Balance Towards Primary Health Care.* Avebury: Ashgate Publishing.

Robinson, R. (2000). Managed health care: a dilemma for evidence-based policy, *Health Economics* **9**(1): 1–7.

Saltman, R.B. (2005). *Primary Care in the Driver's Seat?* John Fry Lecture. London: Nuffield Trust.

Saltman, R.B., Busse, R., and Figueras, J. (eds) (2004). *Social Health Insurance Systems in Western Europe.* Berkshire: Open University Press/McGraw-Hill.

Saltman, R.B. and Bergman, S-E. (2005). Renovating the commons: Swedish health care reforms in perspective, *Journal of Health Politics, Policy and Law* **30**(1–2): 253–275.

Socialstyrelsen (2002). *Komma fram och känna förtroende. – Befolkningens syn på tillgänglighet och fast läkarkontakt i primärvård [Reaching the services and feeling confidence – The view of the population on availability /accessibility continuing relationship with a doctor].* Stockholm: Socialstyrelsen.

Starfield, B. (1998). *Primary Care: Balancing Health Needs, Services, and Technology.* Oxford: Oxford University Press.

Steering Committee on Future Health Scenarios (1993). *Primary Care and Home Care Scenarios 1990–2005.* Dordrecht: Kluwer Academic Publishers.

Van Zwanenberg, T. and Harrison, J. (eds) (2000). *Clinical Governance in Primary Care.* Abingdon: Radcliffe Medical Press.

Van der Schee, E., Braun, B., Calnan, M., Schnee, M. and Groenewegen, P.P. (2003). Public trust in health care: a comparison of Germany, the Netherlands, and England and Wales. Presentation at the European Public Health Association conference in Rome, 20–22 November.

Weber, M. (1947). *The Theory of Social and Economic Organization.* New York: Oxford University Press.

Wildner, M., Den Exter, A.P. and van der Kraan, W.G.M. (2004). The changing role of the individual in social health insurance systems, in Saltman, R.B., Busse, R. and Figueras, J. (eds) *Social Health Insurance Systems in Western Europe*. Berkshire: Open University Press/McGraw-Hill.

World Health Organization (1978). *Declaration of Alma-Ata*. International Conference on Primary Health Care: Alma-Ata, 6–12 September 1978. (http://www.who.int/hpr/NPH/docs/declaration_almaata.pdf, accessed 16 March 2004).

part two

Changing institutional arrangements 83

Changing working arrangements 147

Changing quality standards 201

chapter five

The challenge of coordination: the role of primary care professionals in promoting integration across the interface

Michael Calnan, Jack Hutten and Hrvoje Tiljak

The problem of coordination

The issue of integration and coordination in health care is not new. For many years problems concerning separation and fragmentation of services as well as a lack of communication (Grundmeyer, 1996) and cooperation between health care providers have been discussed in many European countries. However, due to changes in the demands and needs of the population, the search for solutions has become more urgent. The aging of populations leads to an increase in morbidity, especially in the incidence and prevalence of chronic conditions as well as comorbidity. This may lead to a higher demand for health service in general and for more complex, multidisciplinary care in particular. More and different combinations of health services will increasingly be required. Patients who are being treated by more than one care provider are particularly vulnerable to the adverse consequences of inadequate coordination and communication.

Certainly, from the patients' point of view, the integration of care is a crucial element in their evaluation of the quality of care. For example, a study in the United Kingdom (Preston *et al.*, 1999) showed that patients and carers identified five specific issues involved in their experiences across the interface between primary and secondary health care. Four key dimensions were "getting in" (access to appropriate care), "fitting in" (orientation of care to their requirements), "knowing what's going on" (provision of information), and "continuity" (continuity of staff and coordination and communication among professionals). The fifth theme was "limbs" (difficulty in making progress through the system), which was influenced by failures in relation to the other four themes. The concept of progress is central to patients' views of care. It involves both progress through the health care system and progress towards recovery or adjustment to an altered state. It is suggested that the concept of progress may be an appropriate indicator for monitoring health service performance.

The call for increased "patient empowerment" and personalization of care may also have an impact on the need for coordination (Roberts, 1999). A fundamental shift may be required from a service-oriented health care system ("the availability of services to define the kind of care that is provided") towards a more patient-centred approach ("the actual needs of the patient define the kind of care that is provided"). This implies that the provision of care should be organized around and tailored to patients' needs, which requires specific coordinating activities. In addition, the setting in which health care is delivered is changing (from institutional care towards ambulatory care) which may also have implications for the need for coordination of services. This development is enhanced by the introduction of new technologies, especially those that can be used in an ambulatory setting, which means that more severe cases can be cared for at home.

The need, therefore, for enhanced coordination and integration of care is becoming increasingly important. This chapter focuses on the organizational mechanisms that can enhance the role of primary care in coordinating and integrating care. It will be divided into two sections. The first part of the chapter focuses on how the problem of integration (or the lack of it) and coordination manifests itself in different European countries, whether it tends to be associated with certain types of health care systems – NHS model (the United Kingdom), Social Insurance (France, the Netherlands) and Transitional System (Croatia) – and whether it is associated with specific organizational structures, such as the presence of a gatekeeping system. This includes a discussion of the problems of coordination and where they are most evident. The second section deals with solutions the different case study countries (illustrating the different health care systems) have adopted and what benefits the specific solutions have brought, if any.

How do problems associated with coordination manifest themselves in different health care systems?

One important way of characterizing a health care system is to examine whether general practice has a strong central position or not. This organizational feature has numerous implications for the issue of coordination.

Problems with gatekeeping

In countries such as Denmark, the Netherlands and the United Kingdom, GPs have a central position in the health care system. This is mainly based on their role as "gatekeepers". All members of the public (except 5% in Track II in Denmark) are registered with a general practice, the so-called personal list system. The GP is usually the first professional confronted with the patients' problems and the first to decide which kind of services are required. Most drugs are provided only by prescription and often other care providers, such as medical specialists, are accessible only after a referral by a GP. Gatekeepers intend, when possible, to treat patients themselves as long as possible and refer their patients to specialist care only when it is really needed. Furthermore, gatekeepers act as patients' guides through the health care system to ensure that they receive the kind of care that is appropriate. This role of the gatekeeper has been defined as providing navigation and enhancing responsiveness. Their central position enables them to keep medical records of the patients and thus enhance continuity of care.

To sum up, two gatekeeping roles can be identified. First, their control of the use of specialist, hospital or other expensive services, is meant to reduce or restrict health care costs, i.e., GPs act as a mechanism for rationing services. Secondly, they are expected to improve or maintain quality of care through their coordinating role. In this way, GPs are considered as the coordinators of the whole packages of care that is received by a patient, which could improve continuity. Thus, gatekeeping can be seen in a negative light as a mechanism for restricting access to otherwise beneficial care and cutting costs at the expense of the patient. Yet the safety of health care requires that only appropriate care is prescribed and that the system is able to respond to specific individual needs.

Therefore gatekeeping can be seen, at least in theory, as an organizational mechanism to promote integration, although problems can exist in implementing this mechanism (see below). Some studies provide evidence of the effectiveness of gatekeeping (Starfield, 1991; Gervas *et al.*, 1994; Shi *et al.*, 1999; Delnoij *et al.*, 2000; Gross *et al.*, 2000). However, according to Halm *et al.* (1997) it is still largely unproven whether gatekeeping achieves the dual goals of restricting health care costs and enhancing quality of care.

In the United Kingdom in the NHS system, the principal focus has been on problems of coordination across the primary/secondary care (hospital) interface, particularly poor communication due to professional rivalry between hospital doctors and GPs. There has been a continual problem of fragmentation between primary care, community services and social care owing to different systems of governance (Glendenning *et al.*, 1998). This latter problem has only recently been addressed with the introduction of Primary Care Groups (PCGs) and Primary Care Trusts (PCTs) in the United Kingdom.

Problems of communication between care providers are also prevalent in the Netherlands. They result in problems in patient education (patients receive different kind of information), discontinuity in care (waiting times and a lack of a "smooth stream" of patients through the health care system), less efficient use of resources in the provision of care (care providers do not know what diagnostic tests or treatments have already been performed by others, so they repeat them). Several causes for these problems can be identified. One is the organizational boundary between (generalist) primary and (specialist) secondary care Furthermore, the two core disciplines of primary care – general practice and home care – are organized and financed separately. These boundaries are now the main obstacles to the provision of integrated care tailored to the needs of individual patients (see De Roo *et al.*, 2004).

An additional problem is the broad range of tasks that GPs perform (Moll van Charante *et al.*, 2002). It includes preventive activities, acute curative care, care for patients with chronic conditions and sometimes emergency care (out of office). It is difficult to coordinate all these tasks inside and outside the general practice, especially with an average list size of 2 250 patients. A study in the Netherlands showed that the workload of GPs influences the kind of care they provide in daily practice (Hutten, 1998). Busy GPs have shorter consultations with individual patients, carry out fewer technical medical interventions (injections, minor surgery), prescribe medication more often and have higher referral rates to other primary care providers (mainly physiotherapists) than less busy GPs. Furthermore, coordinating activities requires time that is not always available due to high patient loads, more administrative tasks, more time required for continuous medical education and the tendency to work in part-time jobs. Therefore, workload is considered a threat to the position of GPs as gatekeepers in the Dutch health care system.

Problems in non-gatekeeping countries

In other systems general practice has not played such a central role. For example, in the French health care system patients have traditionally had a choice of provider. For ambulatory care, they could visit a GP or a specialist without referral or limitation, either in private practice or in outpatient departments in hospitals. If a physician prescribed tests or care to be performed by another professional, patients could choose the laboratory, nurse or physiotherapist. Although there had been no compulsory registration with a GP, people did have a preferred GP and were generally loyal to their GP with little evidence of "shopping around". There were, however, variations in consulting patterns of care according to social status, with the upper classes tending to favour specialist care, while manual workers preferred to consult a GP.

The lack of such an organizational mechanism in the French system produced problems of coordination and particularly in continuity of care, which was a source of dissatisfaction. This was due to patients having to organize their own journey through the health care system. No professional had formal responsibility for the process of care provided to an individual and the maintenance of his or her health. Moreover, it had become increasingly difficult for GPs to take this role with the development of numerous, highly specialized health care suppliers directly used by patients. Now that the French government has adopted compulsory universal gatekeeping as of 1 January 2005, it remains to be seen whether this new programme will adequately resolve these dilemmas.

There are objective data that indicate that lack of coordination in France can have a negative impact on the quality of care. For example, a national study conducted by the main sickness fund has shown that the medical guidelines for diabetes issued by the National Agency for Evaluation and Accreditation were only partly respected. Only 40% of diabetes patients have an eye examination once a year, with the same percentage having a biological follow-up every six months as recommended. Part of the problem may come from inadequate individual practices; however, the process of care is not managed by the system. It may be that the physician prescribes the tests correctly and advises his or her patient to see an ophthalmologist (and a chiropodist), but that the patient fails to follow this advice. The physician is not in a position to monitor the compliance of his or her patient, however, who may be seeing other physicians for the same illness.

There is growing concern in France that chronic illnesses, involving a process of care necessitating contacts with different professionals in the health care system, are not always adequately managed. In addition to national policies on diseases like diabetes and hypertension, the regional unions of sickness funds carry out surveys on various chronic conditions to evaluate the quality of outpatient care and undertake actions to improve medical practice. The lack of coordination is also a problem in two classic situations: the interface between hospital care and ambulatory care and the interface between health care and social care. As mentioned, it remains to be seen if the current reforms will positively affect these problems.

In central and eastern European (CEE) countries, the importance of one type of practitioner is also less prevalent. Instead, common practice has involved a shift towards *dispanseurs* – specialized clinics for specific health problems. In the late 1980s, before democratization, this approach resulted in two basic types of Primary Health Care (PHC) settings. One is known as 'home of health' or PHC centres, which could correspond to group practice in western European countries. These centres mainly consisted of a group of PHC professionals: GPs and other PHC specialists (paediatricians, gynaecologists), as well as other specialist: internists, oculists, dermatologists, etc. In the former Soviet Union, three PHC practitioners served as the basic PHC structure of so-called 'threeplets'. Their education would be similar to education of internists, paediatricians and gynaecologists, but they worked together as a basic team responsible for PHC service.

A slightly different system was created in ex-Yugoslav countries, where GPs were recognized as basic PHC practitioners. Most of them worked in PHC centres together with other specialists and they played a gatekeeping role within that context. The GPs role included a personal list of patients, keeping an individual medical records of those patients and other administrative responsibilities.

These structures prevented PHC practitioners from becoming individual practitioners offering personal care. Instead, the public perception of PHC practitioners was quite low.

The 1990s transition in CEE countries was characterized by two parallel pathways: (1) recognizing PHC practitioners, mainly as GPs, as a basic element of the PHC service; and (2) privatization of health care. Both movements led to the disintegration of the existing PHC structure and put the GP in a new situation. The GP became the symbol of PHC overall in the professional, medical perspective and at the same time the GP became a private entrepreneur. The coordination role became more evident, but at the same time GPs were allocated important new tasks. Moreover, the coordination role was strongly related to other tasks: financial and organizational, professional development, obligations derived from contractual commitments, and medical educational preference.

The structure of these new PHC settings suggests a broad collaboration, a great amount of teamwork and consequently a need for coordination. However, in the absence of a basic medical professional, the role of coordination was usually allocated to the health care manager or the local health care authority. These managers/co-coordinators were not always medical professionals. This system developed a paradoxical situation in which a group of PHC practitioners worked together but did not collaborate and coordinate their work.

Hospital doctors and consultants gained more public respect. Although the system encouraged good PHC/hospital interface (consultants were working in PHC centres), problems in collaboration emerged from the constant struggle for task allocation and the prolonged battle for public appreciation.

In sum, we can conclude that each of these different systems of organization presents distinct barriers to coordination, as well as a common failure to implement traditional communication channels. The literature suggests that the traditional structural barriers to coordinated care can be characterized in terms of separate management and governance (health and social care are in different parts of the public sectors); different ownership (public/private); atomized and competing providers; professional barriers (rivalries within and between professional groups); and also the problems involved in the implementation and operationalization of coordination instruments (such as delays in referral letters, completeness of patient records and communication between teams).

How different countries have dealt with coordination (country case studies)

The previous section distinguishes between countries with and without gate-keeping systems. However, as will be seen, each of the different countries has in some respects developed different strategies and solutions.

The French experience

There is a long history in France of local initiatives from health professionals to improve coordination among them. Networks were, for instance, organized at the end of the 1980s between hospital physicians and GPs for patients with AIDS. This coordination was particularly necessary since most treatments were initiated or provided in hospitals, and the GPs had to stay in close contact with hospitals in order to treat the patient effectively. Networks were also implemented spontaneously, using the same model, for specific populations, such as drug addicts, people suffering from hepatitis C, and very poor people. The physicians involved were generally GPs with strong social and/or political commitment. The Ministry of Health encouraged these networks with grants, but they were basically functioning according to the general rules for the delivery and financing of health care. The idea of giving one physician the responsibility of managing the care for a patient with a chronic condition ('referring physician') was first envisioned in 1993. At that time, the idea was that it could be either a GP or a specialist, according to the condition and the choice of the patient. This was not implemented at that time, but it was decided that for patients that had serious illnesses which exempted them from co-payments, the physician advisor of the sickness fund should validate a protocol of treatment in agreement with the physician following the patient.

The same reform implemented the *carnet de santé*: the idea was that patients would have a personal health record, which they would show to every physician or health professional consulted, who in turn would update it. The measure was first implemented for the elderly, then extended to the whole population by the 1996 Juppé reform (discussed below).

This regulatory instrument suffered from a double logic and somewhat contradictory objectives. It was an instrument of coordination, but with the primary aim of reducing useless expenses (by eliminating redundant tests and procedures and preventing health care consumers from irresponsible behaviour) rather than with the aim of improving quality.

Presented that way, this measure was more a constraint to patients than a benefit. If the health record had to be shown to all the physicians that a patient was going to see, it would have been difficult, for instance, to consult with a specialist without informing the GP, or to seek a second opinion. Since it was not compulsory (i.e., patients were reimbursed in any case), it did not work.[1]

The 1996 Juppé reform opened up a new opportunity by allowing separate agreements with GPs on the one hand, and specialists on the other. Until then there was a single agreement – the medical profession had always been very careful not to let the government divide them (Wilsford, 1991). A separate negotiation was the benefit given to what was, at that time, the main union of GPs (MG-France), for their support to the 1996 reform.[2] This union promoted a specific re-evaluation of the status of the GP in relation to the specialist, and in 1997 signed an agreement introducing the possibility, for any patient, to choose a 'referring GP'.

In this system (optional for both patients and doctors), GPs who agree to be a referring physician accept commitments: they are paid directly by sickness funds and not by the patient, they keep the patient's medical record, provide continuous service, ensure continuity of treatment, participate in public preventive programmes, follow the recommendations on good practice, and prescribe a certain percentage of generic drugs, etc. In return, for each patient enrolled, the physician receives an annual payment, which was doubled in 2000 to promote the scheme (currently 46 euros, which is fairly generous compared to the average annual fees per patient).

Under this plan the patient is encouraged to consult their GP first (except in emergencies), to consult a specialist only with GP referral, to bring the health record to each consultation and to follow the recommendations of the GP with regard to prevention and screening. This is a moral contract, not an enforced obligation, and there is no link with the reimbursement of care. The incentive to enter the scheme is that patients do not have to pay in advance and then wait to be reimbursed.

The beginning of the scheme was promising. The GP union that signed the agreement strongly advocated the scheme, in spite of the opposition of the other physician unions, and within a few months 12% of GPs had asked to be referring physicians. The number of patients enrolled, though, was much lower (1%).

Then, as is often the case in France, the agreement signed by this GP union and the health insurance funds was legally contested (by the other unions) and cancelled in 1998. Although a new agreement, including the same scheme, was signed in 1998 with the GPs, this time the enthusiasm of the GP union was less clear. In its second version, the scheme was limited to about 10% of GPs and 1% of patients. There had been complaints from GPs who joined the scheme about the administrative workload, and the waiting time to get paid by the sickness funds, etc. The political support of GPs as a whole for this scheme seemed unclear, in spite of the financial incentive. Indeed, the GP union which had signed the agreement was clearly defeated in the elections to the regional physician organizations in 2000.

Another initiative of the 1996 reform opened up the possibility of different forms of networks of providers, on a local basis. The aim of the experiment was to test new forms of coordination between professionals in ambulatory care or between ambulatory care and hospital care. The law gave a 5-year period to experiment, also allowing these networks to experiment with financial rules (tariffs, services reimbursed, remuneration of professionals, etc.). This innovation gave the opportunity to finance elements not taken into account by the prior system of payment (time of coordination and management for health professionals, information systems to share the medical records, etc.), and also to provide new benefits for the population (joint consultations, for instance). A large number of projects were proposed. These projects were promoted by groups of professionals, as well as by pharmaceutical companies and even insurers. Many were targeted at specific subpopulations (the elderly, very poor people) or pertained to specific conditions (asthma, cancer, cardiovascular disease, diabetes) or risk factors (alcohol). Some of the networks already in place sought to gain more financial support by applying to the scheme.

The projects were subject to the prior approval of a commission before they could obtain specific financial rules. This commission was criticized for being slow and discouraging promoters. However, the criteria for funding had not been fixed by law and had to be set up by this commission. There was also a political debate about the projects promoted by the pharmaceutical industry and, even more so, the insurers. The most spectacular was the proposal of a major private insurer who offered to set up a 'managed care-like' organization, i.e. the insurer proposed to provide a comprehensive range of health care services (through a network of selected providers) to a population enrolled on a voluntary basis, and to be funded by a risk-adjusted capitated payment for each patient enrolled. This proposal was rejected by the government.

In a year and a half the commission had accepted 12 projects. At the end of 2001 the annual Act on the financing of health care changed the process in two respects: it created a specific fund to finance the project, and transferred the power to evaluate and accept projects to the regional level (regional hospital agencies and regional unions of sickness funds). Since then, a series of experiments have been initiated in all regions.

The Croatian experience

A prominent issue in PHC in Croatia concerns the policy choice between integration versus coordination. The privatization of general practice in the 1990s (which means GPs have individual contracts with the health insurance fund and individually rent or buy premises for their practices) produced a shift towards less teamwork, less group practice and overall less collaboration. As health insurance funds do not allow joint lists of patients, i.e. group contracts, it is impossible to organize group practices. Individual contracts in PHC are offered to dentists, gynaecologists, paediatricians and GPs. Finally, in 'transitional times' the process of vocational training has not yet been well regulated – resulting in a diminishing number of vocationally trained GPs.

Several efforts have been made to solve the problems of fragmentation and lack of vocational training in PHC. The government as well as the health insurance funds have recognized the problem and developed initiatives to promote group practice and stimulate vocational training. The first problem was which type of group practice is better, monovalent (only GPs) or polivalent (GPs, gynaecologists, etc.)? Closely related to that problem is the type of vocational training that should be stimulated in PHC: only GPs or gynaecologists and paediatricians together with GPs. At this time, vocational training in general practice with the GP as the only contractor in PHC is the most likely option.

Regarding coordination with secondary health care, these initiatives are designed to make task allocations clearer, but tend to create problems in communication/collaboration with secondary care. While there are recent initiatives, most GPs currently work in "given circumstances": single contract, strict list, more or less single practice.

Two new models of coordination can be identified among GPs. Both are products of GPs' awareness that something better could be arranged. One spontaneously created project is the network of 'open-gate practices'. A group of GPs from all over the country have opened the doors of their practices to patients from other general practices. Temporary registration is not a possibility in Croatia and if they fall ill while staying in another city patients can use only emergency departments. If assigned to one of the GPs within the network, patients could use services and get prescriptions from any other GP in the network.

A second new model of coordination in PHC, in Croatia, is the (PHC) policlinic run by GPs. GPs who run these policlinics are working as contractual doctors for a health insurance fund and specialists in polyclinics are working without contract for direct patient payment. It reflects GPs' need to own or rent premises for starting a practice and obtaining a contract with the health insurance fund. However, financing through this contractual arrangement is not sufficient to cover the costs of buying premises. For that reason GPs buy more space and rent it to consultants/specialists. This enables the GPs to cover the costs of investment and also to offer more services to patients. This usually leads to more patients choosing the GP's practice, more patients on his or her list and more money through the contract. The GP can also arrange a different sort of contract to consulting doctors working in his or her clinic. Consultants can be paid a salary and payment for consultation can be collected by the polyclinic owner, i.e. the GP. Also, part of the fee for the service payment of consultants can be collected by the policlinic owner. As services of consultants are paid by patients and not by health insurance there are no limitations on services. GPs can be more secure because expert consultation is available on site and misconduct/malpractice can be prevented. Also, mutual informal education and consultation can be achieved, although no formal education and CME points could be gained though such work.

From the patients' point of view, this model has both positive and negative aspects.

On the positive side, it offers more convenient specialist consultation for patients in remote areas. Mutual consultation and education between doctors reduce clinical errors and an expert team can be formed on site to deal with more complicated conditions. However, on the negative side, most of the services are not covered by health insurance and there is a possibility of unnecessary provider-generated services.

The Dutch experience

In the Netherlands, a distinction can be made between two kinds of strategies. The first is strengthening the gatekeeping position of GPs. The second is the development of new organizational models of integrated care, which is called "transmural care".

Strengthening general practice

In the Netherlands, general practice has been dominated by individual prac-tices. Only recently the percentage of GPs working in partnerships or in health centres has exceeded the percentage of GPs working in individual practice. This implies that individual GPs have a weaker position compared to larger health care organizations such as hospitals, home care organizations and nursing homes. A study by Kersten (1991) showed, for instance, that, despite their pos-ition as gatekeepers, the influence of GPs is rather limited on the care their patients receive in a hospital. Therefore, since the beginning of the 1990s, organizational changes in general practice have been introduced. All general practices are now part of so-called GP-groups (HAGROs). Often these HAGROs (or one of their members) negotiate with hospitals and participate in develop-ment projects in the field of coordination. Furthermore, GPs participate in so-called FTOs: groups of GPs and pharmacists that discuss and coordinate the prescription of drugs. Also, the introduction of practice nurses, who are espe-cially employed to coordinate care for special groups of patients (diabetes, rheumatism) can be seen as a measure to strengthen the central coordinating function of general practice.

Recently the organization of emergency and out-of-office hours care has been changing, especially in larger urban areas. Traditionally this was arranged in small GP groups in which the participating GPs took over the responsibility of each other's patients (the locum system). Now, local large-scale GP services are established in which a limited number of GPs are on duty (during out-of-office hours) for the total population living in a particular town or area. They are supported by a car with a driver, a call centre (often staffed by specially trained nurses) which makes the first selection in patients' calls, and a central building which can be visited by patients.

Transmural care

Since the mid-1990s, serious attempts have been made to create new organizational forms of "integrated care" in the Netherlands. Two committees (Committee for the Modernization of Curative Care and an advisory committee of the National Council for Public Health) formulated new proposals to improve quality and efficiency in the Dutch health care system (Commissie Modernisering Curatieve Zorg, 1994; NRV/CvZ, 1995). In contrast to the implementation of other reforms, no comprehensive programme of reform of change was developed. Instead a bottom-up approach was chosen. The idea was that cooperation and communication between primary and secondary care providers could only be realized at a local or regional level. The process depends to a large extent on direct interpersonal relationships. A number of general changes in the organization and financing of primary care and secondary care were proposed, which could indirectly benefit initiatives for integrated care.

The main problem to solve through integrated care is the (organizational) gap between primary and secondary health care. This can be achieved by the creation of new forms of care – "transmural care" – which breaks down the traditional boundaries between primary and secondary care. The most frequently used definition of transmural care is: care, attuned to the needs of the patient, provided on the basis of close collaboration (cooperation and coordination) between primary and specialized care providers, with joint overall responsibility and the specification of delegated responsibilities (NRV/CvZ, 1995). Close collaboration implies collaboration between health professionals on a formal structural basis (Temmink, 2000). This can be organized in regular meetings between care providers, in which patient-related subjects as well as the preconditions of the transmural care process are discussed. Joint responsibility refers to formal agreements about the transmural care process at an organizational level. Such agreements can be laid down in protocols or guidelines.

There are now many forms of transmural care. Van der Linden (2001) made an inventory of types of transmural care that were established in 1999. She found a total of more than 500 projects which were categorized in seven groups:

1. Specialized nurse clinics for chronic patient sufferers of asthma, diabetes, and rheumatic diseases.
2. Guideline development at national level as well as at regional level for specific diagnoses such as asthma and low fertility. In some areas local guidelines are developed about the patient flows in the organization of care (e.g. discharge protocols, patient information/education guidelines and clinical agreements about the treatment).
3. Home care technology to provide specialist care at home (hospital at home).
4. Discharge planning by the introduction of specialized liaison or transfer nurses.

5. Consultation of medical specialists and use of hospital facilities by GPs (e.g. feedback on the interpretation of the results of diagnostic tests, prescription of drugs and referrals).
6. Rehabilitation wards for patients who require temporary post-acute care after hospitalization (e.g. stabilized stroke patients or post-operative hip patients).
7. Initiatives for streamlining prescription and delivery of drugs.

The organizational structures of these initiatives differ. Some specific forms of transmural care are organized in special groups such as palliative networks and are called "pain teams", which mostly operate in the community. In these kind of organizational units GPs often play a central, coordinating role. First results of some evaluative studies indicate that new organizational forms that increase continuity of care are more cost-effective and lead to higher patient satisfaction, as the needs of individual patients can better be met than in the traditional situation (see, for example, Smelt *et al.*, 1999; Francke and Willems, 2000).

Other forms of transmural care are situated in the hospital. An experiment in this respect is the start of a so-called GP ward in a general hospital. At this ward, patients are treated under the responsibility of the GP. The groups of patients mainly consist of patients who are not fully recovered from day surgery or an operation in a hospital far from the patient's place of residence, "bed-blockers"(non-medical specialist treatment needed or possible and waiting for a place in a nursing home) and other patients who can no longer be treated at home with a low care profile. The participating GPs were positive about the results of this new organizational form (Moll van Charante *et al.*, 2001).

Another successful transmural innovation is the establishment of stroke units in which GPs, home care organizations, hospitals and nursing homes partici-pate. The increase of cooperation and coordination in these units results in better quality of care, better health outcomes, less "bed-blockers" and more cost-effective care compared to the traditional provision of care (Huisman *et al.*, 2001). The stroke unit is best situated in a comprehensive organization including in- and outpatient care (Kwa, 2002).

The "bottom-up" approach has led to regional variations in the provision of health care services. Some regions have only few "transmural" initiatives, while in some other regions so called "chains of care" (*zorgketens*) are formatted. These are regional cooperations of different care-providing organizations, which work together on a formalized or institutionalized basis. The impact of the new transmural initiatives on the gatekeeping position of Dutch GPs is not clear yet. The inventory by Van der Linden (2001) showed that home care organizations, hospitals and nursing homes have a more prominent role in transmural care projects than GPs. Besides, it is unknown how transmural care will develop in the near future. There are still problems regarding the implementation of the (experimental) projects into the daily routine of care provision. The main prob-lems include the financial system, which is not tailored to integrated care, the lack of ICT supports and a shortage of care providers in primary as well as secondary care.

The United Kingdom experience

Over the last decade United Kingdom government policy has placed an increasing emphasis on the notion of a primary-care-led NHS, with an attempt to shift power and resources from secondary to primary care so as to bring planning and provision of care "closer to patients" (Somerset *et al.*, 1999). Initiatives such as fundholding, the total purchasing pilots, Primary Care Groups (PCGs) now Primary Care Trusts (PCTs), and the pilot salaried schemes are all attempts to tip the balance of care further in the direction of the primary and community sector, and away from the hospital sector (Coulter and Mays, 1997). These initiatives have implications for the coordinating role of general practice. Two that are of most significance are fundholding and the introduction of PCGs and PCTs. Fundholding was introduced in the NHS in the early 1990s as a result of the creation of the internal market by the Conservative Government. The introduction of PCGs and PCTs was an initiative taken in the latter part of the 1990s by the Labour Government (Dixon *et al.*, 1998).

The fundholding initiative (Glennerster *et al.*, 1994) allowed general practices to become fundholders and these practices could place contracts for non-emergency care for their patients. With individual patients having no purchasing rights of their own, GP fund holders were to act as proxies, purchasing services on patients' behalf. This initiative, along with other developments in the 1970s and 1980s that enhanced the professional status of GPs (see Calnan and Gabe, 1991), to some extent countered the problems of coordination due to the unequal relationship between GPs and hospital doctors. It attempted to give more power (through control over resources) to GPs in their negotiations with hospital doctors. There is some evidence that fundholding GPs, as proxy consumers, acted in their patients' best interests and strengthened their coordinating role. For example, there is evidence that communication between GPs and hospital doctors improved and fundholding facilitated improvements in services, such as quicker diagnostic test results and shorter waiting times. They were also able to buy in specialist services such as physiotherapy and outreach clinics. However, fundholding was not cost-effective owing to the increased bureaucracy and did create inequalities in access (Coulter, 1995) and there was little evidence that the contracting process actually strengthened the negotiating power of GPs (Baeza and Calnan, 1997). The stimulus for hospital doctors to adhere to fundholders' demands depended on the existence of other alternative sources of supply and provision. In many cases fundholders were loyal and supportive to their local providers rather than shopping around for hospital care (Robinson and Le Grand, 1994; Mays *et al.*, 2001).

One initiative which emerged from the implementation of fundholding was the introduction of outreach clinics in general practice (Abery *et al.*, 1998), which is an example of promoting integration by providing services in primary care that are normally based in hospital. One study (Gillam *et al.*, 1995) evaluated an outreach model of ophthalmic care in terms of its impact on general practitioners, their use of ophthalmology services, patient views and costs. An ophthalmic medical practitioner and an ophthalmic nurse held clinics in the 17 participating practices once a month. The clinic was popular with patients and general practitioners and appeared to act as an effective filter for demand for care in the hospital setting. However, the educational impact of the scheme was limited and the cost per patient serving the outreach clinic was about three times the cost per patient seen in the outpatient clinic.

There have been a number of other initiatives (see Sergison *et al.*, 1997) aimed at improving coordination between primary care and specialist hospital services. One approach has been to allocate a specific coordinating role to a nurse or doctor (O'Leary, 1990; Grahame and West, 1996). Another is setting up an organizational arrangement for shared care for patients with chronic conditions such as diabetes or asthma or for specific services such as antenatal and obstetric care (Tucker *et al.*, 1996). A related model involves follow-up after hospital discharge (Hansen *et al.*, 1992). However, the overall impact of these different initiatives appears to be limited as there is some evidence (Evans, 1996) to suggest that, while primary care-led initiatives in the NHS may have improved communication and increased direct access to facilities, there is little evidence of a shift in resources and services to primary care. Important barriers to change included the attitudes of consultants and the individualistic culture of GPs.

The fundholding system has been replaced by PCGs, which have now become PCTs. The establishment of PCGs and PCTs reflected the clear policy aim of developing integrated care by bringing together primary care with community services and by linking the provision of care with a major responsibility for commissioning (Ham, 2004). A national network of PCGs was established in England in 1999 and PCGs had three core functions: to improve the health of the population in the PCG, to develop primary and community health services within the PCG and to commission secondary and tertiary services for the population in the PCG. However, PCGs were considered to be the first stage of a process resulting in the eventual transition to PCTs (Mays and Goodwin, 1998). PCTs were to be free standing and comprise GPs and community nurses, commissioning services for their populations, and managing the provision of community services such as district nursing and health visiting, while remaining accountable to the local health authority. PCTs had the same functions as PCGs, but with a greater range of responsibilities. Accordingly, PCTs received a unified budget, which represents approximately 80% of the health care budget.

In April 2002 around 300 primary care trusts were formed with strategic health authorities leading the strategic development of the local health community and managing the performance of PCTs and NHS trusts. This left PCTs with the lead NHS role of improving the health of the community, developing primary and community health services, and commissioning secondary care services. Each PCT is run by a board comprising a lay chairman, non-executive director and a minority of executive directors, including the chief executive, the finance director and the director of public health (Ham, 2004). The limited evidence available about the impact of PCGs and PCTs suggests developments in the commissioning of primary and community services, reflecting a desire to initiate alternatives to services traditionally delivered in the secondary sector. Significant progress had particularly been made in commissioning in the areas of community services, primary care and intermediate care (Smith and Goodwin, 2002). However, in the commissioning of acute services, developments have been slower and less significant. This was due in part to the lack of involvement from primary and secondary care doctors and continued poor relations and communication between the primary and secondary sectors (Regen *et al.*, 2001). Evidence from this study (Regen, 2002) also showed that the majority of GPs felt that the added workload associated with PCGs and PCTs had not translated into tangible service improvements in terms of the quality and range of practice services, and that gaining GPs effective involvement in PCTs was proving problematic.

A more recent development (Department of Health, 2004) has been the introduction of practice-based commissioning. From April 2005, practices can receive an "indicative budget" from Primary Care Trusts which they can use to improve the delivery of services. The case study sites where such schemes have been tested suggest patients will have access to alternative pathways of care across primary and secondary care with an emphasis on providing specialist care in general practice. Such an initiative appears to mirror fundholding developed in the early 1990s, although this was within the different context of the quasi-market.

Discussion

This analysis shows clearly that fragmented care and problems of coordination and continuity of care tend to be prevalent irrespective of the type of health care system. In the Netherlands and the United Kingdom, there are still problems of coordination and integration despite the presence of GP gatekeeping and coordinating systems. However, these problems of fragmentation tend to be exacerbated in systems where there is no GP gatekeeping system and the emphasis is placed on "choice", with patients bearing the major responsibility for navigating their own pathway through the health service.

The analysis has also shown the various strategies adopted by four different countries for addressing the problems of fragmentation. One strategy common to all countries was to strengthen general practice, although the driving force behind this policy was as much for reasons of economic efficiency as a concern for patient needs. The introduction of Primary Care Trusts in the United Kingdom, for example, has sought to achieve closer integration between primary care and community health services. An alternative strategy adopted by many countries was to attempt to enhance coordination between primary care and the specialist services, social care and community services. It appears that GPs control the access to the gate but their coordination powers recede after the patient passes the gate. These initiatives included allocating a specific coordination role to a health or social care professional, setting up organizational arrangements for shared care or joint commissioning and introducing services which were usually based in the hospital or social service and transferring them to general practice. The evidence available to assess the benefits of these initiatives is variable, with their success tending to hinge on the willingness of different branches of the medical profession to work together (Evans, 1996).

These organizational changes were typically introduced to strengthen the gatekeeping role, although recent, associated policy initiatives appear to be challenging the basic concept of gatekeeping and particularly continuity of care

(Bosanquet and Salisbury, 1998). For example, in the "new" modernized NHS in the United Kingdom a number of developments have taken place that might be seen as challenges. First, there has been an increase in the points of entry for patients in primary care. Examples of these are NHS Walk-in Centres (Anderson *et al.*, 2002; Salisbury, 2004), NHS Direct (call-in centre) and GPs working in larger organizations, such as cooperatives for out-of-hours care, which are dealing with increasing proportions of the primary care workload. Each of these enables the patient to have direct access to health care and have access to a different health professional.

The second challenge is to the concept of continuity of care. Increasingly, patients do not know the doctors that treat them on a personal basis. This is partly owing to the increase in patients moving or changing doctors, but mainly to the fact that fewer doctors want to work full-time and that practices are generally larger in size. A salaried system has been piloted which, while encouraging GPs to work in deprived areas, is seen by many GPs as a temporary position with little opportunity for patients and doctors to develop a close relationship.

A third challenge in the United Kingdom is the emergence of a specialist role for GPs. GP specialist services such as dermatology have been organized and run by specialist GPs and nurses, providing a substitute for the hospital service. This initiative is targeted mainly at controlling waiting lists. This stands in contrast to the outreach clinics, which emerged from the internal market initiative, where hospital specialists provided clinics based in general practice. In addition, there is a new attempt to involve GPs in local hospitals or community hospitals and what are currently termed "intermediate care systems".

Finally, a fourth challenge is the introduction of the primary health care team and the introduction of nurses (triage) as the first point of contact. In this context GPs are primary care consultants and nurses would deal with a range of activities such as acute care monitoring, health promotion and chronic disease management.

Some of these developments are evident in the new GP contract (Department of Health, 2003; Rowland, 2004), which distinguishes between core activities of GPs "serving people who are ill", additional activities (optional, such as maternity care) and other activities (specialist services), which are provided at PCT level. Thus, increasingly patients would be consulting different professionals for primary care services. This may meet patient demands, or some groups of patient demands, but it challenges the notion of continuity of care. Thus, the new drive for a primary care led NHS may have increased access to primary care and specialist care but it appears to challenge the notion of continuity of care and the coordinating role of the GP. It might be that patients will have to give up the benefits of a "personal" doctor for the advantages of a primary care-based service where the coordinating role is provided through the organization itself. This might be suitable for some types of patients, but for those who value a doctor "who knows you", such as those with chronic illness and multiple illnesses, this development might be seen as an additional barrier to access (Calnan *et al.*, 1994).

These developments, problems and solutions are also evident in other countries where primary care has a central role, e.g. the Netherlands. However, possible general policies for improving coordination, irrespective of the health care system, might include:

- defining the (patient) population beforehand (agreements about diagnostic tests, interpretations, definitions, etc.);
- defining a common package of care activities around the specific needs of a patient group;
- defining shared responsibility and separate responsibilities of the care providing partners;
- creating mutual respect and trust (e.g. by the development of protocols or appointments about the care process);
- establishing clear financial arrangements beforehand (e.g. for the extra time and administrative work related to cooperation and communication);
- improving communication and information facilities (ICT); and
- introducing elements of integrated care in educational programmes (e.g. into continuous medical education).

Notes

1   There is a *carnet de santé* for children, and this is totally accepted, because it helps parents to keep track of all health events of the child and is very useful for both the family and the physicians. But it has no link whatsoever with a cost-containment objective.
2   The other physician organizations were strongly opposed to this reform, which tried to establish a financial ceiling for physicians' expenditure.

References

Abery, A., Bond, M., Bowling, A., McClay, M. and Pope, G. (1998). Evaluation of specialists' outreach clinics in primary care in England, *Quality of Life Newsletter* **16**: 7–8.

Anderson, E., Pope, C., Manka-Scott, T. and Salisbury, C. (2002). NHS walk-in centres and the expanding role of primary care nurses, *Nursing Times* **98**(19): 36–37.

Baeza, J. and Calnan, M. (1997). Implementing quality: a study of the adoption and implementation of quality standards in the contracting process in a general practitioner multifund, *Journal of Health Services and Research Policy* **2**(4): 205–11.

Bosanquet, N. and Salisbury, C. (1998). The practice, in Loudon, I., Horder, J. and Webster, C. (eds) *General Practice under the National Health Service 1948–1997*, London: Clarendon Press.

Calnan, M. and Gabe, J. (1991). Sociology of General Practice, in: Gabe, J., Calnan, M. and Bury, M. (eds) *Sociology of the Health Service*. London/New York: Routledge.

Calnan, M., Coyle, J. and Williams, S. (1994). Changing perceptions of general practitioner care, *European Journal of Public Health* **4**: 108–114.

Commissie Moderniserning Curatieve Zorg (1994). *Rapport Gedeelde Zorg: betere zorg*. Zoetermeer: Hageman BV.

Coulter, A. (1995). Evaluating general practice fundholding in the UK, *European Journal of Public Health* **5**(4): 233–239.

Coulter, A. and Mays, N. (1997). Deregulating Primary Care, *British Medical Journal* **314**: 510–513.

Delnoij, D.M.J., Van Merode, G., Paulus, A. and Groenewegen, P.P. (2000). Does general practitioner curb health care expenditure?, *Journal of Health Services Research and Policy* **1**: 22–26.

Department of Health (2003). *Investing in General Practice: The New General Medical Services Contract: The Stationery Office*. London: Department of Health.

Department of Health (2004). *Practice Based Commissioning: Engaging Practices in Commissioning*. London: Department of Health. (http://www.dh.gov.uk/assetRoot/04/09/03/59/04090359.pdf, accessed 28 October).

De Roo, A.A., Chambaud, L. and Güntert, B.J. (2004). Long-term care in social health insurance systems, in Saltman, R.B., Busse, R. and Figueras, J. (eds) *Social Health Insurance Systems in Western Europe*. Berkshire/New York: Open University Press/McGraw-Hill Education.

Dixon, J., Holland, P. and Mays, N. (1998). Developing primary care gatekeeping, commissioning and managed care, *British Medical Journal* **317**: 125–8.

Evans, D. (1996). *A stakeholder analysis of developments at the primary and secondary care interface*. Institute for Health Policy Studies, University of Southampton.

Francke, A.L. and Willems, D.L. (2000). *Palliatieve zorg vandaag en morgen. Feiten, opvattingen en scenario's [Palliative care today and tomorrow. Facts, opinions and scenarios]*. Maarssen: Elsevier gezondheidszorg.

Gervas, J., Perez-Fernandez, M. and Starfield, B.H. (1994). Primary care, financing and gatekeeping in western Europe, *Family Practice* **11**(3): 307–17.

Gillam, S.T., Ball, M., Pruesad, M., Dunne, H., Cohen, S. and Vaflides, G. (1995). Investigation of benefits and costs of an ophthalmic outreach clinic in general practice, *British Journal of General Practice* **45**: 649–652.

Glendinning, C., Rummery, K. and Clarke, R. (1998). From collaboartion to commissioning: developing relationships between primary health and social services, *British Medical Journal* **317**(7151): 122–5.

Glennerster, H., Matsaganis, W. and Owens, P. (1994). *Implementing GP Fund Holding: Wild Card or Winning Hand?* Buckingham: Open University Press.

Grahame, R. and West, J. (1996). The role of the rheumatology nurse practitioner in primary care: an experiment in the further education of the practice nurse, *British Journal of Rheumatology* **35**(6): 581–8.

Gross, R., Tabenkin, H. and Brammli-Greenberg, S. (2000). Who needs a gatekeeper? Patients' views of the role of the primary care physician, *Family Practice* **17**: 222–229.

Grundmeyer, H.G.L.M. (1996). General practitioner and specialist: why do they communicate so badly? *European Journal of General Practice* **2**: 53–54.

Halm, E.A., Causino, N. and Blumenthal, D. (1997). Is gatekeeping better than traditional care? A survey of physicians' attitudes, *Journal of the American Medical Association* **26**: 1677–1681.

Ham, C. (2004). *Health Policy in Britain: The Politics and Organisation of the National Health Service* (5th edition). Hampshire: Palgrave Macmillan.

Hansen, F.R., Spedtsberg, K. and Schroll, M. (1992). General follow up by home visits after discharge from hospital, *Age and Ageing* **21**(6): 445–450.

Huisman, R., Van Wijngaarden, J.D.H., Scholte op Reimer, W.J.M. *et al.* (2001). Van units naar ketenzorg: stroke service biedt betere zorg voor CVA-patiënten [From units to chain-care: stroke service provides better care for stroke patients], *Medisch Contact* **56**(48): 1765–1768.

Hutten, J.B.F. (1998). Workload and provision of care in general practice. An empirical study of the relation between the workload of Dutch general practitioners and the content and quality of their care. Utrecht: NIVEL (thesis, University of Utrecht).

Kersten, T.J.J.M.T. (1991). De invloed van huisartsen in de tweede lijn [The influence of general practitioners on secondary care]. Utrecht: NIVEL (thesis, University of Utrecht).

Kwa, V.I.H. (2002). "Stroke units" als effectiefste vorm van behandeling ["Stroke units" as most effective form of care], *Pharmaceutisch weekblad* **137**(9): 319–322.

Mays, N. and Goodwin, N. (1998). Primary care groups in England, in Klein, R. (ed.) *Implementing the White Paper – Pitfalls and Opportunities*. London: King's Fund.

Mays, N., Wyke, S., Malbon, G. and Goodwin, N. (eds) (2001). *The Purchasing of Health Care by Primary Care Organisations*. Buckinghamshire: Open University Press.

Moll van Charante, E.P., Ijzermans, C.J., Hartman, E.E. *et al.* (2001). *De huisartskliniek in Ijmuiden: een inventarisend onderzoek [The general practitioner clinic in Ijmuiden: an inventory-making investigation].* Amsterdam/Rotterdam: Instituut voor Huisartsgeneeskunde Amsterdam, Institute of Medical Technology Assessment.

Moll van Charante, E.P., Delnoij, D.M.J., Ijzermans, C.J. and Klazinga, N.S. (2002). Van spelverdeler tot speelbal? De veranderde rol en positie van de Nederlandse huisarts [The changing role of the Dutch general practitioner], *Huisarts en Wetenschap* **45**(2): 70–75.

NRV/CvZ (1995). *Transmurale somatische zorg*. Zoetermeer: NRV/CvZ.

O'Leary, J. (1990). Primary health care. Liaison nursing. Forging vital links in care. *Nursing Standard* **5**(7): 52.

Preston, C., Cheater, F., Baker, R. and Hearnshaw, H. (1999). Left in limbo: patients' views on care across the primary/secondary interface, *Quality in Health Care* **8**(1): 16–21.

Regen, E. (2002). *Driving Seat or Back Seat? GPs' Views on and Involvement in Primary Care Groups and Trusts*. Birmingham: Health Services Management Centre.

Regen, M., Smith, J., Goodwin, N., Mcleod, H. and Shapiro, J. (2001). *Passing on the Baton: Final Report of a National Evaluation of Primary Care Groups and Trusts*. Birmingham: Health Services Management Centre.

Roberts, K.J. (1999). Patient empowerment in the United States: a critical commentary, *Health Expectations* **2**: 82–92.

Robinson, R. and Le Grand, J. (1994). *Evaluating the NHS Reforms*. London: King's Fund.

Rowland, M. (2004). Linking physicians pay to the quality of care – a major experiment in the UK, *New England Journal of Medicine* **351**(14): 1448–1453.

Salisbury, C. (2004). Does advanced access work for patients and practices? *British Journal of General Practice* **54**: 330–31.

Sergison, M., Sibbald, B. and Rose, S. (1997). Skill Mix in PC: A Bibliography. NCRPC, working paper. Manchester: University of Manchester.

Shi, L., Starfield, B., Kennedy, B. and Kawachi, I. (1999). Income inequality, primary care and health indicators, *Journal of Family Practice* **48**(4): 275–84.

Smelt, W.L.H., De Gier, A., Meyer, C., De Bruijn, M., Oudendijk, C. and Van der Kam, W.L. (1999). Huisarts spil in pijnteam: chronische patiënten eerder geholpen [General practitioner at the centre of painteam: prompt care for chronic patients], *Medisch Contact* **54**(48): 1663–1665.

Smith, J. and Goodwin, N. (2002). *Developing Effective Commissioning by Primary Care Trusts: Lessons from the Research Evidence*. Birmingham: Health Services Management Centre.

Somerset, M., Faulkner, A., Shaw, A., Dunn, L. and Sharp, D.J. (1999). Obstacles on the path to a primary care led NHS: complexities of outpatient, *Social Science and Medicine* **48**(2): 213–225.

Starfield, B. (1991). Primary care and health, *Journal of the American Medical Association* **266**(16): 2268–2271.

Temmink, D. (2000) *Transmural Clinics: A Nursing Innovation Explored*. Thesis: Maastricht University. Utrecht: NIVEL.

Tucker, J.S., Hall, M.N., Howie, P.W. *et al.* (1996). Should obstreticians see women with normal pregnancies? *British Medical Journal* **312**: 554–559.

Van der Linden, B.A. (2001). *The Birth of Integration: explorative studies on the development and implementation of transmural care in the Netherlands 1994–2000.* Utrecht: University of Utrecht (thesis).

Wilsford, D. (1991). *Doctors and the State: The Politics of Health Care in France and the United States.* Durham: Duke University Press.

chapter SIX

The impact of primary care purchasing in Europe: a comparative case study of primary care reform[1]

Alison McCallum, Mats Brommels,
Ray Robinson, Sven-Eric Bergman
and Toomas Palu

Introduction and background

Development of purchasing in health care

In recent years several countries have sought to develop organizations that purchase services to reflect strategic health care objectives. These organizations decide which health services to purchase for a population, the terms on which they should be purchased and which organizations should provide them. Potential purchasers include sickness funds in countries with social health insurance systems and local health agencies or municipalities in tax-based health systems. Primary care purchasing occurs where responsibility for a budget, for specialist services or for additional primary care is devolved to primary care practitioners or organizations.

Theoretical benefits of purchasing

The stated advantage of a distinct purchasing function is its focus on population health needs. Purchasing provides opportunities to change historic patterns of service use and reallocate resources to prevent provider capture of the health care agenda. Various incentives associated with devolved decision-making can also improve the flexibility and performance of the health system. Purchasing might enable changes in which the hospital or organization provides services, the balance between in patient and ambulatory care, or the development of clinical rather than administrative quality standards.

Where primary care practitioners or organizations purchase care, several benefits are considered more likely to occur than when sickness funds or local health agencies adopt this role. Primary care purchasing should combine financial and clinical decision-making and provide incentives for GPs to use limited resources more cost-effectively. It should streamline services, making them more patient-focused and influencing the balance of power between primary care and specialist services.

The theoretical benefits of primary care purchasing reflect its flexibility, personal and local scale and lack of bureaucracy. Centralized institutions, particularly those like sickness funds, where efficient claims processing and reimbursement require well-developed bureaucracy, might find it difficult to adopt the necessary flexibility and local responsiveness. Disadvantages for hospitals as purchasers include their larger scale and tendency to reduce the influence and resources available to primary care. Potential exceptions include hospitals with a strong community focus, an emphasis on chronic disease management and access to expert primary care.

The continuum of primary care purchasing in Europe

Over the last 20 years various models of primary health care purchasing have developed. They range from market-based solutions to networks of community-focused organizations. The different models reflect the power of various stakeholders, their reasons for considering primary care purchasing and the prevailing ideology. The most comprehensive examples occur where primary care organizes and finances all aspects of prevention, treatment and care, from community development, drug treatment, diagnostic services and commissioning to specialist medical, surgical and psychiatric care. This is the situation in Britain, where Primary Care Trusts purchase community and specialist services for all but the most complex treatments with a fixed budget.

At the other end of the spectrum GPs influence purchasing indirectly through professional representation on various committees. This tends to occur in health care systems based on social insurance. Between these extremes, budgets for specific services and programmes are devolved. Together these form a continuum of different models of purchasing or devolved budgeting. Table 6.1 illustrates the four main categories.

The range of contracting tools employed in primary care purchasing

The other dimension of purchasing is the sphere of influence within which primary care purchasers operate. This ranges from the ability to shape everyday

Table 6.1 Models of primary care purchasing and devolved budgeting

Model	Main features
Active purchasing	Funds transferred to the primary care budget Degree of organizational autonomy May include financial incentives or risks to encourage different ways of working
Commissioning	Primary care determines nature and content of specific specialist services Indicative budget transferred Formal financial accountability (for example, contract signing) remains with a parent organization
Budget transfer	Responsibility for funding specific services, for example diagnostic tests or pharmaceuticals transferred Limited influence over service delivery
Indirect purchasing	Exercise of representative power or professional influence over purchasing by a third party, e.g. member of group advising social insurance institutions

practice, to plan enhanced primary and community care provision, through to primary care leadership of specialist care redesign.

The purchasing model and sphere of influence affect the nature of contracts as well as similar agreements by primary care purchasers and bodies responsible for overseeing processes. Examples include the availability of information, analysis and expertise to identify and prioritize the care included in contracts, the nature of the contractual relationships, and the mechanisms for enforcing and ending contracts, including the ability to change providers. Effective professional, managerial and financial controls are required to detect unforeseen adverse effects of contracts, to limit financial risks that might disrupt patient care and to reduce gaming.

Evaluating the impact of primary care purchasing

This chapter examines the development and impact of these models of primary care purchasing and commissioning on the organization and development of health services. Sources include published literature and expert opinion. These were appraised using comparative case study methods and cross-case analysis to compare findings across countries and identify lessons that could be generalized.

Evaluation of the success of purchasing experiments in primary care has three elements. First, was the implementation of primary care purchasing successful? Second, did the purchasing experiment achieve the improvements in health service organization, care processes and outcomes that were anticipated? Third, what factors facilitated or constrained the implementation and impact of primary care purchasing? The cases illustrate the continuum from active to indirect purchasing and the range and scope of the initiatives that have developed in each category.

The development of primary care purchasing in England[2]

GP fundholding

Since the 1980s, various reforms have laid the groundwork for primary care purchasing. Preliminary reforms in 1985 and 1990 increased local GP, and thus primary care, accountability before purchasing was devolved (Taylor, 1991; Allsop, 1995; Bloor *et al.*, 1999). In 1991 general practice fundholding was established, and 303 GP practices with patient list sizes of 11,000 or more received budgets to purchase selected services directly for their patients (Glennerster *et al.*, 1994). The standard fundholding budget covered about 20% of the hospital and community health service budget, including most elective surgery (cataract extraction, hip replacements, etc.), ambulatory (outpatient) assessment, diagnosis, treatment and prescription costs. The local health authority purchased all other services, including emergency care. The fundholding budget excluded the GPs' personal income, which was paid separately. Practices could reallocate fundholding savings to other services but not to supplement GPs' income. Although cash limits were applied to health authorities and NHS trusts, and thus non-fundholder purchasing, fundholder overspending was tolerated.

Fundholding evolved (Mays and Dixon, 1996) to incorporate more complex procedures and services, for example cardiovascular surgery and specialized nursing care. Fundholding was also adapted for smaller practices; from April 1996, practices with lists of 5000 or more patients were eligible to apply. Practices with 3000 to 5000 patients could purchase community services included in the standard fundholding budget. This "community" model allowed small, even single-handed, GP practices to become fundholders.

At the other end of the scale, more sophisticated organizations developed. These included practice consortia and multifunds. Here fundholding practices pooled some management functions, achieving economies of scale without jeopardizing the flexibility of fundholding. This combination of initiatives extended fundholding across the range of primary care. The proportion of the population covered by fundholding increased from 7% in 1991 to over 50% in 1997.

Total purchasing pilots

In 1996 selected Total Purchasing Pilots (TPPs) were introduced to purchase all but highly specialist services (Total Purchasing National Evaluation Team 1997). The average first-wave TPP comprised four general practices and 20 GPs and an average patient population of 31,300 (ranged 8100 to 84,700). The second wave included one health authority area covering over 300,000 people. This experiment, unlike fundholding, was independently evaluated for evidence of improved management practice, cost-effectiveness and patient benefits.

GP commissioning

Despite its growth, GP fundholding remained controversial (Robinson and Hayter, 1995). Non-fundholding organizations, called GP commissioning groups, developed as parallel purchasers. They aimed to change primary care and specialist services through collaboration rather than contracting. Although budgets and responsibility for commissioning were devolved to the commissioning groups, technically, contracts were held between the health authority and the provider.

Primary Care Groups and Trusts

Primary Care Groups replaced fundholding and commissioning groups between 1999 and 2002. These organizations were to maintain service improvements introduced by some fundholders and GP commissioning groups but with lower transaction costs and without the fragmentation, duplication and perceived inequities in service development created by fundholding (Department of Health, 1997).

Initially, 481 PCGs were established around local communities. The average population served was 100,000 people, but ranged from 50,000 to over 250,000. Unlike fundholding, PCG membership was compulsory. PCGs were health authority subcommittees with a multiagency governing body, although GPs formed the majority. PCG commissioning occurred within the framework of the local health authority's Health Improvement Programme and in collaboration with other local organizations. Three-year service agreements replaced contracts but monthly monitoring continued.

The four levels of PCG differed in the range and scope of their purchasing. At Level 1, PCGs were commissioning advisors to health authorities. Budgetary responsibility and independence increased up to level 4. Here, PCGs commissioned care for the PCG population and provided community health services. PCGs at levels 3 and 4 became Primary Care Trusts.

In April 2002, Primary Care Trusts were established as independent organizations across England and district health authorities were abolished. PCT chief executives are responsible for ensuring local clinical quality and financial control within a nationally agreed framework. PCTs make primary care the centre of decision-making and local health strategy. They commission all but highly specialist services for populations of around 80,000 to 300,000 and are responsible for 75–80% of the NHS budget. PCTs combine purchasers and provider functions; their structure and requirement to adopt systematic approaches to collaboration are intended to facilitate commissioning of care that is integrated across the health, social care and independent sectors.

Purchasing service redesign

The level of optimism about PCT sustainability varies; calls for a return to local, less bureaucratic organizations than PCTs and recommendations for mergers have both been reported (Honey *et al.*, 2003; Gould, 2004). The establishment of NHS Foundation Trusts promised increased freedom from local control over capital and service development for "high performing" NHS Trusts (Dixon, 2003; Klein, 2003). Although the extent to which Foundation Trusts will be able to function independently of the local health community is unclear; this development, and the proposed increase in emphasis on activity based funding, could reduce PCT scope for manoeuvre and ability to resource community-based services.

Opportunities for practice-level commissioning are intended to deflect criticism of PCTs as stand-alone purchasers, to produce a layered approach to primary care purchasing and increase patient and public involvement. Practice-based commissioning, for example, devolves commissioning to individual practices or to small groups that agree to pool their populations and resources. All practices can participate and receive indicative budgets that take account of activity levels and health needs. Practices are accountable to the Professional Executive Committee of the PCT for their commissioning decisions so their decisions must be justifiable in terms of local objectives. Practice-based commissioning is intended to improve care for patients with common chronic conditions and to help practice teams fund innovation at neighbourhood level (Department of Health, 2004).

Practice-led commissioning is slightly different from practice-based commissioning. It is closer to fundholding in allowing practices to invest in improved care if they make savings. However, the adoption of standard prices, the explicit quality criteria included in the new general practitioner contract, and the financial incentives attached, are intended to focus contract negotiations on quality, the development of tailored services and to reduce avoidable admissions (Lewis, 2004).

Nurse-led commissioning is a related initiative (Department of Health, 2004). The development of nurses as purchasers should remove anomalies over access to community services. Historically, problems have arisen at the boundary between health and social care or health and housing. Here, judgements about the relative benefit of drug and nondrug treatment (e.g. environmental assistance or aids to daily living) have been distorted by perverse incentives associated with the organization and funding of services.

Personal Medical Services pilots

The above reforms emphasized purchasing of specialist services. The evaluation of total purchasing, however, considered that enhancing primary care provision was also important (Mays and Dixon, 1996; Wilkin *et al.*, 1999). Eighty-five Personal Medical Services (PMS) pilots were established in 1998. Further waves have followed. Single-handed practices can now collaborate in a PMS framework that is the provider equivalent of community fundholding (Honey *et al.*,

2003). Primary Care Trusts and participating practices can purchase enhanced primary care and community services tailored to local need. In return for this flexibility, general practice contracts are managed locally rather than being nationally held, locally administered contracts.

Spain: the purchaser/provider split in Catalonia

Spain began its primary care reform in the 1980s. Implementation was measured; areas with lower socioeconomic status were prioritized. Professional education, medical management and improved salaries underpinned the reforms.

Several aspects of Catalonia's health care system differ from elsewhere in Spain. It piloted a purchaser-provider split when the Health Care Organization Law was passed in 1990 (*Llei d'Ordenació Sanitària de Catalunya*, or LOSC). This facilitated integrated care, organizational rationalization and improved regulation in a system in which 60% of beds were owned by private and public organizations not belonging to the Regional Health Authorities (Regional Health Department). Similar diversification of provision was implemented in primary health care. Among the diversified primary care providers a form of fundholding developed in the mid-1990s with the *Entitat de Base Asociativa* (EBA). Here, a team of doctors and nurses receives a budget for a defined population, including salaries, premises, diagnostic tests, specialist referrals and prescriptions. The proportion of the population covered by organizations separate from the Regional Health Authorities (EBA and other public organizations linked to municipalities and religious organizations) is growing as implementation of primary care reform continues. In 2003, the EBA provided 14 out of 346 primary care teams. At the end of 2003, 20% of primary care was provided by teams that are not directly owned by the health department (*Institut Català de la Salut*). Although evaluation of this aspect of the Catalan reforms has been limited, indicators are generally positive. (Violan *et al.*, 2000) Comparison of socioeconomically similar areas of Barcelona also found that service use, practice indicators, quality and drug costs did not vary significantly between the different models of primary care provision, although non-public services employed relatively fewer nurses (Guarga *et al.*, 2000). An external evaluation found that general quality indicators were similar in different models, although EBA teams employed fewer nurses, prescribed less drugs, ordered fewer laboratory tests and referred fewer patients to specialists. On the contrary, health teams managed by non-departmental organizations linked to municipal-religious or private community hospitals were higher prescribers, referred more patients to specialists and carried out more laboratory test. The *Institut Català de la Salut* was in between the two models (Fundació Avedis Don Avedian, 2003). The lack of differences on the quality indicators suggests that the policy of diversifying ownership of the organizations providing primary health care services promoted competition and benefited the whole Catalan community and not only the citizens covered by the pilot projects (Gené-Badia, 2003).

The Russian Federation and the former Soviet Union

The first experiments with primary care funding in the Soviet Union occurred in St Petersburg, Kemerovo and Samara between 1987 and 1991 (Tragakes and Lessof, 2003). Some initially promising findings, for example reductions in hospital admissions, were not sustained. A combination of ineffectual regulation and the financial crisis of the early 1990s appeared to overwhelm the health care system, with primary care suffering most (Tragakes and Lessof, 2003).

Experimentation continues in Samara. Polyclinics are budget holders, providing primary care and purchasing hospital services for a listed population. The budget is based on a capitation formula and includes financial incentives. If inpatient costs exceed the budget (there are some exceptions for complex treatments) the polyclinic must fund the difference. Reform is backed by physician education in primary care, modernization of management and regulation, active collection of health insurance and protection of payments made on behalf of the non-working population. In Samara the proportion of the budget allocated to hospital inpatient care has dropped from 80% in the Soviet era to around 54% and many polyclinics have developed day facilities.

Despite this progress, concerns remain that funding is insufficient to provide modern health care. There are suggestions that enhanced services are available for those able to pay, and additional payments may be requested for services included in polyclinic capitation payments (Tragakes and Lessof, 2003).

Primary care reform in Finland – a continuum within a country

The Finnish Government Subsidy Reform Act of 1993 changed the way that health services were funded and turned municipalities (local authorities) into potential purchasers. The reform enabled municipalities to allocate funds prospectively rather than simply paying for activities that had already been undertaken. At the same time, national taxation became less important; now most health care is funded from local income taxes, without an earmarked allocation for health care. Since the subsidy reforms, municipalities have been able to provide services themselves, with other municipalities, or purchase them from other public or private sector providers.

Despite the opportunities offered by the subsidy reform, few municipalities purchase specific services or procedures actively, for example, by specifying targets, expected levels of activity, or quality. Clinical input into the allocation of funds to specialist care is similarly limited; in many municipalities even the role of the chief physician, who should advise the health and social care board of the municipality about health care provision, is limited to making changes at the margins. Barely a handful of examples exist of primary care professionals being actively involved in purchasing. Most of the examples from Finland that were characterized previously as primary care purchasing, therefore, are actually purchasing by health and social care boards of municipalities (local authorities).

Health centre purchase of community services

Community services for elderly people as well as residents with mental health or substance problems are often purchased from small private and not-for-profit providers, including patient organizations. Since Finnish regulations require that health services delivered by external providers are subject to a tendering process, health centre chief physicians contribute to the design of tenders, with active purchasing of services for these patient groups. Municipalities can also supplement their funding by purchasing mainstream services from not-for-profit organizations. As the profits of the Slot Machine Association (*Ray*) fund most of the costs and activities of most not-for-profit organizations that provide health-related services, municipalities can purchase care from them at less than full cost, thus benefiting indirectly from lottery funding (Myllymäki, 2002).

Purchasing specialist services in primary care

Nilsiä, a rural municipality, provides a typical example of primary care purchasing of specialist services. Primary care holds the budget for health centre diagnostic and treatment services, including a basic laboratory, X-ray facilities and small in-patient units. Most specialist care, however, requires a 50 km journey to the regional centre. To improve local access the health centre (through the chief physician) purchases diagnostic and consultant outreach clinics from the hospital district and private providers. Examples include cardiology, gastrointestinal endoscopy, and speech therapy. The services purchased, however, comprise only around 0.2% of the specialist care budget.

Failed attempt to contract for primary and specialist care

Another rural municipality – Liminka – attempted comprehensive purchasing by tendering its primary and specialist health services (Keisu, 2002). No provider tendered for primary care and only the hospital district offered comprehensive specialist care. Subsequently the municipality contracted with the hospital district for specialist care. Based on this tendering exercise, private providers were more expensive, and purchasing specialist care piecemeal would have increased transaction costs while reducing annual spending by only 0.5%.

Network-based purchasing

Primary care has greatest influence on specialist services where primary care and basic hospital services have been integrated into area-based federations. Here, GPs usually manage the federations and negotiate agreements with the hospital district and private providers for specialist services on behalf of member municipalities. These federations wield the combined purchasing power of the member municipalities and are more able to purchase and deliver care in line with integrated care plans that reflect local health problems (Ministry of Social Affairs and Health, 2002).

Primary health care purchasing in Estonia: primary care budgets for diagnostic services and indirect purchasing

Since 1998, family practitioners (FPs – the preferred translation of the Estonian term for GPs) have undertaken limited fundholding functions. The 2002 virtual budget, for example, comprised 18.4% of capitation fees to purchase selected clinical and diagnostic services that were excluded from capitation funding. A government decree lists the services FPs should purchase: clinical care includes minor surgery and physiotherapy, while laboratory services include routine X-rays, more common endoscopic procedures, and biochemical tests. In 2002, the "budget holding" comprised €3.5 million in total, or €5,000 per FP. FPs contract with providers of diagnostic services and manage the payments but cannot retain funds if they under-utilize diagnostic services. If they pay less than the health insurance list price for services, however, they can retain the savings. Currently, 5–10% discounts on laboratory tests are available. This initiative is designed to develop negotiation, budgeting and planning skills among primary care purchasers and laboratory service providers.

Indirect purchasing in Estonia

Involvement in indirect purchasing complements FPs' fundholding role. FPs participated in the health insurance fund process for commissioning specialist ambulatory care services for the first time for the 2002 contracts. Commissioning was limited to the two major urban areas and selected specialties: orthopaedics, ENT, obstetrics and gynaecology, and ophthalmology. The final decisions reflected cost and quality criteria; FP preferences accounted for 20% of the quality evaluation. These arrangements are still evolving and the health insurance fund has recognized that expansion of purchasing will require improved measurement and further strengthening of governance arrangements.

Linking direct and indirect primary care purchasing with primary care team development in Italy: the Imola project

Italian GPs are gatekeepers but the law forbids them from purchasing treatment for patients. However, indirect purchasing through policy development and implementation is widespread and GPs enjoy strategic influence over health care spending. Drug prescribing and diagnostic tests provide further purchasing opportunities for GPs. One example is the 1997 demonstration project in Imola Local Health Unit, near Bologna (Donatini, 2002).

   Imola has a population of 106,000 and one hospital. All 87 GPs were organized, voluntarily, and with the support of professional organizations, into nine teams covering homogeneous areas. The health unit and GPs designed team objectives to improve quality of care and collaboration. Teams and individual GPs were offered incentives, including finance and facilities. The implementation process included training around the project objectives and reporting system, clinical guidelines, budgeting, team-based agreements, funding for team meetings and professional development. GPs were rewarded for achieving project objectives in their own practice. Maximum rewards were received where the whole team achieved the objective. The project tackled common, important clinical problems such as hypertension. Here, the aim was to make treatment more evidence based, producing 1% shifts in the balance of different drug treatments.

Sweden – failed attempt to introduce primary care purchasing

Primary care has been relatively underdeveloped in Sweden compared with other countries with tax-based health care systems. In the early 1990s, some "model" county councils piloted different models of the purchaser-provider split. In Stockholm and Dalecarlia primary care became part of the purchasing organization to provide expert support to the commissioning process (Bergman, 1994). Purchasing districts in Stockholm averaged 200,000 inhabitants while in Dalecarlia they were coterminous with municipal boundaries. District populations averaged 20,000; the smallest had fewer than 10,000 inhabitants. In Northern Dalecarlia, around Mora district hospital, strategic and collaborative relationships between primary care and hospital specialists improved and helped to integrate services. This is the only obvious Swedish example of primary care doctors participating actively in purchasing (Svalander and Åhgren, 1995).

Primary care no longer purchases specialist services. Political concerns about lack of separation between the purchasing organization and primary care provision means that county council purchasers now contract with family doctors, other specialists and hospitals in parallel. Some consider this an improvement; primary care is more independent of county councils, and has a higher profile. Alternative attempts are under way to improve collaboration between health care professionals and to reform primary care.

Comparing theory and practice

To what extent have purchasing arrangements, as discussed in the previous section, met the expectations of its advocates? This is a difficult question to answer because of the limited available evidence. Primary care purchasing has developed furthest in the United Kingdom, the United Kingdom has experimented with models that cover most of the primary care purchasing continuum and it is here that primary care purchasing has been most widely evaluated. For these reasons, substantial use is made of United Kingdom evidence but, throughout, it has been compared and contrasted with evidence from other countries too.

Evidence of benefits arising from primary care purchasing

The wider organization of the health service clearly has an influential role in determining the extent to which it is possible to devolve budgets to primary care. There is no evidence, however, that a simple relationship exists between the degree to which purchasing initiatives achieved their objectives, the type of purchasing undertaken, and the previous influence of primary care in the health system. Many of the benefits result from opportunities available to primary care purchasers to accelerate the implementation of improvement processes, such as review of prescribing patterns that were already under way. The evidence of the benefits of primary care purchasing can be summarized as follows.

1. Organizational improvement

- Reduced isolation among small practices, facilitating alliances between GPs, respecting single-handed practice while providing the organizational and financial advantages of joint working.
  Cases: Community fundholding (United Kingdom), some PMS initiatives and Imola network (Italy).
- Increased resource allocation and commitment to organizational development in primary care.
  Case: Total Purchasing Pilots and Primary Care Trusts (United Kingdom).
- Primary care reform programme aligned with devolved budgeting.
  Cases: Estonia, Italy, Spain.

2. More flexible service provision

- Expanded range of services in primary care.
- More responsive services – timelier access, test results, electronic communication.
  Cases: United Kingdom – fundholding, commissioning, TPP, PMS pilots, Estonia, Finnish GP Federations, Sweden.

3. Quality of care

- Increased adherence to laboratory guidelines, reducing blood tests by approximately 8% and reducing hospitalization for ambulatory care sensitive conditions like diabetes by 6%.
  Case: Italy – Imola.

4. Improved cost-effectiveness of care

- Limited evidence but linked to availability of financial or professional incentives encouraging, for example, cost-effective prescribing.
  Cases: United Kingdom – fundholding, commissioning, PCG, PCT, Italy, Imola.

5. GP as the patient's agent

- No evidence that fundholders reduced referrals inappropriately, some made wider use of the private sector.

Case: United Kingdom – fundholding and commissioning, Estonia, preliminary results.
- Purchasing used to bypass bottlenecks and reduce waiting times.
  Case: Finland.
- Fundholders and commissioning GPs used extra information about clinical and organizational quality of specialist services to help redesign and reprovide services.
  Cases: United Kingdom – fundholding and commissioning.
- Imola and Samara projects improved population coverage of primary care.
  Cases: Italy, Russian Federation.
- Tentatively positive results from changes in the primary care environment.
  Cases: Estonia, United Kingdom PMS for underserved populations.

6. Increased influence for primary care

- Short feedback loop and budgetary control provided leverage over specialist care and more active management of the interface between primary and secondary care.
  Cases: United Kingdom – Total Purchasing Pilots, Sweden – Dalecarlia pilot, Finland – specialist care in reach and primary care federations, Spain – Catalonian primary care reform.

Problems with the implementation of purchasing

Problems associated with devolved budgeting initiatives include a mixture of foreseeable and unforeseeable adverse consequences of implementation undertaken as planned, as well as subverted, incomplete or unsuccessful implementation.

1. Management and transaction costs

- Decentralization of purchasing, invoicing, processing and monitoring of small contracts and active GP involvement in increased management and transaction costs, 85% of management costs incurred at practice level in TPPs.
  Cases: United Kingdom – most obvious in fundholding and TPPs, but GP time commitment also heavy in commissioning.

2. Direct or indirect financial risk and perverse incentives

- Evidence of indirect risks, for example, reduced ability to purchase care because of specialist services overspending, funding cuts, limited control over specialist referrals because of weak gatekeeping or care coordination.
  Cases: Finland, Russian Federation, Sweden.
- Theoretical direct risk of income reduction following 'inappropriate' purchasing decisions. In practice, risks were limited where primary care provision received dedicated funding, risks limited to additional income, or 'borrowing' from one year to the next allowed.
  Cases: Estonia, Italy – Imola, United Kingdom – fundholding.
- Focus on cost of laboratory tests rather than quality, for example the reliability of results, may encourage family practitioners to contract with services

that use cheaper but less appropriate methods of analysis or laboratories with poorer control systems.
Cases: Estonia, United Kingdom – fundholding.

3. Governance

- Lack of effective sanctions on fundholder overspending despite impact on contracts for non-fundholding practices and squeeze on management resources for developing non-fundholders.
  Case: United Kingdom.
- Professionals may protect their income at the expense of necessary referral, comprehensive service provision and maintaining ethical standards.
  Case: Russian Federation.

4. Adverse impact on equity

- Trend towards shorter elective waits, more consultant outreach, and wider range of service models in fundholding and PMS practices rather than availability being directly related to need. Not found in Catalonia because equity explicitly built into strategy.
- Opportunities for active purchasing, and the service improvements that resulted from tackling bottlenecks in service provision, for example, were possible because of the competence of specific individuals; availability was unrelated to the level of health need and the opportunities of individuals to use alternative services.
  Cases: PMS, United Kingdom – fundholding.

5. Lack of strategic focus

- Certain conditions emphasized over others, e.g. elective surgery over chronic conditions, little evidence of anticipated change of focus from demand to population needs assessment and longer-term development.
- One-year contracts may allow some purchasers (particularly those in urban areas) to disengage from dysfunctional providers but do not provide the stability or the incentives necessary to encourage service redesign or longer-term development.
- Emphasis on current activity and intervention fails to take account of the importance of teaching and research for future patients.
- Cases: Sweden, much of United Kingdom – fundholding.

Factors associated with the failure of primary care purchasing to develop

The health systems of countries that have failed to develop primary care purchasing and devolved budgeting share several characteristics. These may be considered under four headings: alignment of policy and practice; consensus about the role and objectives of primary health care; the primary care infrastructure and operational environment; and financial risk.

Alignment of policy and practice

Devolving budgets to primary care, empowering primary care purchasers and developing a primary care-led service requires direction of policy, resources and professional expertise towards the same objectives. In the United Kingdom, national and local primary care organizations shaped purchasing reforms. Individual champions were complemented by an influential primary care presence in the health care system. Similarly, the long-standing alliance between politicians, professionals and the public in Catalonia, and the creation of co-operative stakeholder relationships in Imola provide one explanation of why reform flourished in these settings. The contrast between cases that illustrate relatively successful and limited implementation of devolved budgeting highlights the importance of professional and political relationships, misaligned policies and organizational factors.

Role and objectives of primary care

The limited implementation of devolved budgeting in Sweden illustrates the failure to clarify the objectives of the initiative, or to address issues such as the GP's role in gatekeeping and coordination of continuing care before purchasing was established. This implies limited consensus between stakeholders about their responsibilities (Delnoij and Brenner, 2000). Specifically, neither the role of general practice nor the involvement of primary care professionals in the development of health policy and strategy at local level were agreed (Svalander, 1999). This became clear when the key players took positions that limited the potential of primary care purchasing. Politicians perceived that having primary care purchasers blurred the distinction between the politicians' and officials' strategic role and the doctors' responsibility for day-to-day health care. Hospital staff worried that, as purchasers, primary care leaders would have greater access to politicians and officials, and thus would receive preferential allocation of resources. GPs held the opposite view, fearing that they would be forced to take financial responsibility for decisions made without their involvement, and that, being close to those who set their budgets; it would be easy for primary care funding to be squeezed.

Infrastructure and operational environment

The power of primary care as a potential purchaser was also weakened in Finland and Sweden by changes to the infrastructure and operational environment that facilitated the development of alternative primary care providers. In Finland, the economically active population is encouraged to use workplace services, and visits to private specialists are partly reimbursed by the social insurance institution. While this weakening of the role of the primary care doctor was probably unintended in Finland, competition was an explicit policy objective in Sweden, particularly in Stockholm. It is difficult for primary care to provide a strategic lead in a health system in which primary care providers compete with each other, and with ambulatory care services. In contrast, separation between the GP as primary care doctor and the individual doctor's strategic role in purchasing organizations has enabled GPs in the United Kingdom to remain purchasers and providers.

Neither the United Kingdom nor the Catalonia experiments suggest that tendering for services is the main obstacle to purchasing. Rather, the problem relates to limitations in the GP's role as gatekeeper and coordinator of care for a designated population. Population-based information about health, disease, health service use, and patient preferences are essential if primary care staff are to base purchasing decisions on evidence. Life long patient records complement population information, providing the link between purchasing decisions for individuals and populations, and the detail necessary for managing care across organizational boundaries. From the utilization review perspective, clinical records provide the evidence required to challenge provider assessments of co-morbidity and limit Diagnosis Related Groups (DRG) creep. In countries where patients can choose their provider by episode, comprehensive records are rare. Where register systems are employed as alternatives, for example in Finland and Sweden, the register fields may limit the information available. This restricts the GP's role as patient agent, care coordinator, and informed purchaser.

The organizational environment, particularly the extent to which policy-making is shared within the health care system, is also important. In Finland, devolved budgets enabled some Finnish health centres to introduce more patient-friendly services. However, GPs in individual health stations (the equivalent of a group practice in the United Kingdom) are rarely consulted over purchasing decisions. Being the agent of the collective patient, therefore, is a struggle. The Finnish case and the problems highlighted in the Russian Federation experiments illustrate the need to establish the GP's role as the patient's agent before introducing purchasing.

Financial risk

Some commentators have suggested that primary care purchasing in the United Kingdom would have been more successful if GPs had borne greater financial risks. Conversely, the cases studied here suggest that the ability to make choices about financial risk taking and to control the size of the risk are more important arbiters of primary care professionals' behaviour. Scrutiny of other United Kingdom initiatives, for example, suggests that GPs (at least the early adopters) have been willing to sacrifice income or time for service improvements in which they believed. For example, many GPs have undertaken more minor surgery or anticipatory care than that for which they were reimbursed. While threats to organizational budgets may have accelerated changes in practice, the financial risks associated with purchasing and innovations have been smaller than those related to purchasing premises or establishing a professional practice in the United Kingdom.

These direct risks, however, have been within primary care's span of control. Purchasing has foundered, however, where there is a perception of uncontrolled financial liability. Where primary care staff's core income has not been protected, for example in the Russian Federation, imperatives to cut costs and maximize income to ensure personal security and organizational survival seem to override those associated with enhancing quality. In contrast, financial risks associated with most devolved budgeting initiatives have related to additional or organizational income.

In a more modest way, the reluctance of Stockholm GPs to embrace purchasing reflected concerns about liability for financial risks that they could not control. Examples include their limited influence over patient use of specialist services resulting from the lack of GP gatekeeping. Similar reservations about expanding purchasing in Estonia reflect family practitioner concerns about taking responsibility for prescribing budgets before funding flows reflect optimal treatment of common, chronic diseases in primary care. At the same time, however, Estonian FPs have expanded the care they provide to children in line with professional and national priorities (Maaroos and Meiesaar, 2004). This illustrates the potential conflict between policy-makers and politicians, whose main reason for introducing primary care purchasing may be ideological, and GPs, whose motivation is likely to combine a wish to improve health care and their own status.

Assessing the impact of primary care purchasing across Europe

The evidence outlined in this chapter illustrates a continuum of primary care purchasing: from the comprehensive purchasing found in the United Kingdom, Catalonia and Finland to the indirect influence and limited active purchasing found in Estonia and Bologna. Across this continuum, purchasing experiments have provided examples of innovation and changes in practice.

Primary care purchasing seems to facilitate modest but important improvements resulting from change at the margin. The establishment of fundholders as small-scale purchasers could facilitate the shift of services to alternative providers without destabilizing the funding base of local specialist services. Fundholders and commissioning groups could also provide more detailed evidence of quality problems than was available to the health authority through routine data collection.

Evidence from the cases suggests that primary care purchasing can act as a lever to streamline decision-making, improving the flexibility, timeliness, and appropriate use of diagnostic services. Where appropriate incentives and regulatory mechanisms exist, prescribing may also become more cost-effective. The alignment of incentives with the objectives of the various stakeholders is crucial. While the Imola project achieved most of its goals, delivering savings, higher quality care, and improving population coverage of treatment, attempts at more complex changes in the organization of primary care were less successful. The level of intensive home care, for example, did not increase significantly, and only just over a quarter of GPs (11 of 41) extended their opening hours. Success, therefore, requires the ability to combine clinical and financial decision-making and to ensure that financial strategy and spending reflects agreed clinical policy and best clinical practice. It seems unlikely; therefore, that purchasing will develop in health systems in which retrospective reimbursement of specialist services predominates.

The purchasing of primary care and community services in Finland has led to more widespread changes in practice than purchase of hospital services. This also suggests that effective purchasing is unrelated to its complexity; these community services require detailed agreements to ensure that patients' needs are met adequately and appropriately. This finding confirms, however, that where purchasers have flexibility and a short feedback loop, it is possible to tailor services more closely to patients' needs.

The achievements of devolved budgeting illustrate the benefits of approaches that involve marginal shifts, incremental improvements and well-chosen incentives. At the level of care groups, clinical directorates or teams, very small changes in investment patterns can achieve modest but important improvements. Centralized health authority-style financial management finds change like this difficult. It may be the ability of Finnish purchasers to effect modest but important changes in investment patterns in primary care and community services, and organizational constraints on doing so for hospital services, which explains the relative effectiveness of purchasing in some settings, and its failure in others.

The Finnish example also provides a limited example of a wider move to link devolved budgeting initiatives to the integration of care for patients with chronic conditions across organizational boundaries. These approaches may have been successful because they enable management theories about devolved budgets to be adapted to fit current theories about clinical practice. The latter include examples of how best to manage primary care demand and acute illnesses within a framework that recognizes the prevalence of chronic disease and the co-morbidity experienced by frequent users of health services.

At a system level, optimizing the balance between encouraging innovation with tools such as devolved budgeting while minimizing the bureaucracy associated with maintaining equitable access and service provision requires careful management. There is some evidence that Primary Care Groups (PCGs) helped extend the apparent benefits of fundholding and commissioning to a wider group of practitioners and patients in the United Kingdom. PCGs were also more democratic organizations. Their elected GP leaders were often chosen for their motivational and negotiation skills. In part, these personal characteristics, the availability of peer information, feedback and educational support limited the potential for free riding by less interested GPs and the dilution of accountability often found in larger organizations. Primary Care Trusts are even larger, designed as complex networked organizations with employed staff, professionals with portfolio contracts and independent contractors providing a mixture of purchasing and provider functions. These are potentially dynamic organizations but in a large organization like the NHS the temptation to create new bureaucracies is always present. Many PCTs have recognized this risk, retaining smaller locality developed during the 1990s, and establishing mechanisms for involving local people in decision-making. (Wilkin *et al.*, 2001; Honey *et al.*, 2003). The relatively smooth transition between organizational forms in the United Kingdom and Spain reflects the detailed attention given to planning and implementation. Without such planning, the tension between flexibility, responsiveness and order may result in unrestrained market conditions replacing centralized structures, as in the Russian Federation, or, as in neighbouring Finland, may produce little increase in flexibility or empowerment and no reduction in bureaucracy.

Despite the mixed picture from the evaluation of commissioning groups (Smith and Shapiro, 1996) and fundholding, positive results from purchasing experiments across Europe reflect the endeavours of a small group of skilled, enthusiastic, influential professionals (and occasionally politicians). These innovators share clear objectives, a commitment to improving services for local people and the opportunity to effect flexible solutions. Sustainable benefit from devolved budgeting, however, requires primary care professionals to look beyond immediate problems and to develop strategic activities such as health needs assessment, service and programme review. The most successful examples in the United Kingdom and elsewhere have been supported by public health and other strategic expertise. In Bologna, Catalonia, and more recently in Estonia, the purchasing experiments have formed part of an explicit regional strategy, supported by detailed objectives and incentives, underpinned by infrastructure development including clinical and organizational governance.

Contextual preconditions for primary care purchasing

The organizational and professional factors associated with successful implementation of primary care purchasing appear to cluster. This suggests that effective primary care purchasing requires the presence of certain organizational and professional conditions.

Organizational factors include a supportive environment that facilitates needs-based purchasing, ongoing responsibility for care, and a clinical, financial and managerial framework within which strategic and operational purchasing decisions may be evaluated. Specific features include:

- designated population based on residence or registered list;
- gatekeeping – non-emergency specialist care based on referral by organization with budgetary responsibility;
- ongoing responsibility for care;
- lifelong clinical records – shared by clinical teams across organizations;
- well-established budgeting system with independent oversight;
- sound systems for independent clinical review and opportunity for development of more comprehensive clinical governance;
- incentives that reward organizational and clinical innovation and improvement.

Professional factors associated with successful purchasing are based on wider recognition of primary care expertise (Audit Commission, 2002; Iles and Sutherland, 2002). These include:

- primary care doctors' education meets international standards for primary care specialists;
- primary care professionals and supportive managers are developed into competent purchasers (Hallin and Siverbo, 2001);

- established primary care role includes negotiation with patients, specialists and managers about individual cases and service developments;
- dedicated time and resources for purchasing activities;
- primary care research infrastructure with support, for example, for patient profiling and more formal needs assessment;
- ethical and professional framework regulates behaviour;
- clear contractual separation between provider and purchasing/strategic role;
- strong primary care identity with primary care trusted to provide most clinical care.

In comparison with the evidence of successful initiatives associated with devolved budgets, problems have existed where some or all of the preconditions for effective purchasing were not established in advance and where few professional, managerial or regulatory controls existed.

In Finland, for example, there is little evidence that primary care practitioners experienced increased authority following the reforms outlined in this chapter. Loss of dedicated budgets and new responsibilities dissipated the management efforts of chief physicians who now compete for resources with other areas of municipal spending and hospital specialties. With their own budgets being cash limited and without the budgetary influence over specialist care enjoyed in other countries, the power of primary care professionals may have actually diminished. At local level, however, there is some cause for optimism. Demonstration projects, most notably the GP-led federations, have enhanced the position of primary care, enabling local services to position tertiary care in a supportive rather than a dominant role.

The Finnish example illustrates that transferring budgetary responsibility without discretion over the nature of care purchased does not enhance the role or prestige of primary care. Primary care fares well if directly funded separately from hospital care. Without dedicated funding, however, secondary care tends to dominate regardless of organizational arrangements.

An increased emphasis on primary care requires more than devolved budgeting. Additional elements include a supportive policy environment, facilitative management, and leaders with well-developed skills in effecting change. Clearly, market mechanisms have a limited role in health systems that value cost control, collaboration between purchasers and providers, and equitable service provision. Injudicious use of market mechanisms may actually reduce the likelihood of successful purchasing by removing tools like gatekeeping, lifelong records, and defined populations leading to weaknesses in education, training, regulation and in governance being overlooked. Instead, active stakeholder involvement and agreed procedures for determining investment priorities are required, backed by well-targeted incentives, sanctions and peer pressure (Robinson and Steiner, 1998; Killoran et al., 1999).

Few countries, however, fulfil all the preconditions for successful purchasing. The limited evidence base also poses problems for countries considering the development of primary care purchasing, and the optimal size of the purchasing organization is also unclear. Specifically, the available evidence does not reveal the most effective mix of flexibility, short feedback loops, sensitivity to locality needs, limited transaction costs and equity of service provision. The evidence is also heavily weighted towards doctors as clinical purchasers; there is little precedent for the "nurse as purchaser" initiative proposed in England although there are some lessons to be learned from the social care literature (Murphy, 2004).

Alternative developments designed to enhance primary care

Several of the cases illustrate that it is possible to change the perception and position of primary care; budgetary freedoms may have facilitated this outcome. Primary care purchasing exists within a broader organizational approach that emphasizes the role of devolved decision-making, with primary care teams responsible for framing the problems their patients face and for designing ways of addressing them. Purchasing specialist care, however, is only one of the tools available to deliver improvement.

Most current and future initiatives now focus on the development of integrated care.

Traditional health service approaches to problems of finance or quality, such as structural reform, have limited effectiveness as a tool for organizational development; sustainable change requires more sophisticated approaches (Walshe *et al.*, 2004).

Most of the evidence suggests that performance reflects competent management and clinical leadership rather than the size of population served (Bojke *et al.*, 2001).

The attempt to match structure to objectives lies behind the preponderance of initiatives that focus on developing integrated care, networking organizations and devolving funding and responsibility. Recent and planned reforms in Finland, Sweden (Borgquist and Lind, 1997), and the United Kingdom encourage developing networks of cooperation in primary care and across ambulatory and specialist care. Within a primary care-led health service, such organizations should facilitate development of leadership and system-level thinking at local level. In Sweden, devolving responsibility for drug costs in primary and ambulatory care to county councils and piloting integrated drug budgets (Läkemedel i förändring, 2001), encouraging 'proximity health care', increasing the number of GPs and improving their specialist training (Prop., 1999/2000: 149) demonstrates the commitment to organizational development. In Västmanland County Council, 40% of GPs are now independent contractors, funded by the county council and supported by strong multi-professional teams. Here, 80% of inhabitants have an ongoing relationship with an 'own GP'. This is almost twice the national rate of 42% (Socialstyrelsen, 2002). Within this development framework, some elements of purchasing may be returning. In the southern district of Stockholm all health centres have been contracted out through a tendering process. Independent hospitals (private and public) may also be able to tender to run health centres. Hospitals, therefore, may become primary care purchasers. These are ambitious proposals, reflecting increased acceptance of the benefits of integrated care and the management theories that combine empowerment of local professionals with development of agreed programmes of care.

The development of networked organizations will require even more sophisticated support, regulatory mechanisms and resource allocation. Specifically, information from patient profiles, actual and expected activity and costs, based on current best practice, should be built into budgets at programme and health system levels. Assumptions will need to be stated explicitly and tested regularly to minimize the risk of new perverse incentives becoming established and distorting practice.

Current thinking views health services as a complex adaptive system. Here, the role of health care reform is to create the optimal balance between order and chaos and allow excellence to emerge. It remains to be seen whether the networked approaches that are developing in many health systems will be any more successful in enabling health services to perform at an optimal level. At a national level, this also places responsibility on governments to ensure that the future structure and organization of health services, and local and national policies are compatible, supported by economic and social development and environments that empower staff and patients.

Notes

1   Spanish documents summarized and translated by Joan Gené-Badia for this section: Violan *et al.* (2000), Guarga *et al.* (2000), Fundació Avedis Don Abedian (2003), and Gené-Badia (2003). The authors are also grateful to Andrea Donatini for helping to find the Bologna case and for providing contacts.
2   Arrangements governing primary care purchasing differ somewhat between England, Northern Ireland, Scotland and Wales. The systems described in this case study apply to England; some, but not all of them, apply to the other countries.

References

Allsop, J. (1995). *Health Policy and the NHS: Towards 2000.* London: Longman.
Audit Commission (2002). *A Focus on General Practice in England.* London: Audit Commission (http://www.audit-commission.gov.uk/publications/genprac.shtml, accessed 22 July 2002).
Bergman, S-E. (1994). *Purchaser-Provider Systems in Sweden.* Spri tryck 250.
Bloor, K., Maynard, A. and Street, A. (1999). *The Cornerstone of Labour's "New NHS": Reforming Primary Care. Discussion paper No. 168.* York: University of York, Centre for Health Economics.
Bojke, C., Gravelle, H. and Wilkin, D. (2001). Is bigger better for primary care groups and trusts? *British Medical Journal* **322**: 599–602.
Borgquist, L. and Lind, J-I. (1997). Förnyelse i sjukvårdssystem – kvalitetsaspekter och besparingspotentialer vid verksamhetsförändringar [Renewal in health care systems – aspects on quality and potentials of saving when changing the activities], *Kommunal Ekonomi* **5**: 21–23.
Delnoij, D.M.J. and Brenner, G. (2000). Importing budget systems from other countries: what can we learn from the German drug budget and the British GP fundholding? *Health Policy* **52**: 157–169.
Department of Health (2004). *Practice Based Commissioning Engaging Practices in Commissioning.* London: The Stationery Office (http://www.dh.gov.uk/assetRoot/04/09/03/59/04090359.pdf, accessed 1 December 2004).

Department of Health (1997). *The New NHS: Modern, Dependable*. London: The Stationery Office.

Dixon, J. (2003). Foundation trusts, *British Medical Journal* **326**: 1344–1345.

Donatini, A. (2002). Personal communication.

Fundació Avedis Don Abedian (2003). *Avaluació de la reforma de l'Atenció Primària i de la diversificació de la provisió de serveis [Evaluation of primary health care reforms and diversification of service provision]*. Barcelona: Fundació Avedis Don Abedian.

Gené-Badia, J. (2003). Todos los ciudadanos se han beneficiado de la política de deiversificación de la gestión de atención primària en Cataluña [All citizens benefited from primary care management diversification in Catalonia], *Cuadernos de Gestión para el Profesional de Atención Primaria* **9**(3): 117–119.

Glennerster, H., Matsaganis, M., Owens, P. and Hancock, S. (1994). *Implementing GP Fundholding*. Buckingham: Open University Press.

Gould, M. (2004). Merger pressures on primary care threaten to blur local focus, *Health Service Journal* **114**: 10–11.

Guarga, A., Gil, M., Pasarín, M., Manzanera, R., Armengol, R. and Sintes, J. (2000). Comparación de equipos de atención primaria de Barcelona según formulas de gestión, *Atención Primaria*, **26**: 600–606.

Hallin, B. and Siverbo, S. (2001). *Jakten på den goda styrningen [The hunt for the good steering]*. Gothenburg: Centre for Analysis of Health Care (CHSA).

Honey, S., Small, N. and Walsh, M.J. (2003). *Being a GP in a Primary Care Trust*. Nuffield Portfolio Report No. 20. Leeds: Nuffield Institute for Health (http://www.nuffield.leeds.ac.uk/downloads/being_a_gp.pdf, accessed 12 October 2004).

Iles, V. and Sutherland, K. (2002). *Managing Change in the NHS. Organisational Change: A Review for Health Care Managers, Professionals and Researchers*. NHS Service Delivery and Organisation (SDO) Research and Development Programme. London: NCCSDO (http://www.sdo.lshtm.ac.uk/publications.htm, accessed 1 September 2002).

Keisu, M. (2002). *Tarjouskilpailu Limingan terveyspalveluista [Tenders for Liminka health services]*. Paper presented at a seminar on competitive tendering from a social and health policy perspective, organized by the National Centre for Research and Development in Social Services and Health.

Killoran, A., Mays, A., Wyke, S. and Malbon, G. (1999). *Total Purchasing. A Step Towards New Primary Care Organisations*. London: King's Fund.

Klein, R. (2003). Governance for NHS foundation trusts, *British Medical Journal* **326**: 174–175.

Läkemedel i förändring [Pharmaceuticals in alteration] (2001). News letter from Federation of County Councils, No. 18 (http://www.lf.se/lakemedel, accessed 22 July 2002).

Lewis, R (2004). *Practice-led Commissioning*. London: King's Fund.

Maaroos, H-I. and Meisesaar, K. (2004). Does equal availability of geographical and human resources guarantee access to family doctors in Estonia? *Croatian Medical Journal* **45**: 567–572.

Mays, N. and Dixon, J. (1996). *Purchaser Plurality in UK Health Care*. London: King's Fund.

Ministry of Social Affairs and Health (2002). *National project on securing the future of Finnish health care. Proposed actions for the renewal of the functional and administrative structures of the service providing system. Working Group report*. Helsinki: Ministry of Social Affairs and Health.

Murphy, E. (2004). Case management and community matrons for long term conditions, *British Medical Journal* **329**: 1251–1252.

Myllymäki, A. (2002). *Kansalaisjärjestöt palvelujen tuottajina ja raha-automaattiyhdistyksen tuki [Citizen organizations as service providers and Slot Machine Association funding]*. Paper presented at a seminar on competitive tendering from a social and health policy perspective, organized by the National Centre for Research and Development in Social Services and Health.

Prop. 1999/2000: 149 (1999/2000) *Nationell handlingsplan för utvecklingen av hälso- och sjukvården.* [Governmental proposal for a national plan for development of health care.]

Robinson, R. and Hayter, P. (1995). Reluctance of general practitioners to become fundholders, *British Medical Journal* **311**: 166.

Robinson, R. and Steiner, A. (1998). *Managed Health Care.* Buckingham: Open University Press.

Smith, J. and Shapiro, J. (1996). *Holding on While Letting Go.* Birmingham: Health Services Management Centre.

Socialstyrelsen (National Board of Health and Welfare) (2002). *Nationell handlingsplan för hälso- och sjukvården. Årsrapport 2002 [National plan for health care. Yearly report 2002].* Stockholm: National Board of Health and Welfare.

Svalander, P-A. (1999). *Primärvården inför framtiden [Primary health care in the future].* Stockholm: Landstingsförbundet.

Svalander, P-A. and Åhgren, B. (1995). *Vad skall man kalla det som händer i Mora? – och andra frågor om styrmodeller. En preliminär uttolkning av fallstudier i sex landsting [A preliminary interpretation of case studies on steering models in six county councils].* Rapport till HSU 2000. Stockholm: Landstingsförbundet.

Taylor, D. (1991). *Developing Primary Care: Opportunities for the 1990s.* London: King's Fund Institute.

Total Purchasing National Evaluation Team (1997). *Total Purchasing: A Profile of National Pilot Projects.* London: King's Fund.

Tragakes, E. and Lessof, S. (2003). *Health Care Systems in Transition: Russia.* Copenhagen: WHO (http://www.euro.who.int/document/e81966.pdf, accessed 3 December 2004).

Violan, C., Elias, A. and Ponsà, J.A. (2000). El modelo catalán de atención primaria [The Catalonian Primary Care Model], *Cuadernos de Gestión para el Profesional de Atención Primaria* **6**: 43–47.

Walshe, K., Smith, J., Dixon, J., *et al.* (2004). Primary care trusts, *British Medical Journal* **329**: 871–2.

Wilkin, D., Gillam, S. and Coleman, A. (2001). *The National Tracker Survey of Primary Care Groups and Trusts 2000/2001: Modernising the NHS?* Manchester: University of Manchester.

Wilkin, D., Gillam, S. and Leese, B. (eds) (1999). *The National Tracker Survey of Primary Care Groups and Trusts: Progress and Challenges 1999/2000.* Manchester: University of Manchester.

chapter seven

The evolving
public-private mix

**Rod Sheaff, Joan Gené-Badia,
Martin Marshall and Igor Švab**

Conceptual framework

Policy change in Europe after 1990 involved a variety of shifts from public to private health care provision, especially in the countries of central and eastern Europe (CEE). This chapter takes a broader perspective than others in this volume, reviewing how the public-private mix has changed not just in primary care but also in the more general area of primary health care, among the mechanisms that coordinate what is a broad mix of related activities.

PHC can be defined as health care which a person can access directly (not via intermediaries) and use while still living at home (Sheaff, 1998). Its backbone is primary care medicine (general practice or the equivalent) but it also includes domiciliary care, paramedical services, pharmacies, workplace health care, self-help, emergency services, ambulances and direct-access hospital outpatient clinics. Before 1990 European health systems were conventionally classified as Bismarckian, Beveridge or Semashko types. Bismarckian systems funded private, charitable and public health care providers through an employment and income-based system of compulsory subscription to not-for-profit sickness funds. In Beveridge systems the national, regional, and/or municipal government owned and managed most health care providers, funding them from general taxation. Semashko systems differed mainly in not permitting private practice alongside public practice, as well as its normative-based system of planning and management (Yugoslavia was an exception – see below). Switzerland never formally adopted the Bismarckian system but a combination of sickness fund and private insurance, subsidies and regulation attained 98% population health care insurance cover by 1990. Furthermore, health systems often mixed these different models. In Spain, for example, general practice operated partly on the Beveridge model with GPs doing 2.5 hours a day consultation in public clinics, but seeing insured and private patients outside those hours.

Coordination of public and private health care providers occurs – or fails to – at three levels. One is the national "macro" level. At the second, subnational ("meso") level, health care organizations with a planning and/or financing function exist either at regional (Canton, *Land*, Departement, Oblast) or at district (e.g. municipality) level. As the third level, providers, including individual free professionals, are the "micro" level of analysis. Despite the term "micro" some primary care providers can be quite large (for instance, health centres in Scandinavia, Portugal and Spain). Primary care providers fall into four categories. Semashko and Beveridge systems have traditionally relied on public providers directly line-managed by governmental bodies. An important health system development has been the management of some primary health centres as "public firms", publicly owned but with similar managerial autonomy to a private firm (see below). Not-for-profit providers range from charities to large institutions which do not distribute dividends to shareholders but in many other respects behave as commercial bodies (e.g. BUPA). Purely private (e.g. for-profit) bodies are the remaining category. It includes commercial firms; however, individual self-employed doctors, or partnerships of doctors, are the commonest form.

The situation before 1990

Before 1990, macro-level coordination of public and private provision occured in a rather negative way in Beveridge systems. Law and regulation demarcated a division of labour between public and private providers. In the few matters where the law, regulation or contract were silent, the public system was not obliged to provide services but private providers could. For English GPs, for example, certifying deaths was NHS work, but certifying health for insurance purposes was private work for which patients would pay the GP. Private practice was regulated by the general legal system and any contracts through which public bodies purchased services from private providers.

Bismarckian systems used two main means of coordinating independent practitioners with the sick funds, the health ministry and other providers. Regular negotiations took place between sick funds, primary care providers, the government and, on occasions, other interested parties (e.g. pharmaceutical firms). In West Germany these discussions were routinized as a permanent institution. Coordination was also achieved by setting common terms, prices and conditions for GP contracts, whether at national (e.g. France, the United Kingdom) or meso level (e.g. the Netherlands, West Germany). Whatever the standard contract did not prohibit was open to conventional private practice.

Superficially, macro-level coordination was simple in Semashko systems. Their principles were universal coverage and equal access for the whole population. There was little room for independent practitioners, or voluntary and charitable health care providers. During a transition period after 1945 GPs were allowed to work in existing health centres or premises that they had previously owned, but as public employees receiving a salary from the state. As the state rapidly built further health centres and polyclinics, these physicians were forced to work there under similar conditions to other salaried employees. The exception was Hungary, where the state built few polyclinics but allowed independent practice throughout the communist period. GPs were allowed to work outside regular hours as independent practitioners (Švab et al., 2000). During the "years of stagnation", illegal private practice (under-the-table payments, bribes, etc.) was ignored in official policy but in reality increasingly tolerated. For senior officials (including health managers) separate *nomenklatura* services also operated (particularly in the USSR), somewhat analogously to private health care in the west. Certain occupations also had separate health services: military and security services, railway and telecommunication workers (Poland) and airline workers (USSR). These parallel systems included primary care.

For Semashko systems, meso-level coordination between the *nomenklatura* and other parallel services and mainstream services was weak. Although private practice was legally forbidden in most communist countries, meso-level authorities silently tolerated some forms of it. Physicians received low salaries, leading to low levels of service and to physicians seeking private income, often through informal payments or illegal practice. For example, in the former Yugoslavia, private dental practice flourished and was known to exist by everyone even though it was legally forbidden. It was quite often run in dentists' homes after working hours for patients who could afford out-of-pocket payments (Švab et al., 2001).

In all three systems, where the same individual did public and private work, the two were coordinated by "fitting in" private work whenever public sector duties allowed. In Bismarckian systems, general practices could subcontract other private providers to undertake, say, out-of-hours cover or paramedical services. Where voluntary and charitable bodies filled gaps in the public service provision (e.g. by providing "hospital-at-home", family planning or hospice services), public and private services were coordinated through referral paths. Beveridge systems also coordinated services by managerial direction.

The Yugoslav system was based on Andrija Štampar's (former President of the Yugoslav Academy of Sciences and Arts) ideas which, although socialist, differed from the Semashko system. Štampar's model emphasized meeting population health care needs through doctors working in the community in close contact with local authorities. Health centres were local hubs for delivering health care, health promotion and prevention. General practice was always considered central, but community nursing was also valued. However, a range of specialist services were introduced after 1950, making health centres very similar to Semashko-style polyclinics, especially in big cities (Zarkovic et al., 1994; Švab et al., 2000).

Different health system architectures accommodate different forms of provider, and therefore a different public-private mix, although there is no simple one-to-one correspondence between provider mix and health system architecture.

The main medical care providers in Bismarckian and some Beveridge systems (the United Kingdom and Denmark) were self-employed doctors contracted to the state or to sickness funds but also permitted to undertake private practice and commonly doing so in France, Greece and Portugal (Geschwind, 1999). Spanish GPs in ambulatory clinics were public employees paid by capitation. Having given 2.5 hours per day consultation at the health centre, they were free to undertake private practice thereafter. Public consultations were overburdened, giving GPs little chance to deliver high quality care. Consequently most citizens had private insurance or visited their own public doctor as private patients. They gained longer consultations while retaining the privileges of public coverage: diagnosis tests, referrals to specialists, prescriptions free of charge or with a co-payment. These arrangements also enabled private insurance companies to offer lower premiums. Teachers and civil servants could, and still can, subscribe to "Muface", a public insurance company. They avoid public ambulatory clinics, use private practice, choose their GP and have free access to specialist care. Muface pays doctors on a fee-for-service basis. In general, though, private practice was more a complement to than a substitute for the public sector in Spain.

Besides generalist doctors, Bismarckian and Semashko systems included specialized doctors working in primary care – most often obstetricians and paediatricians.

In some countries, partnerships developed, with a legal personality distinct from that of private citizens or firms. Most British GPs were in partnerships by 1990 (in Germany fewer: around 25%). Typically these partnerships would have five members or fewer. In England, each partner typically owned an equal share of the capital of the partnership, which they would purchase on entering the partnership and sell on leaving it. Selling lists of patients was made illegal in 1947, but for many years afterwards the cost of entering a partnership would usually include an inflated price for equipment and furniture, ostensibly to purchase the "goodwill". The partners would jointly employ support staff (nurses, receptionists, etc.). Partners usually kept their own personal lists of NHS patients, although they could – and often did – combine their lists. Usually the partners shared at least some of their private practice earnings, sometimes all of them.

Both Beveridge and Semashko systems provided broader service PHC through conventional, hierarchical organizations employing salaried staff. They varied according to what services and professions they included, for instance whether they covered social work (Northern Ireland, Poland), veterinary services (Italy), kindergartens (East Germany), spas (USSR, East Germany), or medicine (provided by independent practitioners instead in some countries). Another variation was whether they were accountable to local government (Italy), the health ministry (Portugal), both of these (USSR), or higher-level health organizations (the United Kingdom). That determined how far operational decisions (about budgets, staffing, repairs, working practices, etc.) were delegated to local managers (e.g. English community health services) or centrally prescribed (USSR); (Burenkova, 1986).

In both Bismarckian and Beveridge systems private provision played a greater role in PHC than in the hospital sector. When not provided by the public sector, nursing and domestic help in the patient's home was provided either by private individuals or, in the case of nursing, employment agencies (private firms). Firms (as opposed to individual professionals and partnerships) rarely provided medical care, but did usually supply pharmaceuticals, equipment and other consumables on a commercial basis (another contrast with the Semashko system).

Main reform trends during the 1990s

The dramatic change after 1990 was the decline of the Semashko system. Reacting against Soviet policy, most CEE governments decided to replace it with "western" practices. In that climate, the larger change of introducing a Bismarckian system or privatization were often more politically acceptable than the smaller move to a Beveridge system. Western governments were also exporting their own health policy models, for instance through the EU PHARE and TACIS programmes. Other international organizations, especially the World Bank, the WTO and the IMF, promoted "Washington consensus" policies of globalizing CEE economies, privatizing wherever possible and dramatically reducing public spending. Their policies helped to generate substantial reductions of public spending on first-line medical care. In Russia, for instance, most polyclinics had difficulty paying even the low official salaries, and could not purchase equipment or consumables. These conditions made western ideas for extracting more health services from given resources doubly attractive to CEE health systems. The Bismarckian model also appeared to offer a way of supplementing state financing with private financing for health care. Not surprisingly, many CEE countries changed primary care financing from public budgets to some form of national health insurance.

During this period, primary care providers saw opportunities to consolidate their incomes and renegotiate their relationship to the state. Virtually all the CEE countries have permitted independent general practice (see Vignette 7.3); however, the proportion of doctors working independently varies between countries. Some countries (e.g. the former East Germany) have made it virtually impossible for a physician not to be a private entrepreneur. In the former Yugoslavia, general practice was already a recognized discipline. Bosnia and Herzegovina, Croatia, and Slovenia relabelled it "family medicine" and improved existing vocational training. Other countries re-introduced general practice as an academic discipline, largely with support from abroad (e.g. Canada, the United Kingdom). Some projects (e.g. in Estonia) were successful, but in other countries (e.g. "the former Yugoslav Republic of Macedonia", Serbia) few changes have taken place. Generally, the policy choice is between either accepting a longer transition period or the coexistence of salaried and independent practice (Lember, 1998; Markota *et al.*, 1999).

Western European countries' economic problems, while nowhere near as severe as in the CEE, still led to health system reform. Britain faced this predicament in the 1970s and by the 1990s Germany, Sweden and Switzerland were also affected (Theurl, 1999; Bergmark, 2000). Initially many western European health systems adopted a "strategy of managerialism" (Flynn, 1992), trying to meet growing demands by exploiting resources more efficiently instead of increasing them or radically restructuring their health systems. The "New Public Management" provided a repertoire of methods: in primary care, its main manifestations were cash-limited budgets (e.g sickness funds negotiating global cash limits with providers), the substitution of cheaper inputs (e.g. by redefining the division of labour between occupational groups and promoting team-based PHC provision), and the introduction of performance indicators and evidence-based medicine. Vignette 7.1 illustrates this with the example of Spain:

Vignette 7.1   Primary health provision in Spain

In the mid-1980s Spain reformed its public health services. The country was divided into subareas of 5,000 to 25,000 inhabitants. Every citizen was assigned a personal doctor and nurse, and received care from a subarea team working in a health centre (in cities) or a local surgery (in rural areas). Teams were composed of GPs, paediatricians, nurses, social workers and a dentist working 36 hours a week for the public sector, acting as gatekeepers and providing preventive, curative and rehabilitative care. Nurses receive a salary while doctors were paid by capitation or salary basis depending on the region. Although doctors may undertake private practice outside working hours, the improved salaries, rising quality of services and prestige of public GPs may explain why private insurance coverage decreased from 20.2% in 1980 to 8.7% in 1990. Compared with the traditional system, the reformed system had fewer GP referrals to specialists, hospital outpatient and inpatient departments and emergency rooms by GPs. Physicians wrote 23% fewer prescriptions for pensioners and 17% fewer for younger patients. Demographic, health or social variables did not explain these differences. Reformed teams complied better with protocols and guidelines for preventive care and follow-up of chronic conditions such as diabetes and hypertension. A comparison of mortality rates for 1984–1996 in three equally socioeconomically impoverished zones of Barcelona showed a clear association between reformed PHC services and a decrease in mortality due to stroke and hypertension. Satisfaction was significantly greater among people using the reformed PHC centres (Gené-Badia *et al.*, 1996; Villabi *et al.*, 1999).

Comparable team-based innovations were promoted in Finland, the Netherlands, Portugal, Sweden, the United Kingdom, and former Yugoslavia in the 1980s.

During the 1990s, two main strategies in response to the economic pressures were to promote competition and substitute private for public provision in primary care. Drawing upon arguments developed by the New Institutional Economics (Niskanen, 1973; Williamson, 1975), and, for health care, Enthoven (1986), proponents of competition also suggested that one alternative to privatization could be reforming public services into public markets. In theory, the resulting "quasi-markets" or "internal markets" could also be opened to private finance and providers. Thus common economic pressures, moderate in western Europe but extreme in CEE, produced rather convergent policies for primary care provision across the continent.

Promoting competition and contestability

In Beveridge and Semashko systems, promoting competition among primary care providers required separating existing organizations into financing and planning levels in contrast with provider levels, and then creating competing providers on the provider side (these distinctions already existed in Bismarckian systems). One purpose of competition was to pay (or penalize) primary care providers in ways that favoured those who contained costs or increased the volume of care for a given budget. One method was to encourage patients themselves to choose between providers, who would then be rewarded for attracting patients (Saltman and Von Otter, 1992). Additionally, the purchasing body could establish benchmarking, i.e. publish ranked "performance" indicators or "league tables" geared to best practice. In England and Wales, for example, experiments are under way to publish comparative data about GPs' clinical services. Even while fundholding was in operation, however, English GPs proved more inclined to work collaboratively than to compete.

Work as well as payments could be transferred between providers. In Beveridge systems, many health ministries promoted competition by reforming their primary care providers into "public firms". These "public firms" have in some cases used their autonomy to adopt service models used in the private sector so as to compete directly with private providers, thus reversing the dynamic of privatization. Conversely, in some countries (e.g. Spain, the United Kingdom), hospital accident departments compensate for deficiencies in primary care services (Rodriguez *et al.*, 2000). The public firm model enables hospitals to turn this into an opportunity to compete for income. In Germany it is proposed to allow university polyclinics to see patients and be paid by sickness funds for doing so – a move which GPs have complained is subsidized public competition, weakening the local medical unions' monopoly (*Ärztliche Praxis*, 9 May 2002; *Die Welt*, 5 October 2001). At least one patient organization has welcomed the proposal for the same reason. The British NHS swiftly copied the idea of convenience clinics (see below) opening 20 experimental free, public-funded convenience clinics of its own, mainly in town centres but at least one in a major airport.

To signal their unwillingness to let new providers enter primary care unless existing providers become more efficient, governments have also begun supporting experimental new organizational forms and models of care such as those illustrated in Vignettes 7.2 and 7.4. English GPs became more receptive to new methods of clinical governance when they began to suspect that otherwise the government would review the entire concept of medical self-regulation in primary care.

Vignette 7.2 Personal Medical Service Schemes in England

Nearly all British GPs are self-employed and obtain most of their income by contracting their services to the National Health Service. Since the NHS began (1948), GPs have provided most primary care services. Since 1997, around 20% of the GPs have exercised a new option to drop the national contract and instead work as part of a Personal Medical Services (PMS) scheme under contract to their local Health Authority or PCT. However, the 1997 legislation also allows non-medical providers to make such contracts. For GPs who do not opt for PMS status, the national contract has been radically renegotiated. It divides GPs' tasks into three categories. All practices have to provide the "essential" services. GPs can opt out of providing "additional" and "enhanced" services, but if they do so their payments are reduced. Then the local Primary Care Trust has either to provide these services itself or subcontract another organization to do so. These proposals thus present an opportunity for new providers, both public and private, to work alongside GPs in delivering such services as chronic disease management, preventative care, home visits and out-of-hours care. Besides facing new competitors, GPs' position as the preferred providers of primary care is being eroded.

All forms of provider competition require meso-level bodies to use contracts, incentives and payment systems that make primary care providers compete over the range and quality of services. Besides new GP contracts in England (Vignette 7.2), Italy and Norway, there have been HMO-like experiments in Germany and Switzerland.

The new forms of contract are also used to apply cash limits (e.g. in Belgium, England, France, the Netherlands; and planned in Germany). In Beveridge systems, governments directly control the purchasing organizations and their budgets. In Bismarckian systems, these ends were achieved by promoting competition among the purchasers to ensure that providers contain costs and introduce new forms of care, and ensure that patients would choose their sickness fund (or other insurer) on the grounds of provider quality and range of services. Such were the Dekker and Simons reforms in the Netherlands, and similar reforms in Austria, Belgium, Germany and Switzerland. Foreseeing the danger of adverse risk selection (insurers "cream-skimming" the most profitable or least costly patients to treat), governments tried to make case-mix differences cost-neutral to sickness funds and PHC providers. In Germany and Switzerland, complex risk structure equalization methods (*Risikostrukturausgleich*) were therefore introduced.

Substituting private for public provision

Privatization across western European primary care has been implemented in two main ways:

(1) Substitution of private for public finance has occurred in some western countries, particularly in the form of increasing co-payments for primary care services. Italy has gradually been extending co-payments for primary care services since the 1980s. In some Bismarckian systems (e.g. France) patients typically buy supplementary private health insurance to cover procedures that do not have full social security cover (Geschwind, 1999). In most of the former USSR Territorial Funds for Compulsory Medical Insurance were created in the 1990s, financed by mandatory contributions from workers and firms. Municipalities pay the subscriptions of non-economically active people.

(2) Privatizing primary care providers has occurred in some countries as part of official policy. Traditionally, of course, Beveridge and Bismarckian systems allowed primary care providers to undertake private and publicly funded work in parallel. In the 1990s, CEE countries accomplished privatization partly by legalizing existing illicit private practice. For example, following new legislation, dentists in the former Yugoslavia were among the first health professionals in that country to embrace independent practice. They declared their existing "secret" practices and have generally continued to work for out-of-pocket payment for the same clientele (Švab *et al.*, 2001). In Spain the market share of private medicine is higher in primary than in hospital specialist care (Urbanos-Garrida, 2001). The German medical networks described below (Vignette 7.6) can collectively pursue private practice.

These two strategies were not always consistent with each other or other policies. For example, evidence-based medicine, the substitution of non-medical for medical staff and the increasing need to coordinate primary health care services all suggest a larger provider unit than the individual doctor. Yet privatization policies worked in exactly the opposite direction when, as in many CEE countries, they involved abolishing polyclinics.

Outstanding innovative experiences

Both competition and privatization have resulted in diversification of primary care providers. However, the resulting fragmentation and competition in the primary care sector did not remove governments' desire to influence the quality of these services and to promote better coordination between general practices, or the local equivalent, and other primary and social care providers. Various primary health care providers themselves often need to collaborate for practical, therapeutic purposes. In the absence of bureaucratic powers of coordination, many governments promoted networks of PHC organizations to compensate for the organizational fragmentation of PHC and to strengthen PHC providers' accountability to government, investors and the public. The following vignettes illustrate this.

New forms of private primary care provision

Apart from independent medical practice, which was an innovation for the CEE countries but not for western Europe, four main new types of primary care provider appeared. Commercial providers exist, but are exceptional. In Britain, one of the few examples of successful commercial providers have been walk-in clinics recently opened in major London railway stations. Patients have consultations without prior appointment on a first-come-first-served basis. Similar private walk-in clinics were started in Swedish cities as early as 1983 (Saltman and von Otter, 1987). Other new forms of private and/or mixed public-private service delivery are: medical cooperatives (see Vignettes 7.3 and 7.4) and collaborations between doctors, other health professions and voluntary organizations (Vignette 7.5).

PHC networks

During the 1990s, the need to coordinate medical care with nursing, para-medical and social care became greater as chronic disease, care of the elderly and substitution for hospital care became more prominent. Where the coordination of PHC services by public bodies has been dismantled or never existed, these trends have made it necessary nevertheless to construct alternative mechanisms to coordinate the public-private mix at local level. Three categories of network

Vignette 7.3   Medical cooperatives in former Yugoslavia

Health centres remain the predominant form of PHC organization but GPs can opt to work as independent solo GPs who refer their patients to specialists. The problem of waiting lists for some specialists is generally solved by making direct out-of-pocket payments to those specialists. However, medical cooperatives as a form of joint venture between primary and secondary specialists do exist in both Croatia and Slovenia, although they are relatively rare. Examples exist of firms owned by GPs and employing secondary care specialists, mostly on a part-time basis or even through a part-time contract. Most frequently, the aim of such a cooperative is to make specialist services more readily available to patients registered with the cooperative. Additional employment of salaried specialists in independent practices has been recognized as a source of concern by policy-makers and hospital managers, but the problem has not been adequately solved. Quite often the cooperatives are a cover for a specialist secondary care, which is one of the most frequent forms of independent and private practice. In some cases established specialists ask to be licensed as GPs only to be able to have patients registered with them and to offer their specialist services to their patients under the title of general practice, which is paid for largely by the state.

Vignette 7.4   Medical cooperatives for out-of-hours services in England

After 1990 English GPs increasingly organized out-of-hours clinics on a cooperative basis. GPs have been formally responsible for providing all-day every-day medical cover for their patients. Previously this requirement was most often met by hiring commercial deputizing services, and in many places it still is. Cooperatives consist of a group of GPs (membership is voluntary) who take it in turns to provide night-time and weekend services for patients of all the GPs in the cooperative. The cooperative pays a fee for this work. All members also contribute money to meet these and other running costs, but these contributions are in turn reimbursed from public budgets. (Thus, an individual GP can either gain or lose money on balance, depending on the sums involved and how much out-of-hours work he or she does.) A few of these cooperatives have gone further, by providing clinic premises which patients can attend and in some places they have taken responsibility for the NHS Direct services described below. Out-of-hours services provided by patients' own GPs appear to be of somewhat higher quality than the commercial alternatives (Cragg *et al.,* 1997), although little evidence yet exists comparing them with hospital emergency departments.

Vignette 7.5   The *Entitat de Base Asociativa*, Catalonia

The Health Care Organization Law (*Llei d'Ordenació Sanitària de Catalunya,* 1990) broke the monopoly of primary care provision by regional public authorities staffed by civil servants. Most hospitals were already owned by organizations belonging to churches, municipalities, regional government or private owners and managed in a similar way to private organizations with more rapid and flexible personnel and financial management processes than in the public sector. Many of these organizations launched primary care services (Martí and Grenzner, 1999; Violan *et al.,* 2000). In the mid-1990s five EBAs (*Entitat de Base Asociativa*) appeared. The EBA is a private for-profit enterprise run by a team of doctors and nurses who care for a defined population. It receives a capitation-based budget for doctors' and nurses' salaries, premises, diagnostic tests, referrals to specialists and prescriptions. A study in Barcelona identified no statistically significant differences in the use of medical services, indicators of clinical practice, or quality and pharmacy costs between three different primary care management schemes; although the *per capita* ratio of nurses was lower in the non-public organizations (Guarga *et al.,* 2000). Breaking the public services' monopoly of primary care was seen as powerful stimulus to promoting quality not only in privately managed organizations but also in the publicly managed regional ones.

have emerged. A "virtual primary care organization" is organized around a care pathway, specific care group or geographically defined population, such as (in the Netherlands) local collaborations of health, local government and voluntary services for the purpose of coordinating primary medical care with paramedical services, nursing home services and social services (Houtepen and Ter Meulen, 2000). German Integrated Care Structures (see Vignette 7.6) and English Primary Care Trusts (Vignette 7.7) are further instances. A second type, found in England, Germany (see Vignette 7.8) and Poland, are professional networks for education, clinical audit and promoting evidence-based medicine (EBM). The third category are policy networks that coordinate independent general practices and other PHC providers in implementing intersectoral "new public health" initiatives (e.g. the WHO Healthy Cities Programme, Health Action Zones in England).

Impact of reforms and innovations

More evidence is available about the organizational impacts of European health care reforms on the range and coordination of providers than about their health impacts or effects on patient satisfaction. Better evidence is available about separate local initiatives than about the effects of privatization and competition policies as a whole.

The evidence is equivocal about the effects of competition as a means of selecting primary care providers and coordination of the private-public mix. A

Vignette 7.6   Integrated care structures in Germany

Several countries have attempted to construct Health Maintenance Organizations (HMOs), tending to favour the Preferred Provider Organization (PPO) and Independent Practice Association (IPA) models (Robinson and Steiner, 1997). In the German and Swiss cases, specific financial arrangements are made with a medical network such as those described above, creating an "integrated care structure" (integrierten Versorgungsstruktur). Selected doctors become preferred providers and negotiate special contractual terms with local sickness funds, side-stepping the usual German arrangements under which the local doctors' union apportions a fixed budget between doctors according to their activity. In some places the sickness fund negotiates a block payment, either for all services, for services to a specific care group, or for new PHC services, such as emergency services and nursing care (Südbaden) and walk-in clinics (Schleswig-Holstein). Other services remain financed under the old system. The largest German network is the Berlin Doctors' Networks (Praxisnetze Berliner Ärzte) which involves industry-based sickness funds. It proved easy to recruit doctors to the scheme but to attract patients it had to offer discounts and recruit further sickness funds (Plassman, 1998).

Vignette 7.7 English Primary Care Trusts

All English GPs must now be members of a local Primary Care Trust. The chair and a majority of seats on the PCT's Professional Executive Committee are elected by GPs, who are independent practitioners. PCTs are becoming responsible for managing PHC (including community health services) for the clinical quality of primary medical care and for commissioning secondary care. However, most GPs are not contracted to PCTs but hold a contract with the Department of Health, such that the PCT has no direct contractual control over them. A minority now work under contract to the PCT (see above) but these contracts are not a strong instrument of control (Sheaff and Lloyd-Kendall, 2000; Sibbald et al., 2001). PCTs may also employ GPs, but very few do so as yet. Consequently the PCT has to influence GPs mainly by using information, knowledge, education, local professional and friendship networks, by making "gentleman's agreements" and by subtle political pressures (Sheaff et al., 2004). PCTs are starting to collect data on the current state of clinical practice and attempting to implement evidence-based guidelines produced by the National Institute for Clinical Excellence (NICE) and other national bodies.

Vignette 7.8 Practice networks in Germany

Practice networks in Germany illustrate the professional network model. Following the 1997 German health system reforms, some independent doctors formed networks, some of which included other professions. Physicians join voluntarily. Some regard the networks' independence as increasing GPs' bargaining power with sick funds (Plassman, 1998). About 160 networks have been created, though some have subsequently dissolved, with sizes ranging from 13 to 1800 doctors (the Berlin Kodex project). Their functions range from communications and advice giving only (e.g. in Bielefeld) to clinical quality management, usually through quality circles (sometimes interdisciplinary) or clinical audit. They also enable doctors to purchase consumables more cheaply (Szecseny et al., 1999) and to share equipment. Some have created combined budgets for medical and non-medical expenses (paramedical services, pharmaceuticals). The network in Münster has also created patient registers for chronic diseases and provides out-of-hours services. Another common activity is to establish cross-referral systems between generalist and specialist doctors within PHC, and to ensure that hospitals provide ambulatory services such as day surgery which are still relatively new in Germany.

number of new forms of primary care provider have appeared. The reforms have also stimulated quality management activity, partly through publicly comparing primary care providers, a corollary of competition. Evidence about what effects these quality management activities actually have upon health outcomes is voluminous, complex and equivocal (Grimshaw *et al.*, 2001), but when a number of different activities occur concurrently, they do appear to promote the practice of EBM and to that extent improve clinical outcomes. Evidence about patient satisfaction is equally indirect. When they are adequately resourced and given sufficient managerial autonomy, public providers in Beveridge systems can improve primary care access and quality, and out-compete private providers. Recent changes in primary health care may also have contributed to a Europe-wide decline in lengths of hospital stay (see Chapter Two). PHC contributes through providing domiciliary care, ambulatory clinics (Germany), "near-patient" diagnostic services (Britain) and "hospital at home" services (France). Although pro-competition policies helped open up PHC to the new kinds of services that were required, these changes largely reflect the new collaborative networks of the kinds outlined above.

Various problems have also arisen. When regulations on sickness funds have been relaxed, for example, a side effect seems to have been to stimulate them to act more acquisitively. Regulatory changes subtly changed the "private" character of some sickness funds from a not-for-profit charity-oriented character to one much (but not completely) like a conventional financial institution. In the Netherlands, sickness funds reacted to competition as much by merging (reducing competition) as by managing providers more assertively. Scope for competition among primary care providers proved to be limited. Unlike inpatient care, primary care has to be provided near the patient's home, and primary care patients tend to value a long-term relationship with their doctor and do not change provider readily (Sheaff, 2001). Provider competition presupposes excess capacity, which exists in CEE and, say, Germany but not everywhere (e.g. there are shortages of GPs in Britain and the Russian Federation). There is evidence that English and German GPs prefer cooperating to competing with each other, and professional networks generally tend to inhibit competition.

As for privatization, reforms in some countries (e.g. Malta, Romania, Russia) have redefined publicly funded primary health care more narrowly. Less medicalized, more socially oriented services such as care of the elderly or disabled, and environmental and occupational health have passed to other ministries whose role is more to oversee private markets than to provide or finance services. Fragmentation has occurred at a time when, as noted, demographic changes, shifts from acute to chronic disease and the substitution of primary for secondary care necessitate closer coordination. In these circumstances, PHC systems have relied on the purchasers to coordinate services and have constructed networks.

When private commercial insurers have made inroads in Bismarckian systems, adverse risk selection has reappeared. Evidence since 1990 repeats this dating back to the 1940s and earlier. Thus in Spain, private insurance appeared to reduce "excess" (i.e. higher than average) consumption of PHC and the insured were disproportionately in one region (Catalonia), the cities and richest classes (Rodriguez *et al.*, 2000). Despite having to offer all adult patients the same premiums, some deregulated Swiss sickness funds achieved profit rates twice as high as others in 1998 by attracting clients with "better" risk profiles (Theurl, 1999). In CEE, the pattern is sharper. Many Russian firms are unable or unwilling to pay sickfund premiums. Whether municipalities can do so depends on their own local tax base, which is small in most Oblasts. Privatization and competition among sickness funds thus appears to have mainly adverse effects on patients in terms of exposing them to great risk selection and thus reducing access to primary care services.

On the provider side, "private" primary care has become an increasingly diverse category. Indeed, assimilating all the new kinds of providers as 'private' obscures important differences. They pursue different goals, respond to different incentives and bring different resources. It might appear that a greater variety of providers increases the risk of adverse selection, or at least differential access to health care. However, in Britain it appears that although GP fundholders succeeded in gaining easier access to hospital and community services for some of their patients (Glennerster and Matsanganis, 1992), there was no reduction in access for non-fundholders' patients (Dowling, 2001). Diversification of providers makes primary care provision more contestable, with the benefits noted above.

Against this, private provision of primary care has in some ways obstructed reform. Independent GPs can choose whether to scrutinize their clinical practice critically or, as the uneven development of practice networks in Germany indicates, not to. Even English GPs, who are obliged to participate in "clinical governance", vary considerably in how actively they do so (Sheaff *et al.*, 2004). Similarly, complications with private pension rights discouraged many English GPs from joining PMS schemes, as did partnership arrangements; a partnership develops at the pace of its most conservative member. Evidence from several countries (Italy, Portugal, Spain) indicates the difficulty in achieving patient satisfaction under Beveridge systems, and in quasi-market systems derived from them, when publicly-employed doctors are free to both practice privately and to manage their own public sector workload. In Greece, the result is under-the-table payments to GPs (Daniildou, 2002). These experiences suggest that in Beveridge systems the underregulated coexistence of public and private practice creates dual standards of access even when the state funds universally free health care.

Reform experience shows that doctors and patients respond to financial incentives (e.g. for patients to accept gatekeeping or a restricted choice of doctor). GPs also respond to the possibility of alternative providers entering primary care. However, these are not the only incentives. The experience of quality management and medical networks suggests that non-financial incentives, such as opportunities to pursue specific clinical interests and making clinical practice transparent to outsiders, can also be effective.

Discussion and policy lessons

Together, the above impacts suggest three sets of policies which counteract each other and wider policy aims (Rhodes, 1997):

- Privatization of primary care purchasing can stimulate adverse selection and thus compromises universal access to PHC.
- Competition and privatization can compromise the policy-responsiveness of primary care organizations.
- By dispersing services among different providers, competition and privatization can compromise the growing requirement for closer coordination of PHC services.

More positively, benchmarking, contestability and competition, as well as giving public providers the latitude and resources to adapt ideas developed elsewhere and to implement their own ideas for innovation, have stimulated existing public providers to offer forms of service that appeal more to patients. There have been the benefits of a spread of evidence-based medicine and the opening of primary care to new providers, organizational innovations and models of care. Hence the value from competition has come less from stimulating micro-level competition between local GPs than from opening up to new providers, new models of care and new forms of organization; in effect, generating a new public-private mix.

What policy implications follow? One is the gradual erosion of the medical monopoly in primary care: a politically delicate issue that may yet trigger resistance to further changes. A second is that competition and patient choice, should not simply be equated with privatization and conventional, commercial markets; or vice-versa. Paradoxically, competition occurs among public primary care providers as well as actors such as sickness funds which are neither fully commercial nor public bodies, while some forms of private primary care provider (e.g. English general practices) display little competition. Although economist orthodoxy asserts that private providers are more efficient than public ones, no evidence of that emerges from the European experience. The corresponding policy implication would be to promote innovation, experimentation and the contestability of provision rather than competition and privatization for their own sake.

Increased diversity of "private" providers raises the question of whether some kinds of privatization are better than others. Many innovations have emerged from the voluntary sector and independent practitioners. The entry of new providers needs to be regulated so as to ensure patient safety and redress, but without creating new monopolies of provision. In Beveridge systems especially, it will be necessary to regulate how providers combine public with private practice so as to safeguard the interests of publicly funded patients. Ensuring policy responsiveness and accountability necessitates making clinical practice more transparent and ensuring that the public bodies responsible for primary care actually obtain the necessary information (and use it). Regulations and contracts will thus need to become more rigid in these matters, but more flexible in others. They also need to be supplemented by more positive methods of coordinating services, for instance by developing primary health care networks.

References

Bergmark, A. (2000). Solidarity in Swedish welfare – Standing the test of time? *Health Care Analysis* **8**: 395–411.

Burenkova, S.P. (ed.) (1986). *Sbornik Shtatnykh normativov uchrezhdeniya zdravookhraneniye.* Moscow: Meditsina.

Cragg, D.K., McKinley, R.K., Roland, M.O. *et al.* (1997). Comparison of out of hours care provided by patients' own general practitioners and commercial deputising services: A randomised control trial, *British Medical Journal* **314** (18 January): 186–88, 190–193.

Daniildou, S. (2002). *Roemer's Law: Does it Apply in Greece?* Paper presented at the Strategic Issues in Healthcare Management conference, University of St. Andrews, 11 April.

Dowling, B. (2001). *GPs and Fundholding in the NHS.* Aldershot: Ashgate.

Enthoven, A. (1986). Managed competition in health care and the unfinished agenda, *Health Care Financing Review*, supplement: 105–117.

Flynn, R. (1992). *Structures of Control in Health Management.* London: Routledge.

Gené-Badia, J., Goicoechea, J., Sadana, R., *et al.* (1996). Primary health care in Southern European countries: an analysis of cross-national experiences, in Goicoechea, J. (ed.) *Primary Health Care Reforms.* World Health Organization Regional Office for Europe. Primary health care reforms, Fifth Forum on Primary Health Care Development in Southern Europe and its Relevance to Countries of Central and Eastern Europe. The Way Forward (Andorra la Vella 3–6 February 1993). Copenhagen: WHO Europe.

Geschwind, H.J. (1999). Health care in France: recent developments, *Health Care Analysis* **7**(4): 355–362.

Glennerster, H. and Matsanganis, M. (1992). *A Foothold for Fundholding.* London: King's Fund.

Grimshaw, J.M., Shirran, L., Thomas, R., *et al.* (2001). Changing provider behavior. An overview of systematic reviews of interventions, *Medical Care* **39**(8), supplement 2: 2–45.

Guarga, A., Gil, M., Pasarín, M., Manzanera, R., Armengol, R. and Sintes, J. (2000). Comparación de equipos de atención primaria de Barcelona según formulas de gestión [Comparison of primary care group management formulas in Barcelona], *Atención primaria* **26**: 600–606.

Houtepen, R. and Ter Meulen, R.T. (2000). New types of solidarity in the European welfare state, *Health Care Analysis* **8**(4): 329–40.

Lember, M. (1998). Implementing modern general practice in Estonia, *Acta Universitatis Tamperensis* **603**: 1–74 (Tampere: University of Tampere).

Markota, M., Švab, I., Sarazin-Klemenčič, K. and Albreht, T. (1999). Slovenian experience of health care reform, *Croatian Medical Journal* **40**(2): 190–194.

Martí, L.J. and Grenzner, V. (1999). Modelos de atención primaria en Cataluña [Primary care models in Catalonia], *Cuadernos de Gestión para el Profesional de Atención Primaria* **5**: 116–123.

Niskanen, W.A. (1973). *Bureaucracy: Servant or Master?* London: IEA.

Plassman, W. (1998). Vernetzte Praxen: Welche Modelle machen Sinn? [Which models make sense?] *Herz* **23**: 64–7.

Rhodes, R.A.W. (1997). *Understanding Governance.* Buckingham: Open University Press.

Robinson, R. and Steiner, A. (1997). *Managed Health Care.* Buckingham: Open University Press.

Rodriguez, M., Scheffler, R.M. and Agnew, J.D. (2000). Update on Spain's health care system: is it time for managed competition? *Health Policy* **51**: 109–131.

Saltman, R.B. and Von Otter, C. (1987). Re-vitalizing public health care systems: A proposal for public competition in Sweden, *Health Policy* **7**: 21–40.

Saltman, R. and Von Otter, C. (1992). *Planned Markets and Public Competition.* Buckingham: Open University Press.

Sheaff, R. (1998). What is "primary" about primary healthcare? *Health Care Analysis* **6**(4): 330–340.

Sheaff, R. (2001). *Responsive Healthcare*. Buckingham: Open University Press.

Sheaff, R. and Lloyd-Kendall, A. (2000). Principal-agent relationships in general practice: the first wave of English PMS contracts, *Journal of Health Services Research and Policy* **5**(3): 156–163.

Sheaff, R., Sibbald, B., Campbell, S. *et al.* (2004). Soft governance and attitudes to clinical quality in English general practice, *Journal of Health Services Research and Policy* **9**(3): 132–138.

Sibbald, B., Petchey, R., Gosden, T., Leese, B. and Williams, J. (2001). *Salaried GPs in PMS Pilots: Impact on Recruitment, Retention, Working Practices and Quality of Care.* Manchester University: NPCRDC (National Primary Care Research and Development Unit).

Švab, I., Markota, M. and Albreht, T. (2000). The reform of the Slovenian health care system: from capitalism to socialism and back, *Zdrav Vestn* **69**: 791–798.

Švab, I., Vatovec-Progar, I. and Vegnuti, M. (2001). Private practice in Slovenia after the health care reform, *European Journal of Public Health* **6**(4): 407–12.

Szecseny, J., Magdeburg, K., Kluthe, B. *et al.* (1999). *Ein Praxisnetz erpolgreich gestalten – Erfahrungen und Ergebnisse aus zwei Jahren "Ärztliche Qualitatsgerieinschaft Ried" [To build a medical practice network successfully – two years operating experience and results of the "Ärzliche Qualitatsgereinschaft Ried"]*. Göttingen: AQUA – Institut fur argewandte Qualitätsforderung und Forschung im Gezundheitswesen (AQUA-Materialen Band VII) (www.aqua-institute.de/projekte_reid.html, accessed 18 August 2005).

Theurl, E. (1999). Some aspects of the reform of health care systems in Austria, Germany and Switzerland, *Health Care Analysis* **7**: 331–54.

Urbanos-Garrida, R.M. (2001). Explaining inequality in the use of public health care services: Evidence from Spain, *Health Care Management Science* **4**: 143–57.

Villalbi, J.R., Guarga, A., Pasarín, M.I. *et al.* (1999). Evaluación del impacto de la reforma de atención primaria sobre la salud [Health impact evaluation of primary care reform], *Atención Primaria* **24**: 468–474.

Violan, C., Elias, A. and Ponsà, J.A. (2000). El modelo catalán de atención primaria [The Catalan primary care model], *Cuadernos de Gestión para el Profesional de Atención Primaria* **6**: 43–47.

Williamson, O.E. (1975). *Markets and Hierarchies*. New York: Free Press.

Zarkovic, G., Mielck, A., Jaohn, J. and Beckmann, M. (1994). Reform of the health care systems of the former socialist countries: problems, options, scenarios, *GSF-Bericht*, GSF (MEDIS) Institut für medizinische Informatik un Systemforschung **9**: 1–163.

chapter eight

Changing task profiles

Bonnie Sibbald, Miranda Laurant
and Anthony Scott

Introduction

Skill mix is a term used variously to refer to: the mix of skills or competencies possessed by an individual; the ratio of senior to junior grade staff within a single discipline; and the mix of different professions within a multi-professional team. General practice shows considerable variations both within and between countries in all three aspects.

General practitioner partnership size is growing in many European countries, with consequent role differentiation among doctors. Nurses are increasingly employed to undertake simple clinical tasks such as taking blood samples and syringing ears. In some countries, notably the United Kingdom, nurses have moved to more advanced roles in first contact care and the management of patients with stable chronic conditions such as asthma, diabetes and cardio-vascular disease. Primary care teams may be further extended through the addition of medical specialists, therapists, or social care workers, as in Finland. Other countries are moving in a similar direction. The United Kingdom, for example, saw a marked rise throughout the 1990s in the prevalence of general practices with a mental health counsellor and "outreach" clinics staffed by hospital-based medical specialists. The Netherlands has introduced policies to enhance collaboration among GPs, primary care psychologists and social workers (Buitink, 2000). The dominant trend is towards a more complex skill mix reflected by larger and multiprofessional teams, and increased role differentiation within teams.

Factors governing change

The factors driving such changes in skill mix are many and complex but may be distilled into the following broad groups:

- wider environment;
- policy;
- payment systems;
- professional regulation and training;
- professional attitudes.

The wider health care environment provides the impetus for change. Rising demand for care, health workforce shortages, and the rising costs of health care provision are powerful factors stimulating the revision of health professional roles. Policy-makers respond by articulating the benefits to be achieved through new ways of working. Payment systems and professional regulatory systems determine whether policy will be implemented in practice. The pace of change is moderated by the extent to which professionals need to be retrained and their attitudes to negotiating new roles.

Wider environment

Population ageing has placed increasing pressure on health care systems throughout the developed world, while, at the same time, medical advances have increased patient expectations. Rising demand and cost of care has led many governments to experiment with cost-cutting reforms. One strategy has been to make GPs the "gatekeepers" to expensive hospital care. A second has been to shift services, such as minor surgery and chronic disease management, from hospitals to general practice. A third strategy has been to shift work from high to low cost health professionals.

Shortages of particular professional groups may additionally accentuate the need to find alternative care providers. In the Netherlands, the United Kingdom, and elsewhere in the developed world, the effective size of the GP workforce has fallen owing to a shift towards part-time working accentuated by the increasing proportion of female doctors (Boerma, 2003). As nurses can be trained more quickly and cheaply than doctors, expanding the nurse numbers and extending their role into the medical arena is seen to be an effective strategy for dealing with medical shortages. Similar arguments may be applied to the use of unqualified health care assistants as substitutes for nurses when the latter group is in short supply.

Policy

Multiprofessional teamwork is a widely favoured strategy for addressing the problems created by rising demand and cost. Good teamwork is thought to enhance the quality of care, constrain costs, and make best use of limited human resources. Quality improvements are sought through the enhanced coordination of care delivery and by the opportunity for specialization within larger teams. Cost savings are sought through economies of scale and scope, and by shifting care from expensive to cheaper health professionals. Better use of scarce human resources is sought by breaking down disciplinary boundaries which prevent professionals being deployed where their skills can best be utilized. Countries such as Italy, the Netherlands and the United Kingdom have been persuaded by such arguments to promote the development of larger multiprofessional teams (Department of Health, 2000; Landau, 2001).

Payment systems

The successful implementation of policy requires payment systems which reward providers for making the desired changes. Where there is no financial advantage for providers, the pace of reform is likely to be negligible.

In the United Kingdom, successive reforms to payment systems for general practice have favoured growth in the size and complexity of general practice teams. The biggest impact was brought about by the 1990 GP contract which gave doctors a budget (i.e. fundholding) with which to purchase the services of community nurses and other health professionals. GPs encouraged primary care nurses to undertake extended roles, largely in the areas of health promotion and chronic disease management (Hirst et al., 1995). The larger practices were best able to find the money and other resources needed to extend nursing roles, and those practices which enhanced their skill mix in this way were best able to meet the new performance targets attracting payment (Baker and Klein, 1991). Thus economies of scale and scope have accelerated growth in team size and complexity. A similar situation prevails in other countries (Nijland et al., 1991; Commonwealth Department of Health and Family Services, 1996).

A closely related issue is whether payers can be billed for the services delivered by non-physicians within primary care teams. In the United States there is considerable variation in whether "mid-level" providers such as nurse practitioners and physician assistants are able to charge for their services or whether the costs must instead be subsumed as a physician overhead. Where mid-level practitioners are able to bill for their services, there is a higher prevalence of such providers (Sekcenski et al., 1994). A randomized controlled trial examining the effectiveness of substituting nurse practitioners for Ontario family doctors concluded that substitution was not cost effective for general practices because payment systems in the 1970s did not enable doctors to bill fully for the services provided by their nurses (Spitzer et al., 1974). In the Netherlands, a covenant was introduced in 1999 to enable GPs to employ nurse practitioners (Ministerie van Volksgezondheid, Welzijn en Sport et al., 1999); but numbers have grown slowly owing to disagreements about the level of reimbursement (De Vries, 2001).

Professional regulation and training

Governments and professional governing bodies specify the scope of practice for the majority of clinical professionals. These regulatory boundaries influence team composition by limiting the opportunities for extending the role of particular health professionals. The ability to substitute doctors for other health professions is constrained, for example, by the drug prescribing rights permitted to non-physicians. The solution is to change the statutes governing scope of practice. England, for example, has extended prescribing privileges to nurses (Department of Health, 2002).

Staff taking on new or extended roles need to be trained for this work. The speed with which skill mix changes can be realized therefore depends on the range of pre-existing skills within a particular health profession and the amount of additional training required to extend those skills. The bigger the gap between existing and desired skills, the bigger the investment needed to achieve change and the slower the pace of development. Central and eastern European countries wishing to move from a hospital-centred to a general practice-centred health care system have had to develop new systems for training doctors as experts in family medicine – a process which takes many years to implement (Gibbs et al., 1999). In contrast, the rapid introduction of nurse-led chronic disease clinics in British general practice was facilitated by the high level of skills already possessed by practice nurses and further supported by the provision of short courses. Even so, the pace of service development in the 1990s often out-stripped the ability of training programmes to equip nurses for these new roles (Atkin et al., 1994).

Professional attitudes

A more pervasive factor affecting the pace of skill mix change is the attitude of health professionals to renegotiating new boundaries between themselves and other disciplines. In the United Kingdom, GPs initially welcomed extended roles for practice nurses where these enabled doctors more easily to fulfil their con-tractual commitments. This, however, conflicted with nurses' views that modifi-cations to their role should be guided by concerns about developing nursing as an autonomous profession which is complementary, not subservient, to medi-cine and medical professionals (Atkin and Lunt, 1996). As the overlap between nurse and physician roles in primary care has grown, GPs have begun to voice concerns that nurses may erode the doctor's role (Wilson et al., 2002). In the Netherlands GPs have been reluctant to introduce nurse practitioners, preferring to use practice nurses who they have themselves trained. For their part, practice nurses are anxious that nurse practitioners might usurp their role (Vogel, 1998).

Mechanisms of change

Skill mix changes may be grouped according to the type of organizational process employed to bring about change.

Within general practice, skill mix change may be brought about through:

- enhancement – extending the role or skills of a professional group;
- substitution – exchanging one type of professional for another;
- delegation – shifting care provision from a senior/higher grade to a junior/ lower grade person within a profession;
- innovation – introducing a wholly new type of worker.

Skill mix may additionally be altered by changing the boundary between general practice and other patient services. This may include:

- transfer – moving the provision of a service to general practice from another health care sector, e.g. substituting general practice for hospital care;
- relocation – shifting the venue of a service to general practice from another health care sector without changing the provider, e.g. running a hospital clinic in a general practice setting;
- liaison – using medical/clinical specialists to educate and support primary care teams in their care of patients.

In practice skill mix change is often complex, involving interdependent changes in a number of these facets. For example, asthma care may be shifted from hospitals to general practice (transfer). In order to support this change, a practice nurse may acquire specialist skills in asthma care (enhancement) enabling her both to extend the range of service provision and reduce the demand on GPs (substitution). Routine tasks formerly undertaken by the nurse, such as patient reception, may in turn be delegated to a more junior nurse (delegation) or a non-clinical assistant (substitution). Hospital-based specialist nurses or doctors may continue to advise and support the primary care team in its management of patients (liaison).

Impact on care: role enhancement, substitution, delegation and innovation

The overarching purpose of skill mix change is to improve health care effectiveness and efficiency. The question is whether it does so in practice. The evidence base for change is generally not robust and has lagged behind service developments. Here we review the impact of role enhancement on health care effectiveness and efficiency, substitution, delegation, and innovation within general practice teams.

Enhancement

Health promotion is one of the principal areas in which nurses working in extended roles have increased the range of services available within primary care. In the majority of British general practices, nurses are responsible for carrying out well-patient health checks and providing lifestyle and other interventions in accordance with agreed treatment guidelines (Atkin *et al.*, 1994). Two large-scale randomized control trials have shown that the benefits to patients of such health promotion do not outweigh the costs (Family Heart Study Group, 1994; OXCHECK Study Group, 1995). The problem is not that nurses are unable to deliver high quality care, but that the treatments they have been asked to deliver are not sufficiently effective (Ebrahim and Davey Smith, 2002).

The situation is more promising in the area of chronic disease management. Here, there is good evidence from controlled trials that the treatments to be delivered by nurses are effective. Case studies show that the quality of care delivered by nurses can be high (Charlton *et al.*, 1991; Renders *et al.*, 2001). However, surveys of nurses working in extended roles suggest that, in reality, many nurses are insufficiently well trained (Atkin *et al.*, 1994). More importantly, there is a dearth of evidence about the overall cost-effectiveness of nurse-led clinics (Scott *et al.*, 1998).

GP roles may also undergo enhancement. Many GPs hold additional qualifications which enable them to provide more specialized services. In the United Kingdom, this is becoming more formal, as GPs with appropriate qualifications may apply to become "GPs with special interests" and so receive patient referrals from doctors in neighbouring practices (Department of Health and Royal College of General Practitioners, 2002). The intention is to expand specialist care in the community and thus reduce waiting times and improve access for patients. The key question which has yet to be answered is what activities will GPs give up to specialize? Does the new balance between generalist and specialist skills result in a more efficient use of resources and increased benefits to patients?

Substitution

The substitution of nurse practitioners for GPs is widespread in the United States and becoming so in the United Kingdom. In these countries nurses are able to undertake advanced training in diagnostics and therapeutics, which enables them to manage a wide range of patient problems without reference to a physician. Such nurses have increasingly been used to provide first contact care for patients presenting in general practice settings. Systematic reviews of the available evidence suggest that these nurses generally achieve as good health care outcomes as doctors and may have superior interpersonal skills (Horrocks *et al.*, 2002).

The substitution of nurses for doctors might be expected to reduce costs. However, research suggests this is not necessarily so. Compared with doctors, nurses have longer consultation times, order more tests and investigations and may recall patients at a higher rate, thus eliminating net savings in salary costs (Venning *et al.*, 2000; Horrocks *et al.*, 2002). From the perspective of the health care economy as a whole, it is generally cheaper to train nurses than it is to train doctors, but savings are again eroded because nurses tend to have lower lifetime workforce participation rates than doctors. The net saving to the state is therefore difficult to predict and may differ between countries and over time.

Delegation

Delegation from senior to junior staff within a profession is not a strong feature of general practice which has a "flat" organizational structure. Nevertheless, when GPs come together to practice in groups there tends to be some degree of differentiation among them in their clinical roles. Female doctors frequently have lead responsibility for managing women's health problems, if only because female patients show a marked preference for female doctors (Chambers and Campbell, 1996). The general assumption is that such role differentiation within teams can enhance the quality of care provision to patients (Landau, 2001).

Innovation

New professional designations are introduced by clinical governing bodies to acknowledge, and then regulate, health workers undertaking new roles which require radical revisions to their training, skills and competencies. The creation of "nurse practitioners", "clinical nurse specialists" and "advanced practice nurses" are good examples. As noted above, such skill mix change centres on revising the work undertaken by existing types of health professionals, so it is arguable whether this should be regarded as "innovation" or "enhancement".

In the United States a unique professional – the physician assistant – has been created. This position is used interchangeably with the nurse practitioner to enhance health service capacity in many areas, notably family practice. Physician assistants are drawn from a wide variety of backgrounds which may include nursing as well as other health or social care workers (Hooker and Cawley, 2003). Research suggests there is little to distinguish nurse practitioners from physician assistants in terms of the quality and scope of their care or cost-effectiveness when used as physician substitutes (Mittman *et al.*, 2002; Hooker and Cawley, 2003). This makes physician assistants an attractive option for expanding workforce capacity when there are shortages of medical and nursing staff (Department of Health, 2000; Hutchinson *et al.*, 2001).

Impact on care: service transfer, relocation, liaison

Skill mix may additionally be altered by changing the boundary between general practice and other patient services. Here we review evidence of the impact of service transfer, relocation and liaison on health care effectiveness and efficiency.

Transfer

Rising demand and cost of care have led many policy-makers to transfer services from hospitals to general practice in an effort to both enhance patient access and constrain expenditure. Good research into the cost-effectiveness of such service transfers is scarce (Scott, 1996; Godber *et al.*, 1997). In particular, evaluations generally fail to take into consideration the wider implications of transferring resources from secondary to primary care. If GP referrals to hospitals decline as a consequence of service transfer then the savings in hospital doctors' time may be used for other purposes. This would only be cost-effective, however, if the benefits of these new activities outweighed the benefits of the service transferred to general practice.

In the area of diabetes a systematic review of available research suggested that the quality of care attained by general practice was equivalent to that provided by hospitals, provided that general practice care was "structured", i.e. patient registers were established, patients were recalled for regular review, and reviews were conducted according to clinical guidelines (Griffin and Kinmonth, 2000). Other research has shown that patients attending general practice clinics report improved access to care and reduced personal costs, largely through reduced travel times. However, the direct costs of care provision may be higher in general practice because practices consume more resources than hospitals in providing the same standard of care (Diabetes Integrated Care Evaluation Team, 1994).

Minor surgery is another service where transfer from hospital to general practice is intended to enhance patient access and constrain cost. This was introduced in the 1990 GP contract in the United Kingdom in which doctors were given financial incentives to undertake minor surgery. Experience showed that the quality of care provided in general practice was initially poor due to inadequacies in GP training, problems in maintaining surgical skills given low patient volume, and inadequacies in the equipment and/or procedures used to sterilize surgical implements (Finn and Crook, 1998). The only controlled study, however, found no differences in health outcomes between hospital and general practice, with patients treated by GPs reporting higher satisfaction and shorter waiting times. The costs of general practice-based minor surgery were also found to be lower than those in hospitals (O'Cathain et al., 1992). Similar results were found for GPs providing diagnostic ultrasound (Wordsworth and Scott, 2002). However, costs were not necessarily "saved" as the failure to divest from hospital activity while increasing care provision in general practice led to an overall increase in service capacity and costs, rather than a transfer from secondary to primary care as was intended (Lowy et al., 1993).

Relocation

Adding specialists to general practice teams might be expected to enhance the quality of care and improve access for patients. These benefits have only partially been realized in England, which has experimented with bringing hospital physicians into general practice to provide "outreach" clinics. A systematic review of research comparing outreach clinics with conventional hospital "outpatient" clinics found that outreach clinics were not cost-effective (Powell, 2002). Although outreach clinics enhanced patient access and satisfaction, clinical outcomes were similar and the costs of service delivery were higher because of increased travel time for physicians and the smaller number of patients seen. Other expected benefits, such as the dissemination of knowledge and skills from hospital specialists to GPs, were not realized, as the two groups rarely interacted.

Mental health problems form a substantial part of the workload for primary care teams in most countries. The United Kingdom and United States have experimented with adding mental health counsellors to general practice teams as a way of both enhancing the quality of care provision and reducing the workload for GPs. A systematic review of available evidence suggests that counsellors are as effective as GPs in the management of patients with minor mental illness – more effective in the sense that patients treated by counsellors recovered more rapidly than did patients treated by GPs (Bower *et al.*, 2002). However, research evidence also shows that other anticipated benefits of attaching counsellors to general practice teams are not fully realized (Bower and Sibbald, 2000). Specifically, the claims that counsellors might generally reduce GP consultations, prescribing, and out-of-hours referrals for mental illness are not well substantiated. Moreover, the costs of care were not lower when counsellors were substituted for GPs in the management of minor mental illness (Bower *et al.*, 2002).

Liaison

Using specialists to advise and support GPs in their care of patients is another strategy for enhancing the skills of primary care professionals and hence the quality of care provision. A number of models for liaison exist. GPs and hospital specialists may enter into "shared care" agreements, which specify the division of responsibility between GP and specialist in the joint management of a patient which the GP would otherwise be unable or unwilling to manage alone. Shared care arrangements have been evaluated in the management of chronic disease (asthma and diabetes). The empirical evidence on cost-effectiveness is mixed. For asthma, shared care used fewer resources (Grampian Asthma Study of Integrated Care, 1994; Eastwood and Sheldon, 1996). There were few differences in clinical and health outcomes, but patients receiving shared care were less satisfied. In diabetes care, most studies reported that clinical and health outcomes were similar to conventional hospital-based care (Greenhalgh, 1994). However, the studies that included costs produced conflicting results. Overall, further evidence still needs to be gathered as results seem to be specific to each context and depend on good communication between specialists and generalists (Eastwood and Sheldon, 1996; Hampson *et al.*, 2002).

Alternatively, hospital specialists may undertake to improve general practice skills through the provision of education or guidance centred on the care of individual patients. A systematic review of available research into this model of working concluded that "educational outreach" appeared "a promising approach to modifying health professional behaviour" (Thomson O'Brien *et al.*, 2002). However, the evidence was not robust. Most evaluations of educational outreach focused solely on prescribing behaviour. Only one study measured a patient outcome and few examined cost-effectiveness. A systematic review of research into liaison working in mental health also concluded that there was a dearth of good evidence on which to base any firm conclusions (Bower and Sibbald, 2000).

Acceptability to patients

How do patients view skill mix change? The answer depends on how their experience of care relates to their expectations – and expectations may vary among individuals, between countries and over time. Campbell *et al.* (2000)

propose that the quality of care for individual patients is determined by *access* (Can patients get to health care?) and *effectiveness* (Is it any good when they get there?). Effectiveness is additionally subdivided into clinical care and inter-personal care in order to reflect the importance of both for patients. Clinical care is concerned with the technical quality of care delivery and asks whether service provision accords with the best available evidence. Interpersonal care is con-cerned with the quality of the relationship between patient and practitioner, which is integral to determining whether care is holistic, humane and person-centred.

Access

Patients report improved access to hospital specialists with shifted outpatient clinics (Griffin and Kinmonth, 2000) and outreach clinics (Powell, 2002) in general practice. Increased specialization among GPs and nurses within general practice teams, together with the addition of other types of health professionals, further increases the range of services and health care expertise available from local general practices.

There are, however, notable disadvantages. Larger team size is known to reduce personal continuity of care and patient satisfaction with access to care. This is because patients find it more difficult to get an appointment with their preferred doctor in larger general practices, although rapid access for acute prob-lems may be easier. Patients favour small practices and full-time GPs, which is at odds with the trend in many countries towards larger team size and part-time work (Schers *et al.*, 2002; Wensing *et al.*, 2002).

Effectiveness

Patient assessments of the technical quality of care are limited by patients' lack of medical knowledge, and hence rarely investigated. Professional assess-ments of the technical quality of care are reviewed above. Although there is a dearth of good evidence, the findings suggest that the quality of care provision is generally not diminished and may sometimes be enhanced through changes in skill mix.

Patients' assessments of the interpersonal quality of their care have been well researched in the area of doctor-nurse substitution, but not other types of skill mix. Systematic reviews suggest that patients rate the interpersonal skills of nurses more highly than those of doctors (Horrocks *et al.*, 2002). The reason for this is unclear and may relate to a number of factors, including nurses' gender, social status, and consultation length. The great majority of nurses are female and females are often regarded as more "caring" than males (Gray, 1982). Nurses tend to have a lower social status than doctors, making them more approach-able to patients. In addition, nurses tend to have longer consultation times than doctors and patient satisfaction tends to be higher with longer consultations (Freeman *et al.*, 2002). It may also be true that nurses, by virtue of their training, have better developed interpersonal skills than doctors.

High satisfaction with nurse care does not, however, mean that patients inevitably prefer nurses to doctors. Patient preferences in most studies are mixed, with some patients preferring to see nurses while others prefer to see doctors (Venning *et al.*, 2000; Horrocks *et al.*, 2002). Preference may be related to the nature of the presenting problem. Laurant and colleagues (2000) found that patients in the Netherlands preferred to see their GP for most aspects of care, although they did favour the nurse for health education/advice and regular health checks. Others have found that nurses are acceptable when the patient believes their problem to be "minor" or "routine" but that doctors are preferred when the problem is "serious" or "difficult" (Drury, 1988).

Impact on professionals

Changing the way people work can win commitment from those professionals for whom new opportunities are created (Leverment *et al.*, 1998). Individuals may feel better supported when they work in teams and good support can offset the stress of high job demand (Calnan *et al.*, 2000). However, restructuring jobs may create losers as well as winners. For example, GPs and practice nurses may view nurse practitioners as unwelcome competitors (Vogel, 1998).

In the context of staff shortages, the reorganization of work can be perceived as work intensification (Leverment *et al.*, 1998) and can lead to working longer, more unsocial hours on a routine basis in order to fulfil new remits (Adams *et al.*, 2000). The transfer of services from hospitals to general practice will increase the primary care workload unless it is adequately resourced (Pedersen and Leese, 1997; Scott and Wordsworth, 1998). Adding nurses to general practice teams may not have the intended effect of reducing GPs' workload (Laurant *et al.*, 2004).

Larger team size increases transaction costs because staff need to spend increasing amounts of time conferring with each other, decreasing the amount of time available for direct patient care (Barr, 1995). A critical point is reached when transaction costs outweigh the benefits of working in groups. Shared patient record systems, to which all team members may contribute and withdraw information, have been advocated as one means to reduce transaction costs (Rigby *et al.*, 1998). Electronic medical records are the preferred option as information can be transmitted quickly to whomever and wherever it is needed. However, developments in this area are often inhibited by the high initial cost of computerization, the incompatibility of computer systems used by different providers, and concerns about the confidentiality of patient information (Keeley, 2000).

Good teamwork is associated with better quality of care (Goni, 1999; Bower *et al.*, 2003) but can be difficult to achieve (West and Poulton, 1997). Redrawing the boundaries between professional groups and established job roles demands excellent human resource management skills. Consultation with key stakeholders, good support for middle managers, and continuity of leadership may help to promote success. Clarification of job descriptions and the introduction of induction programmes (Koperski, 1997) as well as specific training in teamwork (Long, 1996) may also prove helpful. Where steps are not taken actively to manage the transition to multiprofessional work or teamwork, tensions are likely to arise and the desired benefits may not be realized (Landau, 2001).

Conclusion

Skill mix both determines, and is determined by, organizational systems and the wider health care economy. The "correct" mix of tasks and skills that primary care professionals should undertake is therefore heavily dependent on context.

Skill mix change in one part of the system may impact on other parts with unforeseen consequences. When considering changes to task profiles and skill mix, policy-makers need to weigh up and make trade-offs between potential costs and benefits. For example, larger primary care teams may enhance efficiency through improvements in the quality of clinical care, economies of scale and scope, and reduced waiting times for patients. However, this may also increase transactions costs and reduce the continuity of care and patient satisfaction with the interpersonal quality of care.

Policy-makers who assume that task profiles and skill mix can be changed within existing budgets are ignoring the complex realities of health professionals' work. Changing existing tasks and skill mix is likely to increase costs in the short term because services are likely to expand into the new area and existing services will contract much more slowly, if at all. It will not be until the longer term, where new tasks and roles are embedded within new jobs and institutions and where training programmes are changed to reflect these new roles, that gains in efficiency will be forthcoming.

The change in tasks of primary care physicians, and the extent to which they are generalists or are able to specialize, also highlights important trade-offs. Primary care generalists are thought to be the linchpin of a cost-effective health care system as they act as gatekeepers to specialist care. However, where incentives exist for primary care physicians to specialize, what effect will this have on access, on the gatekeeper role, on continuity of care, and on similar hospital-based services? Some countries, with strong primary care-centred health care systems are encouraging their generalist GPs to become more specialized (e.g. the United Kingdom). Other countries, with a strong emphasis on specialist care, are seeking to replace specialists with generalist GPs (e.g. Estonia). This emphasizes the role of context in that these opposite reforms may be efficient in their respective countries.

Whether skill mix change is the most appropriate solution to a perceived problem will depend on the particular context in which change is contemplated. Policy-makers and managers need to carefully analyse the nature of the "problem" they wish to resolve and identify appropriate solutions, taking into consideration the potential wider and long-term effects on the system of care. Optimum team size and composition will vary from country to country and over time, depending on the available mix of health personnel, the labour economy and the priorities accorded to different aspects of the quality of care provision.

References

Adams, A., Lugsden, E., Chase, J., Arber, S. and Bond, S. (2000). Skill-mix changes and work intensification in nursing, *Work, Employment and Society*, **14**: 541–555.

Atkin, K. and Lunt, N. (1996). Negotiating the role of the practice nurse in general practice, *Journal of Advanced Nursing* **24**: 498–505.

Atkin, K., Hirst, M., Lunt, N. and Parker, G. (1994). The role and self-perceived training needs of nurses employed in general practice: observations from a national census of practice nurses in England and Wales, *Journal of Advanced Nursing* **20**: 46–52.

Baker, D. and Klein, R. (1991). Explaining outputs in primary health care: population and practice factors, *British Medical Journal* **303**: 225–229.

Barr, D.A. (1995). The effects of organizational structure on primary care outcomes under managed care, *Annals of Internal Medicine* **122**: 353–359.

Boerma, W.G.W. (2003). *Profiles of General Practice in Europe*. Utrecht: NIVEL.

Bower, P. and Sibbald, B. (2000). Systematic review of the effect of on-site mental health professionals on the clinical behaviour of general practitioners, *British Medical Journal* **320**: 614–617.

Bower, P., Rowland, N., Mellor Clark, J., Heywood, P., Godfrey, C. and Hardy, R. (2002). *Effectiveness and cost effectiveness of counselling in primary care*. Cochrane Review, in: *The Cochrane Library*, Issue 1, Oxford: Update Software.

Bower, P., Campbell, S., Bojke, C. and Sibbald, B. (2003). Team structure, team climate and the quality of care in primary care: an observational study, *Quality and Safety in Health Care* **12**: 273–279.

Buitink, J.A. (ed.) (2000). *De eerstlijns geestelijke gezondheidszorg in perspectief* [Primary mental health care in perspective]. Utrecht/Amsterdam: LHV, LVE, VOG.

Calnan, M., Wainwright, D., Forsythe, M. and Wall, B. (2000). *Health and Related Behaviour within General Practice in South Thames*. Canterbury: Centre for Health Services Studies, University of Kent.

Campbell, S.M., Roland, M. and Buetow, S. (2000). Defining quality of care, *Social Science and Medicine* **51**: 1611–25.

Chambers, R. and Campbell, I. (1996). Gender differences in general practitioners at work, *British Journal of General Practice* **46**: 291–93.

Charlton, I., Charlton, G., Broomfield, J. and Mullee, M.A. (1991). Audit of the effect of a nurse run asthma clinic on workload and patient morbidity in general practice, *British Journal of General Practice* **41**: 227–231.

Commonwealth Department of Health and Family Services (1996). The organisation of general practice, in *General Practice in Australia: 1996*: 107–134, Canberra: Commonwealth Department of Health and Family Services.

De Vries, I. (2001). Praktijkondersteuning (2) [Support in general practice (2)] *Medisch Contact* **56**: 1402.

Department of Health (2000). *The NHS Plan 2000*. London: Department of Health.

Department of Health (2002). *Extending Independent Nurse Prescribing within the NHS in England*. London: Department of Health.

Department of Health and Royal College of General Practitioners (2002). *Implementing a Scheme for General Practitioners with Special Interests*. London: Department of Health.

Diabetes Integrated Care Evaluation Team (1994). Integrated care for diabetes: clinical, psychosocial, and economic evaluation, *British Medical Journal* **308**: 1208–12.

Drury, M., Greenfield, S., Stillwell, B. and Hull, F.M. (1988). A nurse practitioner in general practice: patients perceptions and expectations, *Journal of the Royal College of General Practitioners* **38**: 503–505.

Eastwood, A.J. and Sheldon, T.A. (1996). Organisation of asthma care: what difference does it make? A systematic review of the literature, *Quality in Health Care* **5**: 134–143.

Ebrahim, S. and Davey Smith, B. (2002). Multiple risk factor interventions for primary prevention of coronary heart disease (Cochrane Review), in *The Cochrane Library*, Issue 3. Oxford: Update Software.

Family Heart Study Group (1994). Randomised controlled trial evaluation cardiovascular screening and intervention in general practice: principal results of British Family Heart Study, *British Medical Journal* **301**: 1028–1030.

Finn, L. and Crook, S. (1998). Minor surgery in general practice – setting the standards, *Journal of Public Health Medicine* **20**: 169–174.

Freeman, G.K., Horder, J.P., Howie, J.G.R. *et al.* (2002). Evolving general practice consultation in Britain: issues of length and context, *British Medical Journal* **324**: 880–882.

Gibbs, T., Mulka, O., Zaremba, E. and Lysenko, G. (1999). Ukranian general practitioners; the next steps, *European Journal of General Practice* **5**(1): 29–32.

Godber, E., Robinson, R. and Steiner, A. (1997). Economic evaluation and shifting the balance towards primary care: definitions, evidence and methodological issues, *Health Economics* **6**: 275–294.

Goni, S. (1999). An analysis of the effectiveness of Spanish primary health care teams, *Health Policy* **48**: 107–117.

Grampian Asthma Study of Integrated Care (GRASSIC) (1994). Integrated care for asthma: a clinical, social and economic evaluation, *British Medical Journal* **308**: 559–564.

Gray, J. (1982). The effect of a doctor's sex on the doctor-patient relationship, *Journal of the Royal College of General Practitioners* **32**: 167–169.

Greenhalgh, P.M. (1994). *Shared Care Diabetes: A Systematic Review*. Occasional Paper 67. London: Royal College of General Practitioners.

Griffin, S. and Kinmonth, A.L. (2000). *Diabetes Care: The Effectiveness of Systems for Routine Surveillance for People with Diabetes*. Cochrane Review, in *The Cochrane Library*, Issue 1, Oxford: Update Software.

Hampson, J.P., Roberts, R.I. and Morgan, D.A. (2002). Shared care: a review of the literature, *Family Practice* **19**: 53–56.

Hirst, M., Atkin, K. and Lunt, N. (1995). Variations in practice nursing: implications for family health services authorities, *Health and Social Care in the Community*, **3**: 83–97.

Hooker, R. and Cawley, J. (2003). *Physician Assistants in American Medicine*, 2nd edition. New York: Churchill Livingstone.

Horrocks, S., Anderson, E. and Salisbury, C. (2002). Systematic review of whether nurse practitioners working in primary care can provide equal care to doctors, *British Medical Journal* **324**: 819–823.

Hutchinson, L., Marks, T. and Pittilo, M. (2001). The physician assistant: would the US model meet the needs of the NHS? *British Medical Journal* **323**: 1244–1247.

Keeley, D. (2000). Information for health – hurry slowly, *British Journal of General Practice* **50**: 267–8.

Koperski, M. (1997). *Nurse Practitioners in General Practice: Strategies for Success*. London: Camden and Islington Health Authority/London Implementation Zone Educational Initiative.

Landau, J. (2001). *Organising General Practitioners into Group Practices. The City of and Province of Milan, Italy*. Milan: Bocconi University.

Laurant, M., Hermens, R., Braspenniing, J. and Grol, R. (2000). *De huisarts en de praktijkverpleegkundige in Midden Brabant. Eindrapport: Resultaten effect- en procesevaluatie*. [The general practitioner and the nurse practitioner in Midden Brabant. Final report: results from the effect and process evaluation] Nijmegen: WOK/UMCN.

Laurant, M.G.H., Hermens, R.P.M.G., Braspenning, J.C.C., Sibbald, B. and Grol, R.P.T.M. (2004). Impact of nurse practitioners on workload of general practitioners: randomised controlled trial, *British Medical Journal* **328**(7445): 927.

Leverment, Y., Ackers, P. and Preston, D. (1998). Professionals in the NHS – a case study of business process re-engineering, *New Technology, Work and Employment* **13**: 129–39.

Long, S. (1996). Primary health care team workshops, *Journal of Advanced Nursing* **23**: 935–41.

Lowy, A., Brazier, J., Fall, M., Thomas, K., Jones, N. and Williams, B.T. (1993). Minor surgery by general practitioners under the 1990 contract: effects on hospital workload, *British Medical Journal* **307**: 413–417.

Ministerie van Volksgezondheid, Welzijn en Sport, Zorgverzekeraars Nederland and Landelijke Huisartsen Vereniging (1999). *Convenant LHV, ZN en VWS inzake de versterking van de huisartsenzorga*l [Covenant LHV (National Association General Practitioners), ZN (National Insurance Company) and VWS (Department of Health) concerning reinforcement of primary health care]. Den Haag/Utrecht: 30 June 1999.

Mittman, D.E., Cawley, J.F. and Fenn, W.H. (2002). Physician assistants in the United States, *British Medical Journal* **325**: 485–487.

Nijland, A., Groenier, K., Meyboorm-de Jong, B., De Haan, J. and Van der Velden, J. (1991). Determinanten van het delegeren van (medisch-technische) taken aan de praktijkassistente [Determinants of substitution of (medical) tasks to a practice nurse], *Huisarts en Wetenschap* **34**: 484–487, 499.

O'Cathain, A., Brazier, J.E., Milner, P.C. and Fall, M. (1992). Cost-effectiveness of minor surgery in general practice: a prospective comparison with hospital practice, *British Journal of General Practice* **42**: 13–17.

OXCHECK Study Group (1995). Effectiveness of health checks conducted by nurses in primary care: final results of the OXCHECK study, *British Medical Journal* **310**: 1099–1104.

Pedersen, L.L. and Leese, B. (1997). What will a primary care led NHS mean for GP workload? The problem of the lack of an evidence base, *British Medical Journal* **314**: 1337–1341.

Powell, J. (2002). Systematic review of outreach clinics in primary care in the UK, *Journal of Health Services Research and Policy* **17**: 177–183.

Renders, C.M., Valk, G.D., Griffin, S.J., Wagner, E.H., Eijk, J.T. and Assendelft, W.J.J. (2001). Interventions to improve the management of diabetes in primary care, outpatient, and community settings, *Diabetes Care* **24**: 1821–1833.

Rigby, M., Roberts, R., Williams, J. *et al.* (1998). Integrated record keeping as an essential aspect of a primary care led health service, *British Medical Journal* **317**: 579–582.

Schers, H., Webster, S., Van den Hoogen, H., Avery, A., Grol, R. and Van den Bosch, W. (2002). Continuity of care in general practice: a survey of patients' views, *British Journal of General Practice* **52**: 459–462.

Scott, A. (1996). Primary or secondary care? What can economics contribute to evaluation at the interface? *Journal of Public Health Medicine* **18**: 19–26.

Scott, A. and Wordsworth, S. (1998). The effects of shifts in the balance of care on general practice workload, *Family Practice* **16**: 12–17.

Scott, A., Currie, N. and Donaldson, C. (1998). Evaluating innovation in general practice: a pragmatic framework using programme budgeting and marginal analysis, *Family Practice* **15**: 216–22.

Sekcenski, E., Sansom, S., Bazell, C., Salmon, M. and Mullan, F. (1994). State practice environments and the supply of physician assistants, nurse practitioners, and certified nurse-midwives, *New England Journal of Medicine* **331**: 1266–1271.

Spitzer, W.O., Sackett, D.L., Sibley, J.C. *et al.* (1974). The Burlington randomized trial of the nurse practitioner, *New England Journal of Medicine* **290**: 251–256.

Thomson O'Brien, M.A., Oxman, A.D., *et al.* (2002). Educational outreach visits: effects on professional practice and health care outcomes. Cochrane Review, in *The Cochrane Library*, Issue 3. Oxford: Update Software.

Venning, P., Drurie, A., Roland, M., Roberts, C. and Leese, B. (2000). Randomised controlled trial comparing cost effectiveness of general practitioners and nurse practitioners in primary care, *British Medical Journal* **320**: 1048–53.

Vogel, J. (1998). NVDA wil meer overleg over komst praktijkverpleegkundige. [NVDA wants to confer about the entry of nurse practitioners], *De huisarts in Nederland* **12**: 13–15.

Wensing, M., Vedsted, P., Kersnik, J. *et al.* (2002). Patient satisfaction with availability of general practice: an international comparison, *International Journal for Quality in Health Care* **14**: 111–18.

West, M.A. and Poulton, B.C. (1997). A failure of function: teamwork in primary health care, *Journal of Interprofessional* **11**: 205–216.

Wilson, A., Pearson D. and Hassey, A. (2002). Barriers to developing the nurse practitioner role in primary care – the GP perspective, *Family Practice* **19**: 641–46.

Wordsworth, S. and Scott, A. (2002). Ultrasound scanning by general practitioners: is it worthwhile? *Journal of Public Health Medicine* **24**: 89–94.

chapter **nine**

Changing professional roles in primary care education

Jan Heyrman, Margus Lember,
Valentin Rusovich and Anna Dixon

General practice/family medicine has a central role in health care, helping to keep the focus on the needs of the patient. Both policy experts (Starfield, 1998) and official organizations (WONCA/WHO, 2002), support this view, believing that the balance in health care should shift from supply-driven development to needs and community-driven priority setting. Given that the main challenge for health care is to find and maintain an appropriate balance between quality, equity and cost-effectiveness, it is natural that primary care (PC) is expected to make a central contribution (Boelen, 1999).

Teaching, training and reaccreditation are important instruments in the adaptation of primary care professionals to these new challenges. This chapter evaluates the evolution and impact of professional training in strengthening the role of PC within European health care systems. Education can be seen as the cornerstone of professional self-regulation. We also analyse the role of professional organizations in the development of a new role for PC. To place PC in the driver's seat of the health care system requires professional leadership and support. Professional associations and colleges can play a key role in the critical field of education and training, and more generally, in strengthening the political and professional position of PC.

Main actors and stages in PC education

In 1999, EURACT (European Academy of Teachers in General Practice, the educational board of WONCA-Europe) collected information on the impact of the central players, governments, medical professionals and scientific groups and universities on the different educational stages of the GP profession (EURACT, 1999). The enquiry covered basic medical education, internship, specific training and continuous medical education (CME) in 27 European countries. This chapter maps the power positions of different actors at different stages of the process of medical education and training based on the evidence generated by EURACT and other sources.

Professional organizations

The history and influence of the professional bodies of GPs is not comparable between western and eastern Europe. In some countries of the newly independent states (NIS) of the former USSR they have existed for less than three–five years, in the Baltic countries they were established more than 10 years ago, and in some other countries of central and eastern Europe even longer ago. In most of western Europe, PC professional associations were created from the 1960s onwards. Very little comparative evidence on professional associations has been gathered across Europe to date.

In most European countries professional organizations are the main governing body in continuous medical education and lifelong learning. Undergraduate education is mainly in the hands of universities, but professional organizations also have some influence in the content as well as in the recruitment for internship positions. In between is the crucial period of specialty training, which in four European countries (including Norway and the United Kingdom) is the responsibility of the profession, but in most countries (10, including Belgium, Finland and the Netherlands) this training is organized by academic university departments. In Denmark the state or municipalities have this responsibility. To complete the picture of diversity, in some central, eastern and southern European countries, specialty training in general practice is still in the 'start-up' phase and professional bodies of GPs are weak or absent.

Universities and ministries of education

Basic medical education in Europe is largely the responsibility of ministries and departments of education, with universities providing most core medical training (see Table 9.1). Progressive at the scientific level but rather conservative at the level of health policy, they are generally characterized by a strong dominance of specialist-centred care. Universities and medical schools are also the most important provider of postgraduate specialty training in 10 countries, while independent postgraduate schools are responsible for this in four countries.

Ministries of health

Health ministries are the authority for PC specialist training in most European countries. In more than half of Europe they control CME as well. In all countries where a formal recertification procedure has been established, the health ministries and medical colleges are responsible. In several European countries, the health ministry is also involved in human resource planning in health care.

Table 9.1 The role of government, professionals and universities in PC education

	Specialist training, ST: PC setting	ST: Hospital setting	CME accreditation	CME providers
Belgium	GP	GP	G	U + P + S + PI
Bosnia and Herzegovina	U	H	G	U
Croatia	U	U + H + GP	G	Many different
Czech Republic	PS	H	G	n.a.
Denmark	S	H + GP	P	Many different
Estonia	U	H	n.a.	U
Finland	U	U	G	U + S + G + PI
France	U	U + H	G	S
Germany	P	P	G	P + S + H
Greece	GP	H	G	P + PI
Hungary	U	U + H	G	U
Ireland	GP	S	G	S
Israel	U	H	n.a.	U + HI
Italy	PS	PS	G	P + PI
Lithuania	U	U	G	U
the Netherlands	GP	GP	G	P + S
Norway	P	H	G	P
Poland	PS	H + GP	n.a.	Many different
Portugal	GP	H	G	Many different
Romania	GP	S	PS	GP
Slovakia	GP	PS	G	PS
Slovenia	U	H	n.a.	U + P + PI
Spain	GP	GP	G	S + U + PI
Sweden	G	G	G	G
Switzerland	P	H	G	P + S + H
Turkey	n.a.	U + H	n.a.	P
United Kingdom	GP	S	G	Many different

Source: EURACT (1999).
* G=Governement (national or county level), P=Professional groups, S=Scientific societies (including colleges and GP educational structures), U=Universities as a faculty, GP=GP departments, PS=Postgraduate schools, HI = Health Insurance, PI=Pharmaceutical Industry, n.a.= not available

The number of health professionals and medical doctors by subspecialties is a critical variable in allocating resources and controlling expenditure (see Table 9.2). The number of GPs versus specialists is also important in tracking shifts in the balance of health care towards PC professions.

Private training bodies and the pharmaceutical industry

In the field of PC specialist training, some additional providers of education, such as independent GPs or international support programmes were present.

Table 9.2 Human resources in PC across Europe

	Human resources in PC practices (% of total active GPs)			PC over total medical graduates	
	Trained GP	Inservice training GP	Nontrained GP	Total annual medical graduates	GP annual graduates (% of total)
Albania	3	32	65	175	10
Austria	65	34	1	1100	64
Belgium	100	0	0	700	43
Bosnia and Herzegovina	1	n.a.	99	120	25
Croatia	26	n.a.	74	400	3
Czech Republic	99	0	1	1000	7
Denmark	100	0	0	600	30
Estonia	80	n.a.	20	85	21
Finland	50	0	50	500	18
France	40	0	60	4000	50
Germany	72	0	28	10000	18
Greece	100	0	0	2000	10
Hungary	96	0	4	1000	10
Ireland	45	0	55	n.a.	(75 GPs)
Israel	33	0	67	800	25
Italy	100	n.a.	0	2000	18
Lithuania	71	29	0	650	31
the Netherlands	85	0	15	1500	24
Norway	51	0	49	550	36
Poland	29	0	71	2500	40
Portugal	100	n.a.	0	1100	36
Romania	16	n.a.	84	2500	16
Slovakia	100	0	0	700	11
Slovenia	60	n.a.	40	150	27
Spain	50	0	50	5000	38
Sweden	80	0	20	600	17
Switzerland	98	0	2	600	n.a.
Turkey	2	0	98	4500	3
United Kingdom	75	0	25	4500	44

Note: n.a. = not available. When 'In service training GP' data were not available, they are supposed to be included in "Trained GP" data.
Source: EURACT (2004).

The CME landscape proved the most diverse (EURACT, 1999), as institutions ranging from universities to independent private institutions were involved in professional education. In many countries the major role of the pharmaceutical industry also was notable.

Four models of governance in Europe

Four models of GP education have been proposed based on EURACT (1999) data. However, no country exactly fits the ideal models and some do not fit any model very well.

Regulation-dominated model

This model, existing predominantly in Austria, Germany and some CEE countries (Croatia, Slovenia), is characterized by strong and independent universities and/or an important role for medical associations. Strong regulations regarding basic education and CME are also present. Medical associations also have a central role in postgraduate medical education.

Profession-dominated model

This model, founded in Ireland and the United Kingdom, is characterized by a strong role for GP professional organizations, which are independent and have developed their own pedagogical method. The role of the universities is smaller and departments of general practice usually have strong links with professional organizations. The dominant player in general practice education is the professional organization.

Science-dominated model

The science dominated model exists in the Netherlands and some other northern European countries (e.g. Estonia, Finland). It is characterized by the predominant role of universities, which are responsible for most undergraduate and much postgraduate instruction.

Liberal model

This model exists in Belgium, France, Greece and Italy. It is characterized by independent institutions at the postgraduate level that have links with professional organizations. There is a wealth of different professional and training organizations, which sometimes compete among themselves.

The role of international organizations

The two key international organizations active in European health care are the European Office of the World Health Organization (WHO-Europe), and the European Union (EU). It is worth mentioning the important role given to PC in the Health for All strategy designed by WHO-Europe in 1983, as well as the critical landmark of 1986, when an EU directive was approved recommending the establishment of PC as a specialty in Europe. In 1995, UEMO (*Union européen des médecins omnipraticiens*), the GPs trade union, succeeded in making the EU accept compulsory specialty training for a minimum of two years, which will be expanded to three years in 2006 (UEMO, 1995). In the early 1990s, the WHO started the programme 'Changing Medical Education', which aimed at shifting from 'problem-based' to 'community-based' education. In 1998 it obtained approval from the EU for a document called 'Framework for general practice/ family medicine in Europe' presenting its clear support to PC education development and pointing out the necessary structural conditions and improvements required to realize this goal (WHO, 1998).

Other prominent international organizations active in the European PC sector are the PC professional association WONCA (World Organization of National Colleges and Academies) and its branch WONCA Europe. In June 2002 WONCA developed a condensed document which defined the core competencies of GPs and their role in the health care system. Impressively, WONCA also succeeded in having all European countries adopt it (WONCA Europe, 2002). In 2004 EURACT proposed its first version of 'The Educational Agenda of GP/FM', in which six core competencies were translated into learning objectives; consequences for educational methods, assessment methods were outlined; and a time frame for integration into the educational curriculum was set (Heyrman, 2004).

European support programmes for the development of PC education in CEE and NIS countries are also of vital importance. In the 1990s there were several initiatives involving the World Bank, EU Phare, the WHO, USAID and the Open Society Institute. These provided a wide range of support policies. Their most remarkable achievement has been their capacity-building investment in training people to be leaders of PC education in these countries.

The development of education for family medicine/general practice in Europe

Historically in Europe, two basic models of FM/GP were in use. In France and Great Britain the education of doctors in the nineteenth century was concentrated in hospitals, while in Germany and Scandinavia it was provided in universities (Vuori, 1979; Ko Ko, 1994). Priorities were set by hospitals and science, not by patients or PC. In the United States Abraham Flexner prepared an optimal medical curriculum with a sizeable basic sciences component in 1910.

After the Second World War a massive fragmentation of medical practice into different specialties began. The family doctor remained nonspecialized. PC professionals slowly started to create a speciality as an innovative type of supra-specialist (Starfield, 1998). The first chair of general practice in Europe was created in the United Kingdom in Edinburgh in 1963, followed in 1966 by the Netherlands, and in 1968 by Belgium. These academics created the Leeuwenhorst group, which defined a very wide task profile for PC, ranging from prevention to terminal care. 'Co-operation with other colleagues, medical and non-medical' and 'a professional responsibility towards the community' were mentioned as crucial in their statement on *The General Practitioner in Europe*, which became a central element in many curricula of general practice/ family medicine throughout Europe (Leeuwenhorst Group, 1974; New Leeuwenhorst Group, 1981). By the early 1990s, most PC doctors were already specialists in many western European countries (Boerma and Fleming, 1998), and PC was granted a prominent role within the health care systems in several tax-funded countries as well as the Netherlands.

Developments in eastern and central Europe, with Semashko-type systems, initially went in the opposite direction, with PC having an increasingly subordinate role to subspecialist care. In the late 1980s/early 1990s in most CEE countries it became obvious that specialization had exhausted its limits. More efficient use of resources in the health care system in a time of economic decline was the argument used by international organizations and national politicians to promote general practice (Schepin *et al.*, 1996). At the universities, departments of family medicine were created and selected professionals were sent to western Europe to become PC instructors (Lember, 1996, 2002; Kuznethova *et al.*, 2000).

The role of PC in undergraduate education

General practice/family medicine has a central place in undergraduate medical teaching. As this focus seeks to introduce the community dimension into basic medical education, a first challenge is to obtain an appropriate place as a department in the faculty structure. An enquiry carried out by EURACT in 1997 covered 297 medical faculties, in 26 European countries. There was undergraduate teaching of family medicine in all countries, but only in 191 faculties. General practice was taught at every medical school in 18 out of the 26 countries. The extent and methods of education were quite different. In some countries general practice was an obligatory subject, in others it was not. The bulk of undergraduate teaching in general practice was done in clinical attachments to GPs in the community in most medical schools. Final examinations had been introduced in 14 countries. New, active methods of instruction for the medical undergraduate curriculum have also been developed.

Some documents elaborate on the nature of the GP contribution to basic medical education. The Leeuwenhorst group issued the pioneering statement on 'the contribution of the General Practitioner to undergraduate Medical Education' which stressed the integral, person-centred (versus illness or organ-centred) focus of PC (Leeuwenhorst Group, 1977), and its key role within health care as a profession. From then on, a debate opened on the specific skills or competencies which should be taught by PC undergraduate departments. A publication by Dundee University summarizes the results of this debate in a model for the specification of learning outcomes (Harden *et al.*, 1999), which can be applied to GPs:

- clinical care focus on common, most prevalent diseases;
- teaching communication skills: the key to the patient-doctor relationship;

- teaching organizational skills: GPs are resource managers for their patients;
- teaching professional values: GPs best placed to discuss value choices;
- teaching professional growth: surveying community and patient needs.

An interesting Dutch document (Grundmeijer and Rutten, 1996) defines the possible contribution of PC in the '180 educational endpoints and the 250 problem areas of basic medical education'. It classifies educational areas in three groups:

- content that is best taught by the PC department;
- content that is best taught where PC teaching is by specialist departments;
- content that does not pertain to PC.

Specialist training in general practice/family medicine

A recent overview (EURACT, 2004) shows that European regulations clearly are effective: as of the study's date (2004), in all of the 15 EU Member States and also in at least 13 of the EU accession and pre-accession countries, postgraduate specialist training for general practice/family medicine has been introduced for an average of three years, which is the recommended minimum time frame in Europe since February 2001 (see Table 9.3). The balance between training in a GP setting versus a hospital setting is different in each country. It ranges from three years in a GP setting in Bosnia and Herzegovina to four and a half out of five specialty years in a hospital setting in Switzerland. Almost 40,000 specialist GPs are trained and 10,000 finish the specialty training each year. In two thirds of these countries, there is a local handbook on family medicine available.

The development of PC specialists in Europe has not been an easy task. The design of academic education programmes had to be paralleled by the building of 'in-service training programmes' which would cater to junior doctors as well as enhance the skills of non-trained GPs active in the field. In northern Europe this process started during the 1970s, in southern Europe during the 1980s, and in central and eastern Europe from the 1990s onwards (see Box 9.1).

These developments are surely positive steps in the right direction, but unfortunately often represent more model practices than common examples in many European countries. The quality and the content of the training varies a great deal across Europe. In several EU countries, especially in ex-Semashko countries, there are not enough teaching practices for young GPs and education is still to a great extent hospital-based, with many educational topics delegated to the specialist university departments (Shabrov *et al.*, 2001). In a period of great change these kinds of problems are inevitable. The task of the first chairs in general practice in the region has been to gain acceptance to implement changes. Some authors reported educational changes and relevant research in these countries to be of great importance and interest (Barr and Schmid, 1996). In a next generation, academic GPs could be recruited from the first generation of well-trained GPs.

Table 9.3 Specialty training in European countries: duration (years) by setting

	Duration	GP setting	Hospital setting	Public Health	Content explicit
Albania	2	0.2	1.6	0.2	N
Austria	3	0.5	2.5	0	N
Belgium	3(1+2)	2.5	0.5	0	N
Bosnia and Herzegovina	3	3	0	0	Y
Croatia	3	1	1.2	0.6	Y
Czech Republic	3	0.5	1.3	0	N
Denmark	3.5	1	2.5	0	N
Estonia	3	1.5	1.5	2 weeks	Y
Finland	6	4	2	0	Y
France	3	0.5	2.5	0	Y
Germany	5	2	3	0	Y
Greece	4	0.9	3.1	0	N
Hungary	5	3.5	1	0.5	Y
Ireland	3	1	2	0	Y
Israel	4	2	2	0	Y
Italy	2	0.5	1.5	0.5	N
Lithuania	3	0.5	2.5	0	Y
the Netherlands	3	2	0.8	0	Y
Norway	5	4	1	0.5	Y
Poland	4	2	2	0	N
Portugal	3	2	1	0	N
Romania	3	1.25	1.66	0.09	N
Russian Federation	2	0.2	1.8	60 hours	
Slovakia	3	0.5	2.5	0	Y
Slovenia	4	2	2	0	Y
Spain	3	1.5	1.5	seminars	N
Sweden	5	3	2	0	Y
Switzerland	5	0.5	4.5	0	N
Turkey	3	0	3	0	N
United Kingdom	3	1	2	0	Y

Source: EURACT (2004).

Box 9.1 Retraining in CCEE

With the help of international projects, in different CEE regions the complex integrated process of retraining and structural innovation in PC could be accelerated. For example, in Belarus in 1998–2001, a network of better equipped PC practices was created in the Minsk region supported by the Dutch-Belarussian MATRA project. Model practices were adopted in which young GPs could 'learn by doing' under the supervision of more skilled GPs (Rusovich *et al.*, 2000).

Accreditation and reaccreditation

The combination of declining public trust in the professions and rapid advances in medical practice has led to a demand for doctors to be recertificated. Society has the right to ask for guarantees. Governments in most countries have introduced or are considering implementation of a system with different but parallel names like revalidation, reregistration, relicensing or recertification for doctors. Introducing recertification is not only a technical issue concerned with how to recertify, how often and by whom, but it is also a political issue concerned with the relationship between individual professionals, professional bodies, health care providers and purchasers, regulatory authorities, the state and the public. The traditional assessment tools of recertification are credits assessment, peer review and external inspection or audit. An alternative would be examination, a simpler process to administer but with less external validity. An examination-based approach has been criticized for creating assessment-driven learning (Jolly et al., 2001). In the United States, where mandatory recertification was implemented as early as 1969 by the American Board of Family Practice, difficulties have been reported with devising fair assessment measures based on patient outcomes (Norcini, 1999). It seems there is no proven method for demonstrating physician competence and professionalism (Smith, 2000).

The table below provides an overview of the recertification of GPs in Europe (Table 9.4). It identifies the objectives of recertification, considers the most appropriate methods and finally reflects on the political issues associated with the implementation of recertification. It also deals with newer arrangements such as Continuous Professional Development Planning, which uses newer assessment tools like the personal learning agenda and the individual portfolio.

Objectives, methods and responsible bodies

Recertification firstly aims to ensure that doctors are in a fit state of physical and mental health to practice without endangering their patients. This issue is pertinent in light of studies that highlight problems of alcoholism, drug addiction and stress among health professionals (Firth-Cozens and Greenhalgh, 1997; Weir, 2000; Gossop et al., 2001). Also, when doctors are allowed to practice beyond retirement age, it is important to ensure they are still capable of practicing medicine. Second, recertification aims to ensure doctors are 'up-to-date'. In the context of rapid developments in medical technology, recertification is also concerned with ensuring that doctors' practice is based on state-of-the-art medical knowledge. Third, recertification places increasing emphasis on quality assurance and health care standards. One of the goals is to identify at an early stage those doctors who are underperforming. Other objectives of recertification might be to ensure that doctors abide by high ethical standards, improve patient care and enhance continuing professional development (Buckley, 1999). There may also be unexpressed objectives, for example, the profession may introduce recertification in an attempt to maintain its position as well as control over entry.

Table 9.4 Regulation of recertification in Europe

	Procedure developed	Frequency/ years	Responsible body *	Credit system	Peer group evaluation	Examination
Belgium	Y	3	G+P+U	Y	Y	N
Croatia	Y	6	P	Y	Y	N
Czech Republic	Y	5	P	Y	N	N
Estonia	Y	5	G+P	Y	N	N
Hungary	Y	5	U	Y	Y	N
Ireland	N			Y	N	N
Israel	N		P	Y	N	N
Italy	Y	5	G	Y	N	N
Lithuania	Y	5	G	Y	N	N
the Netherlands	Y	5	P	Y	Y	N
Norway	Y	5	G	Y	Y	N
Poland	N			Y	N	N
Romania	Y	5	S	Y	N	N
Slovakia	Y	5	P	Y	N	N
Slovenia	Y	7	P	Y	N	Y
Spain	N			Y	N	N
Switzerland	N			Y	N	N
Turkey	N			Y	N	N
United Kingdom	Y	5	P	Y	Y	N

*Government (G), Professional (P), scientific societies (S) or Universities (U).
Source: EURACT (2004).

There are different responsibilities associated with the recertification process: setting standards, accrediting CME activities, providing CME activities, inspection and peer review, remedial training, and recertification. For each of these a clear division of responsibility needs to be made to ensure coordination and mutual recognition.

The frequency of recertification depends on a number of factors: whether measures are in place to identify poor practice, whether a doctor has previously failed recertification, the rapidity of developments in a particular field, whether resources are available for recertification, and whether practice is supported by other quality initiatives (e.g. compulsory CME, practice guidelines, prescription information). Some of these factors may justify differential frequency of recertification for different specialties, for doctors at different stages in their careers and for different doctors depending on their background. In practice, in order to ensure consistency across the profession, it is likely that the frequency of recertification will be standardized. However, consideration should be given to the idea of an earlier recall for doctors whose previous appraisal had identified weaknesses in their practice. Standards being developed for mutual recognition of CME activity in Europe could also have a bearing on the frequency of recertification (see below).

Which bodies will be responsible for overseeing the recertification process, setting the standards and inspecting and enforcing them? CME may be provided by universities, hospitals, specialist societies or local health authorities.

Experiences in Greece and Spain suggest that accreditation of these courses and activities should be carried out by a single body (UEMS European Advisory Committee on CME, 2001). Scrivens (2002) makes the distinction between voluntary professional regulation and mandatory state regulation. State regulations usually set minimum standards, whereas professional bodies set high standards to which doctors must aspire. Most countries have a central body responsible for the licensure of all doctors as well as specialist societies which are responsible for the education and training in particular specialist fields. Recertification in most countries will be the responsibility of the licensing body such as the General Medical Council in the United Kingdom, whereas the professional bodies set the standards (e.g. approving CME courses). However, owing to rapid expansion of the number of CME courses, their capacity to ensure that all activities are of high quality is limited. Other conflicts of interest may arise when CME is organized by bodies with commercial interests in PC (such as the pharmaceutical or medical technologies industry).

In the United Kingdom (Box 9.2), purchasing bodies set rules and regulations regarding the practice of doctors under contract and ask for involvement in the recertification procedure. The choice of whether recertification applies to all doctors on the register or only doctors under contract with public insurance has not been totally clarified. In Germany and Switzerland, participation in CME is essential for establishing a contractual relationship with the insurance funds. However, if recertification aims to protect the interests of patients, it should extend to doctors practicing in the private sector. In fee-for-service countries such as Belgium and France, payments differ according to accreditation. Inspections in the Netherlands are carried out by three peers – one who has recently been inspected, one who is due to be inspected and a chairperson (Swinkels, 1999).

Box 9.2   Recertification in the United Kingdom

The proposals in the United Kingdom give the responsibility to the royal colleges and specialist societies for providing guidance on what type of evidence is needed for recertification (Du Boulay, 2000). These organizations are also expected to provide support and retraining for those doctors who fail to meet the standards. GMC has set out the principles of recertification (General Medical Council, 2001). The Royal College of General Practitioners has already published guidelines for good practice which elaborate on these and identify the standards expected of a GP (Royal College of General Practitioners, 2002). In order to evaluate all doctors on a regular basis suitable appraisers need to be selected and trained. These are likely to be peers, thus there are implications of diverting trained personnel away from front-line care. Lay assessors can be used to assess dimensions of care other than technical competency (Southgate and Pringle, 1999) however, doctors are likely to be extremely reluctant to accept appraisal from anyone other than peers.

In the countries of the former Soviet Union a system of five mandatory annual attestations (certification) existed for all physicians. Participating in CME, professional experience, and speciality development were taken into account. All doctors were divided into three qualifying groups and there were small salary differences according to their qualification.

Since the establishment of the European Accreditation Council for Continuing Medical Education (EUACCME) in 2000, mutual recognition of CME for the different specialties (but not for GPs) is possible through the transfer of CME credits between European countries, between different specialties, between the European and North American credit systems and in the case of migration of a specialist within Europe (UEMS European Advisory Committee on CME, 2001).

If free movement of professionals is to be fully realized, then standardized procedures for recertification have to be agreed upon at the EU level. Even if standards are devolved to national organizations, some basic principles and technical aspects would need to be agreed beforehand. Therefore, before CME and recertification are implemented across the EU, a better understanding of the possible consequences is necessary. Evaluation of the impact of recertification (including the comparative advantage of different methods and frequencies of application) would be beneficial in order to see whether the benefits (measured in terms of improved quality of PC) are greater than the costs. To date, there is no specific general practice/family medicine move to mutual recognition of CME activities in a European context.

Political aspects

Public protection from incompetent practice has traditionally been delegated to the profession through the establishment of standards of training, qualifications and codes of practice. The decline in public trust and deference has meant that such structures are no longer deemed to be adequate. Self-regulation in general has been called into question. In light of this, both governments and professional bodies have been acting to ensure public confidence is maintained. Here, the political aspects of the implementation of recertification are briefly considered.

(a) Legislation. If the state is forced to act through legislation, it may be to enhance the powers and scope of statutory self-regulatory bodies or to establish independent bodies to monitor and enforce performance. The introduction of recertification might require amendments to core legislation concerning the licensure of medical doctors and would need the support of the national medical association.

(b) Self-regulation. In order to pre-empt state action, professional bodies in several countries established their own professional development programmes. Much of the political controversy around recertification is within the profession between different specialties vying to control the standards by which they will be judged. PC doctors need to establish their own standards given the generalist nature of PC practice compared to hospital-based specialist practice.

(c) Cost of recertification. In order to ensure that recertification is implemented, the financial responsibility for the cost of recertification must be identified and

budgeted. Direct costs of training and administration are perhaps more obvious but other economic costs, such as time treating patients or recording activities, may have a negative impact on service delivery. A supportive environment for the recertification process will require that managers and health care providers build 'protected time for education, training and appraisals' into service contracts and day-to-day practice. In addition, health care purchasers will have to recognize the need to invest in education in order to ensure that practice is of the highest standard (Du Boulay, 2000). Also the funding of appraisals must be adequate so that resources are not diverted from patient services. The costs of recertification will not be insignificant and will have to be borne somewhere in the system, whether by the professionals, the professional bodies or purchasers (Hayes, 2001). Certainly the costs and benefits of recertification should be evaluated in order to ensure that a sledge hammer is not being used to crack a nut, because the prevalence of seriously underperforming doctors is believed to be low (less than 5%) (Newble, 2001).

(d) Compliance with recertification. In order to ensure that doctors comply with recertification, the sanctions must be clear. In many countries the assumption is that the right to practice will be removed. However, in some countries such as the Netherlands, sanctions are not yet systematically organized and can be imposed at the discretion of the medical societies (Swinkels, 1999). In the United Kingdom if underperformance cannot be dealt with locally then a referral can be made to the GMC, which has the power to remove a doctor from the register (Southgate and Pringle, 1999). Yet if the aim is to improve health care delivery, then a doctor failing to meet recertification requirements must be given support and remedial training. The process must be clearly set out with appeal processes which would stipulate whether the doctor is suspended pending further training, at what point they are irrevocably removed from the register and what criteria might have to be met in order to be reinstated.

The lifelong learning cycle: from continuous medical education to continuous professional development

Lifelong learning, flexibility and adaptability to new roles and challenges has been put forward as the new ideal. This is also true for GPs, although to stay in the mainstream of medical evolutions is very challenging. This is essential, however, if the claim on the driver's seat position is to have meaning. The traditional emphasis on 'continuous medical education' has largely proved to be unsuccessful in changing the competence and daily performance of attendees. Results from the analysis of a broad range of effect studies on different methods (Davis *et al.*, 1995) were very clear: traditional lifelong learning through seminars, retraining weeks and regular reading proves to have almost no impact on changes in practice performance. These educational tools seem to bring some new knowledge, but if the acquired knowledge cannot be implemented quickly, it is easily forgotten. Simply recording attendance at CME does not ensure the fulfilment of the objectives of recertification. It is still possible to be incompetent in practice (Smith, 2000). Participation in CME may be motivated by other incentives (financial and non-financial) such as meeting friends, belonging to the group, networking, free holiday, etc. There is a also danger that recertification provides disincentives for participation in professional development rather than stimulating it (Buckley, 1999).

In a new joint policy document from the quality assurance board and the educational board of WONCA Europe (EQUIP and EURACT, 2003), a plea is made to integrate separate programmes of CME learning and of quality improvement activities into one process. 'The emerging requirements of health care systems focusing on outcome and cost-efficiency combined with new learning paradigms focusing on knowledge, competence and performance, set the scene for Continuous Professional Development Planning. This involves integrating the more traditional options for CME and the more occasional initiatives on Quality Development.' Basic principles are: patient and community priorities concerning health care should be central; CPD should be based on the learners' daily working practices; goals should be set by the GP and/or the practice; and integration should be a continuing process and not a series of sporadic efforts. Central instruments are the personal development plan and the learning portfolio. It should be based on adult learning principles. During the process data should be collected and performances analysed utilizing evidence-based guidelines. To make it a continuous process, practice enabling and reinforcing strategies should be optimized.

The "good CPD guide" (Grant and Chambers, 1999), published by the Joint Centre for Education in Medicine, tries to make CPD an instrument at the structural organization level, clearly managed at trust, PC group or practice level, in pursuit of increased quality of patient care and of service development. Personal Development Plans (PDPs) have to start from individual needs, but should be put in a practice or service context for reinforcement and dissemination and should be discussed with colleagues to form part of the business plan of the clinical unit which makes them open to scrutiny and able to be monitored. These plans should reflect personal interest but should also encompass corporate needs. Practices or PC groups should have a clear written CPD policy and a projected time available, bearing in mind that management of resources is also about better targeting and ensuring value for money. An education-oriented culture should be supported, with a focus on audit, clinical effectiveness and research.

At national government level, a central role in the CPD process should come from recertification bodies and procedures. Traditional CME has a reaccreditation system based on credits that are collectively acquired in seminars or meetings. Their primary goal is that physicians gain professional knowledge. If the focus shifts to competence and performance, the recertification process should be adapted to the new paradigm. This would require a fundamental change from counting credits and monitoring attendance to evaluating personal development plans and monitoring involvement in a quality control process. This would entail expanding the field of accreditation by incorporating a new set of instruments in order to discover what the learning needs are and how they can be met. It is clear that a flexible system of accreditation is important, which would include recertification (competency evaluation) and both practical and professional accreditation (performance evaluation) in a supportive and transparent manner that is overseen by the appropriate national authorities.

At present CPD is more a concept than a reality. Table 9.5 shows the countries

Table 9.5 Features of CME and CPD in Europe

	Compulsory	Responsible body*	Include portfolio/ learning plan	Feedback procedures	Official guidelines
Austria	N	P	N	Y	Y
Belgium	Y	G	N	Y	Y
Bosnia and Herzegovina	N	P	N	N	N
Czech Republic	Y	P	Y	Y	Y
Denmark	N	P+S	Y	Y	Y
Estonia	Y	P+G	N	Y	Y
Finland	N	n.a.	N	N	N
France	Y	P	N	Y	Y
Germany	N	P	N	Y	Y
Greece	N	P	N	Y	Y
Hungary	Y	U	Y	Y	Y
Ireland	N	S	N	Y	Y
Israel	Y	U	N	Y	Y
Italy	Y	P+S	N	Y	Y
Lithuania	Y	S+U	N	Y	Y
the Netherlands	Y	P	N	Y	Y
Norway	Y	G	Y	Y	Y
Poland	N	n.a.	N	Y	Y
Portugal	N	n.a.	N	Y	Y
Romania	Y	P+G+U	N	N	Y
Slovakia	Y	U	N	Y	Y
Slovenia	N	P+S	N	Y	Y
Spain	N	n.a.	N	Y	Y
Sweden	N	G	N	n.a.	n.a.
Switzerland	N	P	N	N	N
Turkey	N	P+U+S	N	N	N
United Kingdom	N	n.a.	Y	Y	Y

Note: *Government (G), Profession (P), Scientific societies (S) or Universities (U); n.a. = not available.
Source: EURACT (2004).

that have not adopted new accreditation systems as a whole, but that increasingly include elements like peer review and other feedback procedures within official guidelines. Individual portfolios that are already utilized in the new curricula for basic medical education and specialty training are still rarely used in continuing medical education.

Conclusions

Globally the specialist-centred care model is predominant in medical universities. In some countries, however, there is more input from GP departments, bringing the community perspective into the curriculum. In terms of the widely accepted specialty training, family medicine as a profession, at least in its documents and position papers, is aware of the changing needs of society, the new emphasis on patient empowerment, and on population-based prevention and screening. Equal access, cooperation and community orientation now serve as the basic cornerstones of the discipline in Europe. To date, what remains unclear is the impact of these principles on the actual content of teaching and training.

In recent decades, general practice has gained a more central position in most European health care systems, owing to its strong position as the first line of care as well as its emergence as a scientific discipline and as a specialization in academic research. National and international organizations of GPs have played a leading role in achieving this, as has the corresponding financial support and other resources dedicated to promoting general practice. Increasingly, official procedures for accreditation and reaccreditation are being introduced as quality guarantees that will further strengthen PC physicians as professionals. The realization of this goal will also require a number of political factors: changes in legislation, delegation of implementation to self-regulating bodies, estimation of the direct and indirect costs of recertification, designation of penalties and sanctions to be imposed for non-compliance, clear allocation of responsibilities for funding and implementation, and adoption of common EU standards. The methods adopted should also be easily incorporated into doctors' daily work and cause minimal disruption to service delivery. To bring continuous education in better balance with the competence and performance in daily practice, a new emphasis is needed on Continuous Professional Development Planning as the content and control system for the future. At present this is still mainly a topic for publications and seminars, as it has not yet been integrated into the field of daily practice. Yet, as an ideal to strive for it seems quite promising.

The academic and professional groups in the 'forefront' countries of general practice development will need to ensure continuous adaptation to new professional and patient needs. Countries that were 'late adopters' will be faced with the enormous task of changing practice, training and teaching all at the same time. Small, incremental change is the only realistic way to implement changes of this scope in these countries. Accreditation and recertification mechanisms will be essential in order to ensure recognition of general practice as a specialty. Inertia, resistance from the specialists and other 'competing' PC providers such as paediatricians should also not be underestimated. Implementing changes will require appropriate human and financial resources. The newly founded professional associations of general practitioners and the wide social support of measures that seek to better meet the needs of the community can serve as an engine of reform in countries with health care systems in transition. Strengthening the position of the professional bodies of GPs is thus crucial for the sustainability of PC-driven health care reforms.

References

Barr, D.A. and Schmid, R. (1996). Medical education in the former Soviet Union, *Academic Medicine* **71**: 141–145.

Boelen, C. (1999). Adapting health care institutions and medical schools to societies' needs, *Academic Medicine* **74**(8): S11–S20.

Boerma, W.G.W. and Fleming, D.M. (1998). *The Role of General Practice in Primary Health Care*. Copenhagen: WHO Regional Office for Europe.

Buckley, G. (1999). Revalidation is the answer, *British Medical Journal* **319** (7218): 1145–1146.

Davis, D.A., Thomson, M.A., Oxman, A.D. *et al.* (1995). Changing physician performance. A systematic review of the effect of continuing medical education strategies, *Journal of the American Medical Association* **274**(9): 700–705.

Du Boulay, C. (2000). Revalidation for doctors in the United Kingdom: the end or the beginning? *British Medical Journal* **320**(7248): 1490.

EQUIP and EURACT (2003). Continuing professional development in primary health care: Quality development integrated with continuing medical education (http://www.equip.ch/groups/cme/rep/CME_QD.pdf, accessed 3 March 2004).

EURACT (1999). *Position on Specific Training of General Practitioners in Europe*. Leuven: European Academy of Teachers in General Practice (EURACT).

EURACT (2004). *EURACT Statement on Selection of Trainers and Teaching Practices for Specific Training in General Practice*. Tartu: European Academy of Teachers in General Practice (EURACT).

Firth-Cozens, J. and Greenhalgh, J. (1997). Doctors' perceptions of the links between stress and lowered clinical care, *Social Science and Medicine* **44**(7): 1017–1022.

Flexner, A. (1910). Medical education in the United States and Canada. A report to the Carnegie Foundation for the advancement of teaching. Boston: Carnegie Foundation for the Advancement of Teaching, Bulletin 4.

General Medical Council (2001). *Good Medical Practice*. London: General Medical Council (http://www.gmc-uk.org/standards/good.htm, accessed 3 March 2004).

Gossop, M., Stephens, S., Stewart, D. *et al.* (2001). Health care professionals referred for treatment of alcohol and drug problems, *Alcohol and Alcoholism* **36**(2): 160–164.

Grant, J. and Chambers, E. (1999). *The Good CPD Guide: A Practical Guide to Managed CPD*. London: Joint Centre for Education in Medicine.

Grundmeijer, H. and Rutten, G. (eds) (1996). *Leerdoelen in de huisartsgeneeskunde [Educational objectives in GP health care]*. Utrecht: De Tijdstroom.

Harden, R.M., Crosby, J.R., Davis, M.H. and Friedman, M. (1999). AMEE Guide No. 14: Outcome-based education: Part 5 – From competency to meta-competency: a model for the specification of learning outcomes, *Medical Teacher* **21**(6): 546–552.

Hayes, S. (2001). GMC's proposals for revalidation. Appraisal is helpful only if done well, *British Medical Journal* **322**(7282): 358.

Heyrman, J. (2004). *Educational Agenda*. Leuven: European Academy of Teachers in General Practice EURACT.

Jolly, B., McAvoy, P. and Southgate, L. (2001). GMC's proposals for revalidation. Effective revalidation system looks at how doctors practise and quality of patients' experience, *British Medical Journal* **322**(7282): 358–359.

Ko Ko, U. (1994). Education for medical practice for tomorrow, *Medical Education* **28**: 54–61.

Kuznethova, O.U., Yaremenko, L.N. and Frolova, E.V. (2000). Postgraduate education of family physicians in Saint-Petersburg – History, development and perspectives, *Russian Family Doctor* **1**: 13–17.

Leeuwenhorst Group (1974). *The General Practitioner in Europe. A Statement by the Working Party appointed by the Second European Conference on the Teaching of General Practice*. Dublin: Leeuwenhorst Group.

Leeuwenhorst Group (1977). *The Contribution of the General Practitioner to Undergraduate Medical Education*. Statement by the Leeuwenhorst Group. Dublin: Leeuwenhorst Group.

Lember, M. (1996). Family practice training in Estonia, *Family Medicine* **28**: 282–286.

Lember, M. (2002). A policy of introducing a new contract and funding system of general practice in Estonia, *International Journal of Health Planning and Management* **17**: 41–53.

New Leeuwenhorst Group (1981). *A description of the work of a general practitioner. A revised statement by the Leeuwenhorst Working Group.* Dublin: New Leeuwenhorst Group, November 1981 (http://euract.org/html/doc003.shtml, accessed 3 March 2004).

Newble, D. (2001). GMC's proposals for revalidation. Purpose of revalidation process must be agreed on, *British Medical Journal* **322**(7282): 358.

Norcini, J.J. (1999). Recertification in the United States, *British Medical Journal* **319**(7218): 1183–1185.

Royal College of General Practitioners (2002). *Good Medical Practice for General Practitioners.* London: Royal College of General Practitioners.

Rusovich, V., Boerma, W.G.W. and Schellevis, F. (2000). Going ahead with the primary care in Belarus, Pilot project in Minsk region, *Medizina* (Belarussian) **1**: 15–17.

Schepin, O.P., Dmitrieva, N.V. and Korotkih, R.V. (1996). Theoretical and organizational aspects of primary health care in Russia, *Problemy Sotsialnoi Gigieny Istoriia Meditsiny* **2**: 3–7.

Scrivens, E. (2002). Accreditation and the regulation of quality in health services. Regulating entrepreneurial behaviour in European health care systems, in Saltman, R.B. Busse R. and Mossialos, E. *Regulating Entrepreneurial Behaviour in European Health Care Systems.* Buckingham: Open University Press.

Shabrov, A.V., Dosenko, M.S. and Yubrina, I.V. (2001). Family medicine tutors training as a component of educational process in general practice, *Russian Family Doctor* **4**: 56.

Smith, R. (2000). Should GMC leaders be put to the sword? No, doctors must work together, *British Medical Journal* **321**(7253): 61.

Southgate, L. and Pringle, M. (1999). Revalidation in the United Kingdom: general principles based on experience in general practice, *British Medical Journal* **319**(7218): 1180–1183.

Starfield, B. (1998). *Primary Care: Balancing Health Needs, Services and Technology.* Oxford: Oxford University Press.

Swinkels, J.A. (1999). Reregistration of medical specialists in the Netherlands, *British Medical Journal* **319**(7218): 1191–1192.

UEMO (1995). *Consensus Document on Specific Training for General Practice. European Union of General Practitioners Reference Book 1995/96,* 65–69. Stockholm: European Union of General Practitioners (UEMO).

UEMS European Advisory Committee on CME (2001). *Update on Structure of National CME.* Brussels: European Union of Medical Specialists (UEMS). (http://www.uems.be/eaccme.htm, accessed 20 May 2002).

Vuori, H. (1979). *Lääketieteen historia [Medical history].* Jyväskylä: Gummerus.

Weir, E. (2000). Substance abuse among physicians, *Canadian Medical Association Journal* **162**(12): 1730.

WHO (1998). *Framework for Professional and Administrative Development of General Practice/Family Medicine in Europe.* Copenhagen: WHO Regional Office for Europe.

WONCA Europe (2002). *The European Definition of General Practice/Family Medicine 2002.* Singapore: World Organization of Family Doctors (WONCA) (http://euract.org/html/page03a.shtml, accessed 3 March 2004).

WONCA/WHO (2002). *Improving Health Systems: The Contribution of Family Medicine – A Guidebook 2002.* Singapore: World Organization of Family Doctors (WONCA).

chapter ten

Managing primary care behaviour through payment systems and financial incentives

Stefan Greß, Diana M. J. Delnoij and Peter P. Groenewegen

Introduction

This chapter assesses the influence of payment systems and financial incentives on primary care doctors. This is a broad topic and not a new one. There is a veritable mountain of theoretical and empirical literature on the influence of payment systems on physician behaviour generally. Moreover, it is also clear that the actual impact of payment systems and their incentives are greatly dependent on health system context as well as other (non-financial) incentives. Although the literature on payment systems for physicians in general and GPs in particular has been very helpful in writing this chapter, it also has a drawback: the emphasis is on the pure effects of payment systems. However, we should be aware that payment systems only work within and in interaction with a broader institutional context. Specific elements of health care institutions that work well in their original institutional context turn out to be useless when transferred to other health care systems. Also, the stability of institutional arrangements influences whether or not certain elements work.

Payment systems and financial incentives are important but other incentives are also relevant. One of our arguments in this chapter is that the incentives of payment systems probably get too much attention, not because they are the most important in steering the behaviour of health care professionals, but because they can be more easily manipulated than other incentives.[1]

The main focus of this chapter is to describe the (potential and real world) effects of payment systems and financial incentives on the behaviour of primary care doctors. In order to answer this research question we first analyse the intended effects of payment systems and financial incentives (section two). However, actual effects depend not only on the behaviour and value systems of physicians but also on context-based incentives which counteract those embedded in the payment system. Therefore, the next step is to analyse the potential interaction of health system context and payment systems (section three). In section four we describe the effects of payment systems and financial incentives on providers, patients and society on the basis of empirical studies of (changes in) payment systems (in other words: we describe the real effects). In the final section we draw some policy conclusions from our findings.

Our analysis is based on an extensive literature review which has been conducted in spring and summer of 2002. Where appropriate, we illustrate our findings with country examples.

Intended effects of payment systems and financial incentives

We focus on the most common payment systems and their intended effects. Each system can be distinguished by the type of unit which is being paid for.

In *fee-for-service* systems payment is made for units of service. In theory physicians and patients could negotiate the price for individual services at each point of contact. In fact fee-for-service systems are usually based on fee schedules which classify physicians' activities with varying degrees of precision.

Physician income in *fee-for-service* systems is determined by the number of services multiplied by the price of services. In general, fee-for-service is intended to allow physicians to react in a flexible manner to patients' needs and also grants them a high degree of autonomy. However, interventions by health authorities or health insurers aimed at containing costs or shifting relative prices of services are likely to have direct effects on clinical decision-making (Groenewegen and Calnan, 1995). Financial rewards are directly connected with work performed. Fee-for-service systems still are widespread in Europe and quite popular with the medical profession. Table 10.1 shows that only some countries rely entirely on fee-for-service (for example Belgium, France and Luxemburg). In other countries physicians are paid fee-for-service for groups of patients (for example, patients with social health insurance in Germany and patients with private health insurance in the Netherlands).

In *capitation*-based systems payment is made for individual patients. The provider is paid a specified sum of money for the care of individual patients for a specified period of time. Patients usually have to register with individual physicians or groups of physicians. Payment is independent of the extent of services individual patients require. Ideally payments to physicians are risk-adjusted for differences in morbidity of patients in order to reduce incentives for risk selection. In fact payments mostly vary according to the age of patients but are usually not so fine-grained as to reflect differences in service utilization. In some countries there are also payments for patients who live in deprivation areas (see Box 10.2). Physician income is determined by (risk-adjusted) capitation multiplied by individual patients enrolled with the physician. There may be limits as to the maximum number of patients enrolled with one physician and/or degressive capitation payments above a threshold of patients. Capitation is intended to ensure access to primary health care services for every registered patient. Furthermore, incentives for supplier-induced demand are reduced and incentives for continuity of care are increased. In European primary care capitation-based systems are not as common as fee-for-service systems (see Table 10.1). Mostly, the capitation payment is combined with some fee-for-service payments.

In *salary* systems the physician is paid for units of time. Remuneration is independent of the volume of services and independent of the number of patients. Salaried providers work within a defined schedule; in some countries they are allowed to treat patients privately after hours. Physician income is determined by the content of the employment contract. Salaries mostly depend on the physician's qualification and his or her task profiles and provide a high degree of income security to physicians. Salary systems are still predominant in the transitional countries in central and eastern Europe although they are increasingly being replaced by other payment systems. A salaried payment system is intended to combine basic income security for physicians with high accessibility for patients. Salaried payment in eastern Europe is substituted by capitation and fee-for-service. However, salaries are still widespread in Portugal, Scandinavia, and Spain (see Table 10.1).

While fee-for-service, capitation and salary are the three basic payment systems for GPs, there are several varieties of each. One of the most interesting varieties is *integrated capitation*. Integrated capitation systems combine a capitation payment for services delivered by different providers or at different levels of care. In contrast to simple capitation other expenditures such as prescription drugs, specialist services or even services in secondary care can be incorporated in integrated capitation payments. GPs may even act as fundholders by purchasing hospital care for their patients.[2] Thus, physician income is determined by integrated capitation payments multiplied by registered patients minus payments to other providers or to other levels of care. Integrated capitation is intended to provide even better incentives for continuity and comprehensiveness of care. At the same time it requires well developed mechanisms for the allocation and monitoring of capitation payments. So far integrated capitation systems have not been very successful in Europe.

Mixed payment systems come in three varieties. The first is that GPs are paid according to a mixed system for all their patients, mostly consisting of a basic payment (salary or capitation) and additional payments to provide incentives for certain tasks. Target payments are used to provide incentives to reach predefined levels of services, such as parts of the population taking part in screening programmes. Function payments are used to reward physicians for services not included in their basic contract, such as providing out-of-hours emergency services. Here the payment system is mixed at the level of patients (for examples see Box 10.1). The second variety is that GPs get paid according to a different system for different patient groups, e.g. according to insurance status. Here, the system is mixed at the level of GPs (for an example see Box 10.2). The third variety of mixed payment system is that some GPs are salaried and others paid fee-for-service or capitation. Here, the mix is at health care system level. Espe-

Box 10.1   Mixed payment systems at the level of patients

Throughout several reforms the payment system for GPs under the NHS in the United Kingdom has maintained the principle of capitation payment that had been used since long before 1948. Today, the payment system of GPs in the United Kingdom consists of a complicated mix of allowances, capitation payment, target payments, and fees-for-services (Department of Health, 2002). As a result of the introduction of target payments for preventive activities there has been a remarkable growth in the number of nurses working in general practices. These practice nurses take up health promotion, along with a whole range of other tasks, for example in the field of care for the chronically ill (Atkin *et al.*, 1994; Hibble, 1995).

Very recently the Italian Government has reformed the payment system of GPs in the NHS. GPs in Italy are self-employed and receive a capitation payment, with a maximum of 1,500 patients per GP. The capitation now has a variable part (30%) and a fixed part (70%). The variable component is defined by individual Health Authorities (HAs) which first have to define priorities which can then be linked to GP performance via the variable component of the capitation payment. A recent study found that so far 61 health authorities (of 196 health authorities in Italy 162 replied to a questionnaire) have defined targets for the variable component. Targets are mostly related to costs for drugs (42 HAs), costs for hospital admissions (31 HAs) and costs on diagnostic and lab tests (13 HAs).[3] So far there is no information on the outcome of these performance-based payments (Vendramini, 2002). However, we know from experience of other countries that health care expenditure can decrease when primary care providers have incentives to curb costs for drugs or hospital admissions (Wilton and Smith, 2002).

cially in the second and third variety, GPs may not show the behavioural effects of the pure payment systems; in the second variety because there may be forces against differential treatment of different patients by the same GPs; in the third variety because one group of GPs may be the dominant one, setting the norms for the other group. The incentives of salaried service with regard to working hours, for example, work out differently in a system with predominantly salaried GPs or in a system with predominantly fee-for-service GPs.

Table 10.1 provides an overview of GP payment systems as of 2004 in the 15 countries of the European Union and five pre-accession countries. From Table 10.1 it is clear that most countries have a mixed system, and that in more than half of these cases the payment is mixed at the level of patients or GPs. This implies that GPs in those countries are not exposed to "pure" incentives.

There has been a clear trend in Europe towards mixed payment systems. In theory mixed payment systems (at GP level) can combine the advantages of several payment systems and avoid their disadvantages. However, even in United States Managed Care organizations, most payment systems are relatively

Box 10.2 Mixed payment systems at the level of GPs

Financial incentives and payment systems in German primary care differ quite significantly depending on the insurance status of patients. All primary care physicians in Germany have a mix of privately and socially insured patients. Physicians receive fee-for-service payments for both privately and socially insured patients. However, there are different fee schedules for each type of patient. Providers are allowed to charge much higher fees for privately insured patients than for socially insured patients. The difference may be even larger if patient and physician agree to refrain from applying the (private) fee schedule. The fee schedule for patients with private health insurance is partly based on the fee schedule for patients with social health insurance. However, since private health insurers do not have any contractual relations with primary care physicians, this fee schedule is issued by ordinance by the Federal Government while the fee schedule for socially insured patient is jointly determined by peak organizations of providers and sickness funds. Since there is no budget for services which are provided to privately insured patients, physicians try to compensate for stagnating or even decreasing income from sickness fund patients by treating privately insured patients. As a consequence, preferential treatment of these patients is quite common and health care expenditures of private health insurers for ambulatory care are skyrocketing.

simple in order to ensure low administrative costs and high transparency. These limits of payment systems underscore the importance of non-financial methods of motivating physicians – such as screening and selection, explicit prescription of desired performance and monitoring of compliance (Robinson, 2001).

Interaction of payment systems and financial incentives with health system context

In general, it is very difficult to separate the analysis of financial incentives from the general context of the health care (financing) system. Thus, experiments made with financial incentives in one country and the results obtained may not be reproduced straightforwardly in another country unless major structural reforms are undertaken. It must also be kept in mind that other non-financial incentives such as mandatory practice guidelines affect physician behaviour and possibly income (Chaix-Couturier *et al.*, 2000). Specifically, payment systems set financial incentives for the behaviour of physicians. However, the method of payment is only one factor determining the outcome of primary care for patients. Therefore, it is difficult to determine whether the behaviour of primary care providers correlates with particular payment methods. Additionally, it would be impossible to reform payment methods without taking into

Table 10.1 GP payment systems as of 2004 in 15 EU Member States and selected accession states

Country	Payment system	Remarks
Austria	Mixed at patient level	Voucher system, which ties patients to one GP for a 3-month period. Payment consists of a flat rate per 3-month period (regardless of the number of services required) plus fee-for-service (Hofmarcher and Rack, 2001).
Belgium	Fee-for-service	(Kerr, 2000)
Denmark	Mixed at patient level	Capitation (about one third of their income) and additional fee-for-service (Vallgarda *et al.*, 2001).
Finland	Mixed at health system level	In "regular" health centres (the previously dominant system): salary, sometimes with bonuses, plus extra payments for certificates of health. In "personal doctor" centres (now covering about 55% of the population): salary (60%), capitation (20%), fee-for-service (15%), local allowances (5%) (Järvelin 2002).
France	Fee-for-service	(source: authors)
Germany	Fee-for-service	Fee-for-service according to a Uniform Value Scale (EBM) which ties the reimbursable "points" to the global budget negotiated with the sickness funds (Busse, 2000b).
Greece	Salary	In addition to their salaries, many doctors receive fee-for-service from private practice (Tragakes and Polyzos, 1996).
Ireland	Mixed at GP level	Patients under GMS (General Medical Services; about 30% of the population) are listed with a GP who receives an age/gender dependent capitation fee. The rest of the population is privately insured under Voluntary Health Insurance and pay fee-for-service, after which they are (partly) reimbursed (source: authors).
Italy	Mixed at patient level	Capitation plus fees for specific services and rewards for effective cost containment (Donatini *et al.*, 2001).
Luxembourg	Fee-for-service	(Kerr 1999)
the Netherlands	Mixed at GP level	Capitation for publicly insured patients (61%) and fee-for-service for privately insured patients (39%). (source: authors).
Portugal	Mixed at GP and health system level	Payment systems: Public sector → salary (plus private – fee-for-service – practice for 50% of GPs). Independent contractors → fee-for-service (Dixon 1999).

Table 10.1 *Continued*

Country	Payment system	Remarks
Spain	Mixed at health system level	"Traditional" model (independent, single-handed GP) → capitation. "Primary Care Teams" (dominant model; health centres) → salary (Rico, 2000).
Sweden	Mixed at health system level	In public health centres (86% of GPs) → Salary + fee per patient (Hjortsberg and Ghatnekar 2001). GPs working as private contractors (but paid via taxes as well) are paid through capitation (40–70% of income) and a smaller fee per patient consultation.
United Kingdom	Mixed at patient level	Payment consists of capitation (50% of the income), allowances, fee-for-service and performance related payment (Robinson, 1999).
Accession countries		
Czech Republic	Mixed at patient level	Reimbursement consists mainly of capitation plus fee-for-service (about 30% of income) for "desirable" services (Busse, 2000a).
Hungary	Mixed at health system level	GPs have four employment options. The majority (77%) work on a contract basis with local government and receive a capitation fee; 21% work in salaried employment of local government; 3% are independent contractors with the Health Insurance Fund, under capitation payment; and a few GPs are employed by hospitals. (Gaál *et al.*, 1999)
Poland	Capitation	(Karski and Andrzej, 1999).
Slovakia	Mixed at patient level	Payment consists of a capitation fee (60% of income) and fee-for-service (40%) (Hlavacka and Skackova, 2000).
Slovenia	Mixed at health system	Primary care doctors work in salaried employment or as private practitioners paid on a fee-for-service basis (Albreht *et al.*, 2002).

account the health system context in primary care (De Maeseneer *et al.*, 1999). Basically, in primary care the most important factors of health system context consist of the way financial access to health services is organized (benefits-in-kind versus benefits-in-cash; formal and informal user charges versus free access), the process of referral to secondary and tertiary care (extent of the gate-keeping role for primary care providers) and the allocation mechanism of patients towards providers of primary care (fixed patient lists versus free choice of providers for patients).[4]

Fee-for-service payments financed by private health insurers are usually combined with benefits-in-cash and reimbursement for privately insured patients.[5] In tax-financed or contribution-based systems the extent of user charges is smaller and benefits are granted either in cash or in kind. However, in health care systems with fee-for-service payment there is no gatekeeping role for primary care providers. Also, patients usually have free choice of providers and are not on a fixed list of primary care providers. As a consequence, the position of GPs as the doctor of first contact with the health care system providing continuous, comprehensive and coordinated care is quite weak. Furthermore, access for patients is hindered by user charges and by reimbursement mechanisms.

Capitation payments are usually funded through taxation or social health insurance contributions and not through private health insurance premiums. User charges and benefits-in-cash are much less common than in fee-for-service payment systems. Capitation implies fixed lists of patients and thus limited choice of providers for the patient; a choice that is restricted further by the fact that GPs under capitation payment are also usually gatekeepers to specialized care. As a consequence GPs have a strong position as providers of primary health care by evaluating patients' needs or urgency for access to secondary or tertiary care. Access may be hindered by risk selection strategies due to non-risk-adjusted capitation payments. Furthermore, under capitation payment physicians may feel encouraged to provide preventive services, since they reduce future costs (Boyden and Carter, 2000; Gosden *et al.*, 2001). And because GPs under capitation payment have fixed patient lists, they are theoretically in an excellent position to provide services that are targeted towards the population.

The most complex payment system with regard to health system context is integrated capitation. On a significant scale it was found in Europe only in the United Kingdom's fundholding scheme. At least in theory it can also be applied in social health insurance systems. GPs have considerable incentives to reduce patient access to secondary and tertiary care, which in turn increases incentives for risk selection inherent in simple capitation payments. On the other hand, integrated capitation on the basis of risk-adjusted capitation payments greatly increases incentives for interdisciplinary coordination of care through active disease management beyond the boundaries of primary care.

Salary payments for GPs are usually funded through taxation and less frequently through contributions. Mostly patients are not registered with individual GPs but are required to receive their primary health care at specific health centres or polyclinics. The attending physician may differ from contact to contact. Formally there are low or no user charges but in several transitional countries informal user charges ('envelope money') are still quite common. Furthermore, the low level of remuneration in these countries increases the incentives for the development of parallel systems of private care (100% user charges). This in turn can undermine the functioning of the official salaried system even further.

Figure 10.1 Incentives of payment systems and of the health system context for central values of primary care.

Payment System	Health System Context			Incentives for central values of primary care				
	User charges, benefits in cash	Fixed patient lists	Gate-keeping function of GPs	First contact	Accessibility	Continuity	Comprehensiveness	Coordination
Fee-for-service (Integrated)	Yes	No	No	0	–	–	–	–
Capitation	No	Yes	Yes	+	+[1]	+	+	+
Salary	No	No	No	0	+[2]	–	+	0

Notes: + positive incentives, – negative incentives, 0 neutral.
[1] Negative incentives in case of non-risk-adjusted capitation payments.
[2] Negative incentives in case of (informal) user charges.
Source: partly adapted from De Maeseneer *et al.* (1999).

Figure 10.1 summarizes the incentives of fee-for-service, capitation, integrated capitation and salary based on their intended effects, health system context and central values of primary care as described by Starfield (1996) and Boerma and Fleming (1998):

- primary care should be the first point of contact for people with (new) health problems.
- primary care should be continuous and comprehensive.
- primary care should be the co-ordinator of care in other parts of the health care system.
- primary care should be accessible to patients, irrespective of their age, gender or illness, and to other health care providers.

Real world effects of payment systems and financial incentives

Impact on provider behaviour

First of all, it should be noted that most of the available literature focuses on the intended effects and economic incentives of payment systems. Furthermore, most empirical studies on the actual effects of payment systems do not satisfy high methodological standards and criteria (De Maeseneer *et al.*, 1999; Chaix-Couturier *et al.*, 2000). Those that do fulfil these criteria find effects that are smaller quantitatively than may be expected (Gosden *et al.*, 2001).

But, all in all, the available evidence clearly states that payment systems do influence physician behaviour (Gosden *et al.*, 2004). However, from an economic point of view, physicians do not only try to maximize income and minimize their workload. Their utility function also consists of other non-price elements such as ethical restraints, professional standards which may dilute or even completely remove incentives for physicians to provide ineffective care merely to increase their income and thus limit supplier-induced demand.[6] Thus, payment systems do not always have the same effects on physician behaviour (Jegers *et al.*, 2002). However, two trends can be deduced from available studies (De Maeseneer *et al.*, 1999; Chaix-Couturier *et al.*, 2000; Gosden *et al.*, 2001; Gosden *et al.*, 2004).

The first trend is that under fee-for-service payment systems doctors tend to delegate fewer tasks to other health care providers than under (integrated) capitation or salary payment systems. This is not surprising since fee-for-service payment systems contain incentives to maximize income by maximizing self-produced services which of course also entails longer working hours.[7] Health authorities or health insurers try to counteract the trend for the expansion of services under fee-for-service systems by setting (negotiated) budgets for primary care services. They also try to steer provider behaviour by changing relative prices for services, for example by reducing relative prices for technical procedures and by raising relative prices for time-consuming individual counselling. While fee-for-service payment systems increase activity of physicians, they also allow for a high degree of flexibility (Engström *et al.*, 2001). Fee-for-service systems are more open to fraud than other payment systems, since GPs can claim for services they have not provided. Although fraud certainly runs contrary to professional standards it is not unheard of in fee-for-service systems.

The second trend is closely related to the first one. While there may be "underdelegation" in fee-for-service systems there may be "over-delegation" in salary and capitation systems. In capitation in fact there are incentives to encourage physicians to withhold care, resulting in undertreatment for patients. GPs can reduce their workload without reducing their income by referring their patients to other providers and can increase income by increasing the number of patients on their lists (Lynch, 1998). Salaried physicians are able to use free time to treat private patients in order to augment their income and physicians under capitation can maximize income by increasing the number of patients on their patient list. For physicians in capitation systems with badly risk-adjusted payments it is profitable to attract favourable risks (health care costs for the individual are lower than captitation payments for the individual) and actively to discourage non-favourable risks (health care costs for the individual are higher than capitation payments for the individual). However, this kind of behaviour is severely restricted by ethical restraints and so far there is little evidence of it in Europe (Lynch, 1998). While risk-adjusted capitation payments are technically and administratively complex, they greatly reduce incentives for risk selection in situations where ethical restraints against risk selection may be less effective (Hutchinson *et al.*, 2000).

Impact on access and patient satisfaction

In fee-for-service systems the combination of free choice of providers and the trend towards underdelegation both contribute to the fact that patients consume more services than in capitation or salary payment systems. Patients often visit several GPs in the course of the same illness and GPs may apply different diagnostic and therapeutic procedures. Non-compatible therapeutic procedures (e.g. different medication resulting in a dangerous combination of drugs) may endanger the health of the patient. However, without evidence on patient health status and clinical outcomes it is unclear if the increased consumption of services itself is hazardous or beneficial for patients (Gosden *et al.*, 2001).

Capitation payment systems provide a higher degree of coordinated care for the patient (Engström *et al.*, 2001). Since they have to enrol with a specific GP and GPs usually coordinate other levels of care, information on the patient needs is much less fragmented than in fee-for-service systems. Of course, owing to fixed patient lists and the gatekeeping function of the GP, free choice of providers is restricted. However, usually patients are free to enrol with another GP after a specified period of time. While this mechanism increases choice options for the patients, it opens up opportunities for risk selection by GPs in (integrated) capitation systems. Although this behaviour is quite uncommon in Europe, there are incentives for GPs to force unfavourable risks to look for other physicians. This behaviour would eradicate the advantages of capitation systems with regard to continuous and coordinated primary care for the group of patients needing it the most.

In salaried systems patients often complain about discourteous physicians. This behaviour probably reflects low motivation of providers who have very limited opportunities to increase income.[8] Moreover, private practice may not only financially but also professionally be more rewarding. Especially in underfunded health care systems in central and eastern European countries patients have to resort to informal co-payments in order to obtain the attention and the resources of the physician.[9]

Of course these often substantial user charges disadvantage patients with lower income who may not be able to pay additional money for ostensibly free services. Thus, the two central functions of salaried payment – income security for physicians and free access for patients – are often not realized in underfunded health care systems with salaried physicians in primary care.

Impact on costs

Policy-makers believe that payment systems are crucial for reaching general health policy objectives at a system level – such as increasing efficiency, responsiveness and equity of health care but also for reaching cost containment objectives. However, not every payment system is suitable for reaching all objectives at the same time.

In theory, price and volume of services in fee-for-service systems are open-ended. Therefore, fee schedules and budgets are supposed to influence the mix of services as well as price and volume. Transaction costs are high for negotiating fee schedules, monitoring for fraud, controlling budgets and of course for settling individual bills of individual providers – either directly with the patient (benefits-in-cash) or with health authorities or health insurers (benefits-in-kind). Fee-for-service systems may still be preferred to other payment systems due to a high degree of choice for patients. However, this choice option creates higher health care costs due to less coordinated and less integrated care. These costs are financed by user charges for patients and/or through higher taxes, contributions or premiums.[10]

Transaction costs of capitation payment systems are lower than those of fee-for-services systems since payment is based on individual patients – which is simple to calculate – and not on individual services. Regulation costs especially of integrated capitation may be high due to the necessity of the development and refinement of risk adjustment formulas. However, capitation systems tend to have a containing effect on health care costs (Delnoij *et al.*, 2000) and provide a stable financial environment for physicians while at the same time there is less choice for patients.

Salaried payment systems have very low transaction costs since physicians receive predetermined payments for units of time according to their qualification and tasks. Furthermore, these payments are easy to account for in a budgetary sense – which may be the reason why they are frequent in tax-financed systems. However, societal costs of underfunded salaries can be quite substantial. If physicians feel they have to augment their income by treating private patients and/or raising informal user charges of patients's trust in the system is eroded. However, it is important to note that this erosion of trust may not be caused by a specific payment system (in this case salaries) but by the underfunding of the health care system. Obviously, policy-makers tend to prefer salaries if they want to keep tight or even underfunded budgets – precisely because salaries are easy to administrate and to control.

Policy conclusions

Payment systems and financial incentives do influence the behaviour of primary care providers. However, how exactly and to what extent depends on a number of other influences such as ethical and professional constraints and health system context. Thus, the experience of one country with payment systems and financial incentives cannot easily be reproduced in another country – even if there is a high degree of cultural and institutional similarities.

Much has been published on effects of payment systems and financial incentives on (primary care) physician behaviour. However, most of these publications cover the intended and expected effects of payments systems and financial incentives only. Moreover, empirical evidence from studies with high methodological standards is scarce. Accordingly, policy-makers should be very careful about the distinction between intended and actual effects. The methodological standards alone probably make the results of studies into elements of payment systems less applicable. The available evidence suggests that fee-for-service payment systems tend to increase the volume of services provided to patients. This tendency towards overprovision may be harmful for patients and costly to society – which is the reason why health authorities and/or health insurers try to limit the volume of services. Fee-for-service payment systems are usually combined with a free choice of physicians which increases opportunities to choose for the patient but in turn also decreases incentives for a well coordinated primary care system. Policy-makers should be aware of this trade-off. Primary care providers paid by salary or capitation in underfunded health care systems have high incentives to either privately treat patients and/or to raise informal user charges. Both practices can endanger access to primary health care for those people needing it most. Thus, policy-makers should be careful to provide adequate funding for salaried primary care physicians in order to reap the potential advantages of salaries – high income security for primary care physicians, high accessibility for patients and low transaction costs for society.

There is a trend towards underprovision of services in capitation payment systems. Since capitation payment systems are usually combined with fixed patient lists and a gatekeeping function of the primary care physician, they also restrict opportunities of choice for patients. At the same time they provide large incentives for providing comprehensive and well-coordinated primary care and have low transaction costs for society. However, policy-makers should make sure that they adjust capitation payments for the morbidity of individual patients in order to minimize incentives for the physician to raise income by selecting risks. This is especially true in integrated capitation payment systems where primary care physicians act as fundholders for services in secondary care or for services provided by other care providers.

Alternatively, the idea of gatekeeping might be at odds with the preferences of modern and self-conscious health care consumers. We should think about ways to reconcile these two aspects. For one, the increasing scale of general practice makes it possible for patients to have more choice within the panel of GPs working in one practice. The issue of gatekeeping as restriction of consumer freedom could be solved in the way Denmark did, with its two insurance types, one giving more freedom but asking more cost sharing and the other restricting freedom in return for no cost sharing. One danger of the coexistence of a dual system (which – by the way – does not seem to apply to Denmark) is that those willing to accept restrictions on their freedom of choice are usually a healthy selection from the population. This is, for example, the case in Health Maintenance Organizations in the United States and it also seems to be the case in Switzerland (Colombo, 2001).

Payment systems are not the most influential factor that steers professional behaviour, but the one that is easiest for policy-makers to modify. This being the case, policy-makers should make sure that – if they cannot resist the urge to reform doctor's payment systems – at least the financial incentives for different providers are aligned. If you combine capitation payment for GPs with salaried specialists (as in the United Kingdom), you risk having waiting lists for specialist care. If you combine capitation payment for GPs with fee-for-service payment for specialists, you run the risk of excess referrals and high expenditures for specialist care – though the comparatively low referral rates of Dutch GPs do not support this hypothesis (Fleming, 1993). It is exactly this type of empirical "exceptions" to common sense expectations about the effect of payment systems that underlines the basic argument with which we started this chapter: payment systems work within and in interaction with a broader institutional context. This institutional context can reinforce or counteract the incentives embedded in payment systems. Therefore, we should try to research the effects of payment systems as part of configurations of health care system elements.

Notes

1   However, it is important to note that our chapter is still very much focused on finan-cial incentives for primary care doctors – although we take into account health system context. We mention other incentives – such as working conditions or career opportunities – only marginally and where appropriate, since extensive treatment of them would constitute another chapter. For an overview on non-financial incentives see Chaix-Couturier *et al.* (2000).

2   The revitalization of the fundholding idea in the British National Health Service is called Practice-Based Commissioning. From April 2005, individual GP practices are given the opportunity to hold budgets for primary and secondary care of their patients. Primary Care Trusts themselves will continue to be legally responsible for the contracting process, but any savings which result from managing referrals more efficiently will be shared between practices and PCTs, with all of those savings being reinvested into patient care (Department of Health, 2004).

3   Interestingly enough, some GPs opted not to have any incentives linked to their targets. They refused payment related to their performance since they consider fulfil-ling these targets as part of their job anyway.

4   Of course there are non-financial incentives which also influence physician behaviour. According to De Maeseneer *et al.* (1999) they can be grouped into factors referring to patient characteristics (number and type of disease, acute versus chronic diseases, diagnostic versus therapeutic procedures and ability to pay), personal char-acteristics of the physician (age, gender, experience, qualification) and his or her organizational environment (individual versus group practice, level of local competi-tion, volume of activity).

5   In most European countries tax-financed or contribution-based systems exist as well as private health insurance – and primary care providers realize income from different sources via different payment systems.

6   This is nicely illustrated in a recent Norwegian study (Grytten and Sörensen, 2001). The study compared fee-for-service primary care physicians and their salaried colleagues with regard to their response to increased competition. Neither of the two groups of physicians increased their output as a response to an increase in physician density. This could be expected for the salaried group while it provides evidence against the inducement hypothesis for fee-for-service physicians.

7   Incentives for physicians to induce demand are of course only effective if marginal cost for the production of health care services is less than marginal income. Another pre-condition is uncertainty about the appropriate treatment – if there are standard-ized and well-documented guidelines it is much more difficult to induce demand for physicians (Flierman and Groenewegen, 1992). Finally incentives for supplier-induced demand are higher if there is oversupply of primary care physicians – physicians may have low workload and may try to reach their target income. See also Gosden *et al.* (2001).

8   However, a recent study from the United Kingdom shows that GP morale and job satisfactions do not necessarily have to be lower in salaried systems than in capita-tion/fee-for-service systems. Salaried contracts in the United Kingdom are associated with lower stress levels, higher satisfaction with income and hours of work and the same levels of overall satisfaction as those of non-salaried GPs (Gosden *et al.*, 2002). This trend is an example of the fact that payment systems can have different effects depending on whether they are the dominant system or not. Salaried GPs in the United Kingdom are a small minority and the situation would probably be quite different if all GPs in the United Kingdom were salaried.

9   For example, the formal remuneration of physicians in Poland is relatively low and

provides few pecuniary incentives to work. Remuneration is poor not only in comparison with other sectors of the economy but also vis-à-vis the rest of the public sector. The average monthly salary in the health sector in 1996 was 84% of the average salary for the public sector. Salaries are often supplemented by payments for private sector consultations and by informal out-of-pocket payments which constitute an important source of earnings for providers. According to a study estimating health care expenditures in Poland for 1994, informal payments by patients to physicians contribute to as much as double of the physician's salary (Chawla *et al.*, 1998). A more recent study estimates that 40% of health care expenditures are still financed by informal payments (McMenamin and Timonen, 2002).

10 This development is illustrated by the "Managed Care Backlash" in the United States. The market share of fee-for-service health care plans is rising again – with more choice of providers but higher user charges and/or higher premiums (Draper *et al.*, 2002).

References

Albreht, T., Cesen, M., Hindle, D. *et al.* (2002). *Health Care Systems in Transition: Slovenia*. Copenhagen: European Observatory on Health Care Systems.

Atkin, K., Hirst, M., Lunt, N. and Parker, G. (1994). The role and self-perceived training needs of nurses employed in general practice: observations from a national census of practice nurses in England and Wales, *Journal of Advanced Nursing*, **20**(1): 46–52.

Boerma, W.G.W. and Fleming, D.M. (1998). *The Role of General Practice in Primary Health Care*. London: World Health Organization.

Boyden, A. and Carter, R. (2000). *The appropriate use of financial incentives to encourage preventive care in general practice*. West Heidelberg, Centre for Health Program Evaluation, Research Report 18.

Busse, R. (2000a). *Health Care Systems in Transition: Czech Republic*. Copenhagen: European Observatory on Health Care Systems.

Busse, R. (2000b). *Health Care Systems in Transition: Germany*. Copenhagen: European Observatory on Health Care Systems.

Chaix-Couturier, C., Durand-Zaleski, I., Jolly, D. and Durieux, P. (2000). Effects of financial incentives on medical practice: results from a systematic review of the literature and methodological issues, *International Journal for Quality in Health Care*, **12**(2): 133–142.

Chawla, M., Berman, P. and Kawiorska, D. (1998). Financing health services in Poland: New evidence on private expenditures, *Health Economics*, **7**: 337–346.

Colombo, F. (2001). Towards more choice in social protection? Individual choice of insurer in basic mandatory health insurance in Switzerland. Labour Market and Social Policy Occasional Papers No. 53. Paris: OECD.

De Maeseneer, J., Bogaert, K., De Prins, L. and Groenewegen, P.P. (1999). A literature review, in Brown, S. (ed.) *A Literature Review. Physician Funding and Health Care systems – An International Perspective*. London: The Royal College of General Practitioners: 18–32.

Delnoij, D.M.J., Van Merode, G., Paulus, A. and Groenewegen, P.P. (2000). Does general practitioner gatekeeping curb health care expenditure? *Journal of Health Services Research and Policy*, **5**(1): 22–26.

Department of Health (2002). *Primary Care: GPs' Fees and Allowances and Superannuation* (http://www.doh.gov.uk/pricare/fees.htm, accessed 13 May 2002).

Department of Health (2004). *Practice Based Commissioning. Engaging Practices in Commissioning*. London: Department of Health Publications (http://www.dh.gov.uk/assetRoot/04/09/03/59/04090359.pdf, accessed 21 October 2004).

Dixon, A. (1999). *Health Care Systems in Transition: Portugal*. Copenhagen: European Observatory on Health Care Systems.

Donatini, A., Rico, A., D'Ambrosio, M.G., *et al.* (2001). *Health Care Systems in Transition: Italy*. Copenhagen: European Observatory on Health Care Systems.

Draper, D., Hurley, R., Lesser, C. and Strunk, B. (2002). The changing face of managed care, *Health Affairs*, **21**(1): 11–23.

Engström, S., Foldevi, M. and Borgquist, L. (2001). Is general practice effective? *Scandinavian Journal of Primary Health Care*, **19**: 131–44.

Fleming, D.M. (1993). *The European Study of Referrals from Primary to Secondary Care*. Amsterdam: Thesis Publishers.

Flierman, H.A. and Groenewegen, P.P. (1992). Introducing fees for services with professional uncertainty, *Health Care Financing Review*, **14**(1): 107–15.

Gaál, P., Rékassy, B. and Healy, J. (1999). *Health Care Systems in Transition: Hungary*. Copenhagen: European Observatory on Health Care Systems.

Gosden, T., Forland, F., Kristiansen, I.S. *et al.* (2001). Impact of payment method on behavior of primary care physicians, *Journal of Health Services Research and Policy*, **6**(1): 44–55.

Gosden, T., Forland, F., Kristiansen, I.S. *et al.* (2004). Capitation, salary, fee-for-service and mixed systems of payment: effects on the behavior of primary care physicians (Cochrane Review). *The Cochrane Library*, Issue 1, 2004. Chichester: John Wiley & Sons.

Gosden, T., Williams, J., Petchey, R., Leese, B. and Sibbald, B. (2002). Salaried contracts in UK general practice: a study of job satisfaction and stress, *Journal of Health Services Research and Policy*, **7**(1): 26–33.

Groenewegen, P.P. and Calnan, M. (1995). Changes in the control of health care systems in Europe. Implications for professional autonomy, *European Journal of Public Health*, **5**(4): 240–244.

Grytten, J. and Sörensen, R. (2001). Type of contract and supplier-induced demand for primary physicians in Norway, *Journal of Health Economics*, **20**: 379–393.

Hibble, A. (1995). Practise nurse workload before and after the introduction of the 1990 contract for general practitioners, *British Journal of General Practice*, **45**(390): 35–37.

Hjortsberg, C. and Ghatnekar, O. (2001). *Health Care Systems in Transition: Sweden*. Copenhagen: European Observatory on Health Care Systems.

Hlavacka, S. and Skackova, D. (2000). *Health Care Systems in Transition: Slovakia*. Copenhagen: European Observatory on Health Care Systems.

Hofmarcher, M.M. and Rack, H. (2001). *Health Care Systems in Transition: Austria*. Copenhagen: European Observatory on Health Care Systems.

Hutchinson, B., Birch, J.H.S., Lomas, J., Walter, S.D., Eyles, J. and Stratford-Devai, F. (2000). Needs-based primary medical care capitation: Development and evaluation of alternative approaches, *Health Care Management Science*, **3**: 89–99.

Järvelin, J. (2002). *Health Care Systems in Transition: Finland*. Copenhagen: European Observatory on Health Care Systems.

Jegers, M., Kesteloot, K., De Graeve, D. and Gilles, W. (2002). A typology for provider payment systems in health care, *Health Policy*, **60**: 255–273.

Karski, J.B. and Koronkiewicz, A. (1999). *Health Care Systems in Transition: Poland*. Copenhagen: European Observatory on Health Care Systems.

Kerr, E. (1999). *Health Care Systems in Transition: Luxembourg*. Copenhagen: European Observatory on Health Care Systems.

Kerr, E. (2000). *Health Care Systems in Transition: Belgium*. Copenhagen: European Observatory on Health Care Systems.

Lynch, M. (1998). Financial incentives and primary care provision in Britain: do general practitioners maximise their income? in Zweifel, P. (ed.) *Health, the Medical Profession and Regulation.* Boston/Dordrecht/London: Kluwer Academic Publishers.

McMenamin, I. and Timonen, V. (2002). Poland's health reform: politics, markets and informal payments, *Journal of Social Policy,* **31**(1): 103–18.

Rico, A. (2000). *Health Care Systems in Transition: Spain.* Copenhagen: European Observatory on Health Care Systems.

Robinson, J. (2001). Theory and practice in the design of physician payment systems, *The Milbank Quarterly,* **79**(2): 149–77.

Robinson, R. (1999). *Health Care Systems in Transition: United Kingdom.* Copenhagen: European Observatory on Health Care Systems.

Starfield, B. (1996). Is strong primary care good for health outcomes? in Griffin, J. (ed.) *The Future of Primary Care: Papers for a Symposium held on 13 September 1995.* London: Office of Health Economics.

Tragakes, E. and Polyzos, N. (1996). *Health Care Systems in Transition: Greece.* Copenhagen: European Observatory on Health Care Systems.

Vallgarda, S., Krasnik, A. and Vrangbaek, K. (2001). *Health Care Systems in Transition: Denmark.* Copenhagen: European Observatory on Health Care Systems.

Vendramini, E. (2002). Budgets for general practitioners: an Italian survey, Paper presented at the European Health Management Organization Conference in Gdansk, 26–28 June, 2002.

Wilton, P. and Smith, R. (2002). Devolved budgetary responsibility in primary care, *European Journal of Health Economics,* **3**(1): 17–25.

chapter eleven

Improving the quality and performance of primary care

Richard Baker, Michel Wensing and Bernhard Gibis

Introduction

Two features distinguish methods for improving quality and performance in primary care. The first is the relatively rapid adoption of quality enhancing systems throughout western Europe during the past 15 years, followed by the start of their introduction in central and eastern Europe (CEE), in the context of a pan-European trend towards a more important role for primary care in health services. The second is the extent of diversity in the choice of systems and approaches. In the first section of this chapter, we define what we mean by improvement of quality and performance. We then outline some of the methods of quality improvement employed in primary care in Europe, and summarize evidence about the effectiveness of these methods. Progress in different countries is then considered, with countries being placed into one of three groups according to the level of development of quality improvement systems. We then discuss trends towards the emergence of common European standards and the growing importance of patient involvement in quality improvement activities. In the final section, we consider the implications of these trends and reflect on the requirements for successful quality improvement programmes in primary care.

An outline of the characteristics of health systems and health service reforms in different countries is not included since these are described in detail in other chapters. Also, we do not deal with the use of high-level strategies to influence the quality of care, for example, purchasing arrangements, managed competition or regulation. Our focus is on the first-line clinical and preventive care delivered by GPs, primary care nurses and nurse practitioners, and the teams in which they work. Since primary care professionals have a varied but often central position in health care systems, sound quality improvement processes in primary care are of wide importance.

Quality and quality improvement

Among the many definitions of quality in health care, one proposed by Donabedian (1980) is particularly helpful: "quality is a property of, and a judgement upon, an element of care". The concept of judgement is the key to understanding the meaning of quality – different judges will come to different conclusions, according to their own preferences and priorities. Donabedian suggested that the judges could be categorized into three groups, and in this chapter we will call these groups patients (to include all current, past and potential future users of health care), professionals (all health care professionals) and planners (to include policy-makers, funders and managers). But patients, professionals and planners cannot be expected always to agree on the desirable features of care.

The balancing mechanism lies in the mix of professional regulation, national legislation and health service polices and guidelines that govern clinical practice (Baker, 2001; Baker and Grol, 2002). These explicit statements are supplemented by implicit codes of behaviour that circumscribe the relationship between doctors and society. The societies in which we live, therefore, make the ultimate decisions about whose concerns have priority, or in other words, who has the authority to define particular elements of quality and set standards of performance. The process of adoption of quality improvement methods and programmes in European primary care illustrates not only the varying natures of our different societies, but also three general trends – the first involves the gradual replacement of the implicit codes governing professional/patient relations with explicit rules and regulations, the second involves a more equal sharing of power between the three judges of quality, and a consequent reduction of power among professionals, and the third involves the increasing status of the GP within health services in most countries.

From the 1980s onwards a variety of quality improvement methods have been taken up by primary care professionals (Grol *et al.*, 1994; Grol *et al.*, 1997), and in most European countries various methods are being used and supporting structures have been introduced. However, the extent to which the trends towards explicit codes and power transfer have occurred has varied. The principal influence on this process has been the level of development of primary care services in each country, with those countries with more developed primary care being first to introduce quality improvement programmes. Additional influences include cultural attitudes towards professionals in different countries, the unpredictable occurrence of serious adverse events in health care, the structure of health systems and the place of primary care in those systems and the existence of coherent leadership within the profession of family practice.

Quality improvement methods share three key elements. The first is the specification of desired performance, either in the form of clinical guidelines, care pathways, review criteria or clinical policies. The second element consists of various ways of changing clinical practice. Numerous approaches have been used, all with variable degrees of success. They include lectures, small group education, one-to-one educational outreach visits, audit and feedback, reminder systems, computerized decision support, and patient mediated interventions such as guidelines for patients or training to increase patient assertiveness in consultations. The third element is measurement. Performance must be measured in order to determine whether improvement has occurred, and to what extent, so that further strategies to change performance may be appropriately targeted. Usually performance is measured before the use of change strategies, and again afterwards, and this process is often depicted as a cycle – the quality improvement cycle (Figure 11.1).

Since change is unpredictable, measurement often has to be repeated several times, and in recent years attention has turned towards the introduction of monitoring systems to collect data about aspects of performance on a continuing basis. The improved availability of performance data is increasing pressure for public disclosure of the performance of providers and also making possible the use of techniques borrowed from industry such as control charts, and it is likely that such developments will become widespread in the near future (NICE, 2002).

The diffusion of quality improvement in primary care throughout Europe

In 1981 the Regional Office for Europe of the World Health Organization (WHO) launched a Model Health Care Programmes and Quality Assurance initiative. Although some localized quality improvement activities had been undertaken by small numbers of primary care professionals before then, it was from this point that quality improvement in health care began to be regarded as an important topic by leaders of health professions and the planners of services in Europe.

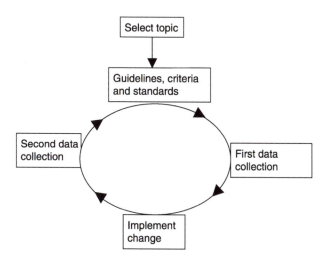

Figure 11.1   The quality improvement cycle

Health professionals have taken a lead in promoting quality improvement. For example, in 1994 the European Union of General Practitioners (UEMO) issued a statement on quality improvement which advised governments and the EU to commit to implementing quality improvement systems for general practice that included adequate resources for the creation of support structures, education on quality improvement, and the employment of a variety of specific methods (UEMO, 1997). The document argued that quality improvement should be a "priority for all GPs, a part of their normal professional life, and actions should be taken urgently to promote such an attitude". The European section of the World Organization of National Academies and Colleges of General Practice and Family Medicine (WONCA) established the European Working Party on Quality in Family Practice (EQuiP) in 1992 under the chairmanship of Richard Grol and with members drawn from six countries. By 2002, EQuiP had delegates from 27 European countries, including many of the reformed nations of CEE.

Acceptance by policy-makers of the need for quality improvement systems in primary care was signalled by in recommendation R (97)17 of the Council of Europe issued in 1997. This advised the 44 member countries of the Council (as of 2004) on the establishment of quality improvement programmes in health care, including primary care. The conditions highlighted as important to establishing quality improvement were policies, including laws, regulations and mission statements; structures, including local and national committees and boards; and resources, including staff to undertake specific quality improvement activities, time and money for professionals and teams, education and tools such as computer facilities.

The progressive introduction of quality improvement in an increasing number of countries has had two elements – the introduction of national policies and funding to create quality improvement programmes of various types and the use of a growing number of specific methods.

Methods used and evidence on their effectiveness

In this section we outline the more commonly used quality improvement methods, and consider their effectiveness. A wide variety of quality improvement methods are available, and different methods have been more or less popular in different countries (Table 11.1). Surveys undertaken by EQuiP in the early and mid-1990s provide some information (Grol *et al.*, 1994; Grol *et al.*, 1997), although more recent data about activities are limited. Chart audit and patient surveys were common in both 1991–2 and 1994–5 as means of collecting data, but by 1994–5, a growing number of countries had improved computer record systems that supported computerized monitoring of performance. With regard to methods of changing performance, written educational materials, courses and CME, and small group education tended to be used most commonly (Table 11.2). However, CME methods are relatively ineffective in promoting changes in performance and we do not discuss them in detail here.

The research literature shows that quality improvement can be effective in primary care, but also that none of the methods is always effective (Table 11.3).

Table 11.1 Methods used to collect performance data in European countries in 1991–2 and 1994–5

	1991–2 (n=17)*		1994–5 (n=26)**	
	N	%	N	%
Outcome or morbidity data	14	82.4	20	76.9
Data on utilisation/costs	13	76.5	19	73.1
Patient surveys	14	82.3	18	69.2
Chart audit	14	82.3	14	53.8
Computerized monitoring	–	–	14	53.8

Sources: Grol *et al.* (1994), Grol *et al.* (1997).

Table 11.2 Methods used to implement change in performance in European countries, 1991–2 and 1994–5

	1991–2 (n=17)		1994–5 (n=26)	
	N	%	N	%
Written educational materials	17	100	26	100
Courses, CME	17	100	26	100
Small group education	17	100	25	96.2
Peer review groups	12	70.6	15	57.7
Practice visits	10	58.8	13	50.0
Continuous quality improvement/ quality circles	8	47.1	11	42.3

Sources: Grol *et al.* (1994), Grol *et al.* (1997).

Passive education, such as written materials and courses, tends to be less effective, while multifacted interventions tend to be more effective. These conclusions are consistent with the wider research literature on quality improvement strategies (Bero *et al.*, 1998).

Quality circles/peer review groups

Although the term "quality circle" is used in industry to refer to a specific type of group convened within the framework of total quality programmes, in primary care in Europe the term is used synonymously with peer review groups. Typically, peer review is undertaken by a group of 5–10 professionals who meet together at regular, intervals over an extended period (Grol, 1994). The activities undertaken include setting criteria, data collection, evaluation of each other's work, and making specific arrangements for achieving change in performance. The first experiments with peer review groups took place in the Netherlands in the early 1980s. Initial experience was positive, and the Dutch Association of

Table 11.3 Reviews of continuing education and quality improvement in primary care

Author	Area (number of studies)	Conclusions
Buntinx et al. (1993)	Preventive and diagnostic test ordering (26)	Varying effects: 5–50% improvement on volume measures. Reminders appear to be more effective than feedback on adherence to clinical guidelines.
Hulscher et al. (1999)	Prevention (58)	Post intervention differences between intervention and control groups varied widely within and across categories of interventions. Most interventions were found to be effective in some studies, but not effective in other studies.
Lancaster et al. (1998)	Smoking cessation (unclear)	Clear improvement of process of care. One in 50 patients who received advice to stop smoking decided to stop smoking.
Wensing et al. (1998)	All areas included (61)	Information transfer alone was effective in 2 out of 18 groups, whereas combinations of information transfer and learning through social influence or management support were effective in 4 out of 8 and 3 out of 7 groups respectively. Information linked to performance was effective in 10 out of 15 groups, but the combination of information transfer and information linked to performance was effective in only 3 out of 20 groups.
Worrall et al. (1997)	All areas included (13)	Six studies involved reminder systems, while the others used small group workshops or education sessions. Five out of 13 studies showed significant effects on patient outcomes.

GPs decided to make participation in peer review groups a compulsory part of a quality assurance and recertification scheme.

Experience in the Netherlands has influenced the adoption of peer review groups in other countries. For example, the successful CME groups in Ireland have gradually evolved to include peer review activities (Boland, 1991), and quality circles were introduced in Germany from 1993, where moderators have received training and a substantial national programme is now operational (Gerlach and Beyer, 1998). However, in Germany concerns have arisen that some groups are not adequately moderated and the efforts of the regional associations to support the groups differ markedly. Participation has been voluntary and the methods used by the circles are variable and have not been adequately monitored (Gerlach et al., 1999).

Peer review groups may be particularly suited to countries in which primary care is largely provided by solo GPs. The regular group meetings enable such practitioners to meet their peers and exchange ideas. In countries in which large primary care teams predominate, other quality improvement systems tend to be preferred. There is limited evidence on small group quality improvement as a single strategy, but it suggests that it can be effective. Studies on the improvement of prevention in primary care showed effects in the range −4% to +31% (Hulscher *et al.*, 1999). Training health professionals to help patients stop smoking resulted in higher numbers of patients who received advice on smoking, made appointments about stopping, etc. (Lancaster *et al.*, 1998).

Practice visiting

Practice visiting has been implemented in several countries. The experience in Sweden offers an example. Data are collected in preparation for the visit and after the visit feedback is provided to promote reflection. Although the activity involves several professionals at once, and takes time, it is reported as being beneficial, and as overcoming the isolation that can sometimes occur in primary care (Eliasson *et al.*, 1998).

In the United Kingdom, practice visits were introduced in the 1970s in order to assess those practices that wished to undertake the training of new GPs. In 1990 the Royal College of General Practitioners introduced a system of awarding fellowships by assessment of performance to GPs who could demonstrate particularly high standards. Explicit criteria were developed, and the method of assessment involved observation of the doctor consulting (usually on videotape) and a visit to the practice to assess procedures and interview the doctor. This system has since been developed for the award of membership of the college. The Quality Practice Award (QPA) is a further method intended for primary care teams who wish to achieve recognition of high-quality patient care. The practice submits evidence to the college about aspects of its performance, and an assessment visit is undertaken. A development of this approach involves the engagement of the practice team in a development programme (Macfarlane *et al.*, 2004).

Experience of schemes such as these suggest that practice visits can serve to challenge practitioners and teams to review and improve their performance, and an international team is evaluating a system intended for wide use in Europe (Elwyn *et al.*, 2004). They also provide some recognition of high standards. In enabling the exchange of ideas, they represent one alternative to peer review groups in those countries in which group practice is common. Two studies on prevention in primary care showed a large difference in effects (5 and 44% change) (Hulscher *et al.*, 1999). A review of this approach in all health care sectors identified three studies, which showed a range of effects of 24 to 50% (Thomson *et al.*, 1998).

Guidelines

In most countries arrangements are in place to produce national guidelines in order to influence the performance of primary care professionals. GPs in the Netherlands were among the first to introduce national guideline development programmes and their experience is an example of what can be achieved.

Clinical guidelines currently comprise the core of the quality improvement activities of the Dutch College of General Practitioners (NHG). Since 1989 about 70 national guidelines have been developed on a wide range of diseases and complaints (Timmermans and In 't Veld, 2001). A structured development procedure is used, which combines systematic assessment of the research evidence and the judgement of experienced GPs. The guidelines are updated on a regular basis and published in the scientific journal of the Dutch College. The college supports the implementation of the guidelines by developing a range of materials, including cards that summarize the content of the guideline, packages for individual and group education, knowledge tests, written patient information materials, an electronic prescribing system, and practice visits by trained practice consultants (Timmermans and In 't Veld, 2001). The guidelines are also used in the vocational training of GPs. A large study in 1999 showed that adherence to the guidelines was overall 67%, with considerable variation across GPs, consultations and specific recommendations (Spies and Mokkink, 1999). In recent years, a recognition that guideline implementation and quality improvement have taken too much of a top-down approach has prompted the college set up a service to identify GPs' needs at local level, provide advice and stimulate local learning and improvement.

The Netherlands illustrates one model of guidelines development in which health professionals take the lead. In some other countries, governments have set up national agencies to provide guidelines, and generally cost-effectiveness of clinical interventions is taken into account rather than merely effectiveness. Thus, the governments in these countries see guidelines as being a mechanism to minimize expenditure on relatively ineffective treatments, and to ensure equity of access to effective care.

Audit

Audit has been defined in various ways. The broadest definition, and the one most commonly assumed by health professionals, has been framed as "a quality improvement process that seeks to improve patient care and outcomes through systematic review of care against explicit criteria and the implementation of change" (NICE, 2002). This view of audit adheres closely to the quality improvement cycle (Figure 11.1) and incorporates the use of a wide range of activities to implement change, from simple educational interventions to revision of systems of care. A narrower definition of audit limits the term to the collection of data about performance. Research evaluations of the effectiveness of audit generally adopt this definition, and restrict the method of implementing change to feedback of data about performance to health professionals.

Audit projects led by health professionals themselves have been shown to achieve both participation and improvements in aspects of care in Denmark (Munck et al., 1999) and Sweden (Melander et al., 1999). This experience has also been applied in Iceland and Norway (Munck et al., 1998). Audit has played a major role in quality improvement activities in the United Kingdom from 1991. The combination of new health service policy, a limited amount of funding and local structures to provide leadership and encouragement, led to the participation of most health professionals in primary care in audit projects.

General practices have reported taking part in a median of three projects each per year, with changes in care being implemented in two-thirds of the audits (Hearnshaw *et al.*, 1998a). Most audits were concerned with aspects of clinical care.

Audit with feedback can (but does not always) lead to improved performance, but the evidence indicates that the effects are often small. A review of 22 studies on the improvement of prevention in primary care showed the effects of audit and feedback lay in the range of 4 to 26% improvement (Hulscher *et al.*, 1999). A review of test ordering, which covered all health care sectors, showed that feedback led to changes in 13 out of 21 studies (Solomon *et al.*, 1998).

Quality management techniques

Since primary care providers are usually very small organizations, commercial quality improvement methods have required some adaptation prior to use in this sector. Nevertheless, there are examples of projects in which these methods have been evaluated, for example in the Netherlands (Geboers *et al.*, 1999) and the United Kingdom (Hearnshaw *et al.*, 1998b). More recently, some countries have begun to introduce collaborative programmes, working in partnership with the Institute for Healthcare Improvement in Boston (http://www.ihi.org). The National Primary Care Collaborative in the United Kingdom is an example. By 2004, this had engaged 5000 general practices caring for 32 million patients in introducing shorter waiting times and other improvements, making this the largest health improvement programme worldwide (National Primary Care Development Team, 2004). Almost certainly, these methods will be used more widely in the future.

Another initiative is the establishment of accreditation schemes in German ambulatory health care. Accreditation (called practice certification in Germany) schemes are aimed primarily at specialist care, but increasingly GP practices will seek accreditation with respected bodies. So far no validated accreditation system has been established in Germany for GP ambulatory health care and various for-profit and not-for-profit institutions offer products. These are mainly based on the DIN-ISO model adapted to the requirement of small private practices, or the EFQM model, which is a European adaptation of the Malcom Baldridge award.

National policies on quality improvement in primary care

In the EQuiP survey of 17 European countries in 1991–2, six had national policies on quality improvement in family practice (Denmark, Iceland, the Netherlands, Norway, Sweden, the United Kingdom) (Grol *et al.*, 1994). The policies involved national governments and professional organizations, and included funding and legislation. Seven countries had policies under development (Finland, Germany, Hungary, Ireland, Israel, Portugal, Spain), and four countries neither had a policy nor plans to develop a policy (Belgium, the Czech Republic, France, Italy). The respondents to this survey were asked about factors they believed were required in order to implement quality improvement, and the factors most frequently cited were resources including money and staff, and support structures such as professional committees; education on quality improvement techniques; policies that included leadership from planners and professional bodies backed by political and financial support; research into effective methods of quality improvement; activities to increase interest and motivation towards quality improvement among GPs; clinical guidelines; and collaboration between European countries to exchange ideas and experiences.

The survey was repeated in 1994–5, this time including 26 countries (21 from Europe, plus Australia, Canada, Hong Kong, New Zealand and the United States) (Grol *et al.*, 1997). It was evident that in a relatively short time, progress had been made in many countries. Sixteen countries reported having national boards and networks for quality improvement, 11 had specific training programmes and 10 had a legal framework addressing quality improvement in one way or another. In 20 countries, academic and professional organizations were providing a lead in promoting quality improvement in primary care. Despite these signs of progress, the study confirmed that quality improvement activities were, at that time, a relatively new endeavour in most European countries. No country had reached the point at which quality improvement had become a normal part of daily work for primary health care professionals. The most commonly expressed need in order to increase quality improvement activity (mentioned by 10 countries) remained resources such as financial support, extra time or dedicated staff. The creation of a positive attitude towards quality improvement among GPs was mentioned by respondents from eight countries; education, political support and rewards or incentives were each mentioned by five, and four mentioned a need for better indicators and quality improvement tools.

In general, policies emerged at an earlier date in the countries of Scandinavia and western Europe in comparison with the CEE countries. In the following section, we present brief outlines of progress in selected countries, grouped into those countries that were first to introduce quality improvement systems (the first wave), those that quickly followed suit (the second wave), and those now in the process of introducing quality improvement systems. For the most part, we draw on reports from EQuiP.

The first wave

By 1992 all the countries in this group had made considerable progress in introducing national policies on quality improvement in primary care, supported either by local structures, a legal framework or formal accreditation systems. They also tended to have well-developed primary health care systems associated with high professional status for GPs, including for example national colleges or associations and established training schemes. For example, in 1992, the proportions of GPs who were members of national colleges were: Denmark 100%, Finland 70%, Iceland 95% the Netherlands 90%, Sweden 95%, and the United Kingdom 60% (Grol *et al.*, 1994). In most of these countries, the initial policies have been further developed in recent years, involving both more expenditure on quality improvement and greater obligations on GPs and practices to take part. Thus, quality improvement systems have increasingly become integral features of health services.

Denmark

By the early 1990s Denmark had a national policy, local structures and an accreditation system, and many GPs were taking part in audit projects. In 1995 a new agreement between the Danish Association of General Practitioners and the National Health Insurance was reached that included a charter on quality improvement. Funding was made available and local authorities set up quality improvement committees. The committees were tasked with developing local policies and leading practical projects. Plans were also agreed for the development of national guidelines (Jensen, 1996), and the college of GPs began development of national guidelines in 1998–9. The guidelines have been used in the context of local groups of which all GPs are members. Quality development activities are funded locally, with a range of projects including outreach visits to practitioners. In addition, a system for coordinating care across the boundary with hospitals has been established (Olesen and Jensen, 1999).

Finland

Although a national policy was only partly operational by 1992, a legal framework was under development and formal accreditation was in operation. Professionals had become interested in quality improvement in the late 1980s, and a national training project was instituted in the mid-1990s, the training being delivered through health centres. A national policy statement was issued in 1996, all providers being encouraged to formulate a policy on quality improvement. Guidelines for GPs became available from 1991 in electronic form (Makela, 1996). The national recommendations on quality management were updated in 1999, and they advised health care organizations to develop regular patient feedback, provide continuing education for staff, and make use of guidelines. National projects undertaken by health centres include a continuing review of care for people with diabetes and another for those with hypertension.

Iceland

A national policy on quality improvement emerged at an early stage, associated with a formal accreditation scheme, and promotion by government and professional organizations. Activities included annual practice plans and target setting, and work with patient groups. In the mid-1990s a quality development committee was established, and computerized records introduced. The Icelandic College of Family Physicians has a Quality Council, which has the task of organizing activities. These have included the promotion of local quality circles and the conduct of a patient survey (Gudmundsson and Mixa, 1998).

The Netherlands

Quality improvement in primary care has been initiated and coordinated by the profession, encouraged by the government. Since the 1980s, professional organizations have national programmes for the development and implementation of clinical guidelines and for continuing education through peer review groups. Laws have been established that arrange professional autonomy, patients' rights on informed choice, and quality management in health care organizations (1996 Quality Law, or *Kwaliteitswet*). The law on professional autonomy prescribes a required level of quality improvement that is needed for recertification as a professional. The law on quality management is relevant for practices with two or more GPs. It requires that the practice publish annual quality reports to account for the quality of care delivered and for efforts to improve quality. A GP can meet the requirements of these laws by participation in the profession's quality improvement programmes. National policies on quality improvement have been agreed upon at special, five-yearly conferences in which organizations of health care providers, patients, insurers and the government participate.

Sweden

By 1992 Sweden had begun to implement a legal framework for quality improvement activities, had a national policy, local structures and an accreditation scheme. Training on quality improvement became widespread following new legislation in 1994. Extensive use was made of a collection of methods for quality improvement, contained in a Quality Tool Box developed by EQuiP (Persson, 1995). A National Board was established in 1997, backed by new legislation, to allocate funds to county councils for quality improvement activities that included audit. The legislation required local systems to include methods for responding to patient views and complaints, and ways to ensure the clinical competence of professionals (Persson, 1997).

The United Kingdom

A few GPs began to undertake audit from the 1970s, and by 1983, the Royal College of General Practitioners had adopted a goal that within 10 years, all GPs should incorporate standard setting and performance review as an integral part of their professional lives. 1991 saw the introduction of local organizations (medical audit advisory groups) to support and facilitate audit by all GPs and primary health care teams. Limited funds were provided to enable these groups to function, although participation in audit was voluntary. In 1998, a new mandatory system – clinical governance – was introduced, that incorporated audit into a wider collection of quality improvement activities. At the same time, a national body for guideline development was created. Since then, other national agencies have been set up to lead developments in patient safety (Rubin *et al.*, 2003) and address poor performance among a limited number of doctors. In 2004, a major development in quality improvement took place. A new incentive-based contract for general practitioners was introduced, payment being linked to the achievement of targets for the care of selected conditions and assessment of patients' experiences (Department of Health, 2003). This is probably the most advanced example to date of explicit codes defining quality of care and the transfer of power to determine quality from professionals to planners.

The second wave

In these countries, systems for quality improvement were less well developed in the early 1990s, but substantial progress has been made since then. The proportion of GPs who were members of national colleges in 1992 tended to be lower in most of these countries in comparison with those in the first wave (for example, Belgium 40%, France 15%, Ireland 95%, Israel 25%, Italy 0%, Portugal 55%, Spain 30%).

Austria

Quality circles were first introduced in 1994, and spread widely under the leadership of the Austrian Society of General Practitioners (Glehr, 1997). Leaders of quality circles have received training by the society, and a survey of GPs has shown that they regard involvement in quality improvement as necessary. Guidelines have been developed for use by the quality circles (Glehr, 1999), and a survey of quality circle members has confirmed doctors' positive views about them.

Belgium

Guidelines and peer review groups have formed the basis for the quality improvement system in Belgium since approximately 1995. The review groups have been supported through training of group leaders, instruction manuals, and evaluation procedures. Participation in peer review groups is mandatory in order to obtain accreditation. In addition, some national audits have been performed, for example on care of people with type 2 diabetes. Self-registration or audit of aspects of performance by GPs has been established for some years, and national congresses on quality improvement have been held.

France

The National Agency for the Development of Medical Evaluation (ANDEM) was created in 1990 to develop guidelines and methods for the evaluation of services, including methods for audits (Doumenc and Lafont, 1997). However, at that time, there was no comprehensive national policy, legal framework or local structures for quality improvement activities. In 1997, ANDEM was succeeded by the National Agency for Accreditation and Evaluation in Health Care (ANAES), which subsequently established local support services for quality improvement in all regions of the country in 1999. These local services were given responsibility for raising awareness among local doctors and initiating audits. Programmes were established for education about quality improvement and the development of guidelines. (Samuelson, 1999) From 2002, programmes for both GPs and specialists were established to support voluntary participation in self-assessment activities. Local leaders have been trained, and given quality improvement tools to support their work. At the same time, teaching about quality improvement has been introduced to the medical undergraduate curriculum throughout the country.

Germany

Quality assurance issues are mandated in the Social Code Book 5 for public health care and through the recommendations of the German medical association for private health care. Despite limited funds for the support of quality improvement activities, primary care professionals have increasingly initiated projects. These have included guideline development and quality circles; 1600 quality circles were discovered to be in operation in 1997 (Gerlach and Szecsenyi, 1997). Among other professional organizations, the German Society of General Practice has established a programme for the development of guidelines (Gerlach and Szecsenyi, 1998).

The latest developments (such as practice accreditation initiatives and disease management) show that in public health care quality improvement initiatives for GP care are changing from a rigid and mandatory approach to quality management. The use of a balanced mix of mandatory directives and stimulation of voluntary initiatives has been regarded as important.

Ireland

For many years CME groups have been active throughout Ireland. The Irish College of General Practitioners now has a Quality in Practice Programme that has established a distance learning programme and supports the local CME groups. Guidelines have been developed, and during 1999, progress was made in developing CME groups into quality improvement or peer review groups (Boland and O'Riordan, 1999).

Italy

A limited number of guidelines had been produced by 1996, generally by specialist societies. Since then, a larger number of guidelines has been published, and interest in evidence-based medicine has grown rapidly. Local and regional quality development programmes became included in professionals' agreements with health authorities from 1997. The Italian Quality Assurance Society has promoted peer review and quality circles, and the society has a primary care unit. In addition, several large regional quality improvement projects have been undertaken.

Portugal

A considerable degree of progress has taken place in Portugal over a relatively short period of time. The Ministry of Health established a Central Department for Promotion and Quality Assurance, which has provided vigorous leadership as well as practical support. It has instituted several programmes, including for example a project to monitor outcome indicators in health centres or to improve patient satisfaction. Guidelines were also being developed (Pisco, 1997). A health strategy was launched in 1998 with the aim of initiating a new, patient centred culture that would include a total quality health care system. The MoniQuOr project (Assessment and Monitoring Organizational Quality in Health Centres) has been one element of the strategy, and has involved the assessment of all primary health care centres. Prizes have been offered to health centres providing the highest levels of service.

Switzerland

A small number of quality circles were introduced in the early 1990s, and by 1995 180 circle leaders had been trained. A law came into force in 1996 under which care providers were obliged to implement quality improvement programmes. Aspects of these programmes could be delivered by professional organizations, and activities included peer review groups or quality circles and the development of guidelines (Kuenzi and Egli, 1996). The first national guideline project was launched in 1997, and addressed low back pain.

Third wave

The third wave is mainly composed of CEE countries. The pre-existing systems based on the Shemasko model lacked incentives to improve quality, but this issue is now being addressed in health service reforms. Practice management has also been poorly developed, and this is being rectified, one benefit being improved ability to undertake quality improvement at the practice level (Jack *et al.*, 1997). Furthermore, quality improvement has been regarded as an aid to raising the often low status of GPs in the health care system, e.g. Bulgaria (Goranov and Balaskova, 1998) and Slovakia (Jurgova, 1998).

Croatia

The development of a quality improvement programme is recent. Mandatory recertification for doctors and a patients' complaints system were the first elements. Professional bodies initiated a national society for quality assurance in health care in 1998, and at that time voluntary quality improvement activities among family doctors were increasing, including for example, audits and quality circles (Tiljak, 1998a). Project facilitators have been trained in quality improvement techniques, and experience has been rolled out to other professionals through workshops and conferences (Tiljak, 1998b). Assistance in training professionals in quality improvement methods has been obtained from experts in the Netherlands.

Czech Republic

Progress in the Czech Republic has generally been in advance of other CEE countries. An accreditation system was in operation in the early 1990s, and the country was the first from CEE to have representation in EQuiP. This was followed by several local quality improvement projects, but the principal task from the early 1990s was the establishment of the general practice profession. University departments and training programmes underwent development, and towards the end of the 1990s quality improvement initiatives had begun to include guideline development and a variety of implementation methods.

Estonia

In Estonia, training for GPs was instituted in 1991 and the Estonian Society of Family Doctors was established in the same year. By 1995 the society was organizing meetings on quality improvement (Lember, 1996). Interest in the use of quality improvement methods has extended to investigation of patient satisfaction with primary care (Polluste *et al.*, 2000).

Poland

In the reforms that followed the collapse of communism in Poland, a College of Family Physicians was established in 1992. Quality improvement activities have not been the first priority during these changes education and professional development have come first, but quality improvement is now gaining more importance, and is being introduced into daily practice (Windak, 1998). Representatives from Poland participated in the first International Summer School on Quality Assurance in General Practice in 1994, these individuals later taking a leading role in the development of activities in Poland. Although an early attempt to establish peer review groups failed, quality improvement projects on topics that included upper respiratory tract infection and hypertension were implemented (Windak *et al.*, 1998). A National Centre for Quality Assessment has recently been established, and early work has included preparation for a patient survey.

Slovenia

Following the declaration of independence in 1991, reforms have been implemented in the health care system. Primary care had been established under the previous regime, with the provision of premises and the creation of the Slovene family medicine society in 1966. However, vocational training was slow to arrive. Interest in quality improvement has increased in the last decade and courses and teaching materials were readily available from 1994. Attitudes towards quality improvement are positive among family doctors. Participation in peer review is now obligatory, and the number of projects undertaken by primary care professionals to evaluate their own care is increasing (Kersnik, 1997).

Turkey

In Turkey, reforms have progressed slowly over several decades, the general aim being to strengthen primary care. Family medicine is still a relatively new discipline and has had to establish itself within the health care system. Vocational training has been introduced, university departments of general practice established, but quality improvement is at an early stage (Basak and Saatci, 1998). Activities initiated during 2001 included the administration of a patient survey to more than 1000 patients, and the creation of a core group to define the standards for record systems.

Emerging trends

The previous section has demonstrated that quality improvement systems are being introduced into primary care in most European countries, although at different speeds in different groups of countries, largely dependent on the level of development of the profession of general practice. In this section, we briefly consider two early trends that can be detected, particularly among those countries that embarked on quality improvement first. The first of these is the development of common standards of care and quality improvement systems, and the second is the increasing role of patients in policy-making and the assessment of quality.

Common European standards

As with the development of quality improvement within countries, at an international level initial steps have been taken in the field of vocational training, and in the EU, common standards for training have been agreed. Developments with regard to clinical care are at an early stage, and most activity has been led by professional bodies. Several European collaborative groups have emerged, with a shared interest in a particular condition, such as diabetes or coronary heart disease. The aim of these groups is to share ideas and generate support for improved care. Some groups have issued guidelines. One such example is the recommendations of the joint task force on prevention of coronary heart disease (Wood et al., 1999). However, although these were developed by professionals, the majority were specialists rather than GPs. A statement on improving care across the interface between primary and secondary care has been issued (Kvamme et al., 2001), and ideas about a common European view on aspects of quality improvement have been proposed, for example a statement from EQuiP on the role of indicators (Lawrence and Olesen, 1997).

Although many national governments have developed and promoted national clinical guidelines, they have not begun to agree common European guidelines. There are obvious reasons why this should be the case. Since different countries have different health care systems and different levels of resources devoted to health care, the uniform application of common clinical standards across Europe would be virtually impossible. However, in the long term it is likely that some degree of commonality will emerge in the health care systems of Europe and common guidelines or standards will then be possible. It is also conceivable that pressure from professionals and patients in those states that spend less on health care will accelerate this process.

Patient involvement

The agreement of common European standards is at an early stage, but progress towards greater involvement of patients is more advanced. This suggests the existence of a general social movement across Europe for greater empowerment of patients, and increasing limitations on the power of professionals. At the level of individual patients, it is now widely accepted that doctors and nurses should actively seek to involve patients in their own care. General practice has proved amenable to this development, since it has itself developed a perspective on the doctor-patient relationship that placed emphasis on the patient's perspectives and circumstances: the so-called patient-centred clinical method. At policy level, policy-makers in many countries have responded to the pressure of patient's organizations to review complaints systems and to create structures to enable patients or their respresentatives to take part in decisions about the design of services. Typically, such developments are most advanced in the countries in the first wave group described above, and in these countries national guideline development programmes place importance on the involvement of patient representatives in the agreement of guideline recommendations. The United Kingdom is one example.

Surveys of patient opinion have also become highly popular, among both planners and professionals. Large numbers of patients in Europe have been asked in recent years about their views on the primary care services available to them. The design of valid survey instruments requires expertise, and several standard instruments are now available and have been widely used. One example is the general practice assessment survey (GPAS) that seeks patients' views of general practice services (Bower *et al.*, 2002), another is the consultation satisfaction questionnaire (CSQ) concerned specifically with consultations in general practice (Baker, 1996), and a third, the patient career diary, is concerned with the process of referral from general practice to specialist care (Baker *et al.*, 1999). An international collaborative group of researchers and GPs, associated with EQuiP, have developed a European standardized questionnaire for patient evaluations of general practice (EUROPEP) (Grol and Wensing, 2000). This instrument was developed from the start in an international context. The questionnaire (23 items) focuses on patient priorities for general practice, which had been established through surveys among patients in different countries (see Box 11.1) (Grol *et al.*, 1999). The final version has been translated into 15 languages: Danish, Dutch, English, Finnish, French, German, Greek, Hebrew, Icelandic, Norwegian, Portuguese, Slovenian, Spanish, Swedish and Turkish.

Survey studies in 16 countries in 1999–2000, and including more than 25,000 individuals, showed that patients generally had positive evaluations of general practice care. For most aspects, 80% of more of patients felt that the care

Box 11.1 Top-10 patient priorities regarding general practice in Europe

- Time in the consultation to listen, talk and explain
- Quick availability in emergencies
- Confidentiality of patient information
- Information about the illness
- Opportunity to talk about health problems
- Possibility of making an appointment at short notice
- GP goes to courses about new medical developments
- Preventive services
- Critical evaluation of medication and advice
- Adequate explanation of diagnostics and treatment

received was good or excellent, although considerable variation was found within countries. For instance, a further analysis showed that patients in practices with few practitioners and few other care providers had more positive evaluations of the availability of general practice (Wensing *et al.*, 2002). In a series of studies in the United Kingdom, Baker (1997) has shown not only that patients prefer smaller practices, but also that many professionals and planners have preferred larger practices, and as a consequence the proportion of large practices has increased. Thus, investigation of patients' views cannot be assumed to lead to patient involvement in policy-making. Additional methods are required to ensure that patients or their representatives take part in decisions about the design and delivery of services. The further development of patient involvement is likely to depend on the wide introduction of practical methods suitable for use at the local level, such as citizens' panels, community consultation groups, or representation in policy-making bodies. Although isolated examples of such local iniatives can be found in some countries, they are as yet uncommon.

Conclusions and future developments

In this chapter, we have seen how quality improvement policies and methods have become widely adopted in primary care in Europe at the same time as the profession of general practice has become established and primary care in general has been given a more important role in health services. The extent to which quality improvement has been introduced, however, has varied between countries. The process appears to depend first on the creation of a profession of general practice, with both formal training programmes and national leadership from within the profession itself, generally in the context of a college or association. Once this stage has been reached, some professionals explore quality improvement methods and then take on the role of convincing others to follow their lead. In due course, planners recognize the opportunity presented by a vigorous general practice profession to expand the role of primary care services, and an integral feature of this development is the introduction of formal and funded systems to enable quality improvement activities to function. The process started earliest in the countries of western and northern Europe, but was quickly taken up in southern Europe. It has also found its way into the reforming health care systems of CEE, although developments in many of these countries are at an early stage. The United Kingdom has advanced in this direction more than most countries, as illustrated by the work of the state-funded National Primary Care Development Team and the 2004 contract for general practitioners based on explicit quality targets.

If we return to the definition of quality outlined at the beginning of this chapter, it may be surmised that the evolution of quality improvement is a consequence of the shift in the authority to judge the quality of care from professionals to patients and planners. However, it has in reality been a more complex process. The standing of the profession of GPs had to be improved in almost all countries before quality improvement began, indicating that first of all, GPs had to acquire some authority over quality and standards. Once GPs had acquired authority, some among them recognized that the authority should be shared with planners and patients. The specification of the responsibilities of professionals for participation in quality improvement in laws or regulations is an example of the replacement of implicit codes (in this case, GPs are assumed to act to maintain or improve quality) by explicit rules (GPs are obliged to maintain or improve quality) as described at the beginning of this chapter. The introduction of quality improvement can also be regarded as one aspect of the sharing of authority with planners. As discussed above, patients have yet to be involved in quality improvement beyond merely the completion of questionnaires and therefore the next stage of sharing authority with patients has only begun to take place.

Methods of patient involvement have been largely limited to surveys, and any effect of these activities on the quality or design of services is difficult to detect. A more fundamental change is required before a genuine sharing of authority with patients can be achieved. The public disclosure of information about the performance of services – or individual health professionals – may be one element of the initiatives required to bring this about. Greater patient access to information about the management of disease may be another element, for example the provision of guidelines to the public. Permitting patient access to their own clinical records is another potential element. The role that local consultation systems might play has been outlined above. However, despite the availability of these approaches, little progress is discernible, even in the first wave group of countries.

Another challenge is that of achieving genuine improvements in care. Despite the wide adoption of quality improvement activities, convincing evidence about their impact on the quality of care is difficult to find. Research evidence has shown that some methods can sometimes lead to improvements, but the goal of routine achievement of change in the context of primary care quality improvement systems has not been attained. The explanation may lie in a failure to identify the most effective approach. If this is the case, all that is required is to introduce a new approach shown to be promising in another context. The hunt for a new technique that will ensure success is an old one in the young field of quality improvement research, and the most recent example is that of the theory of complex adaptive systems (Plsek, 2001). It is too early to judge whether this approach will indeed prove the solution to the challenge of changing performance, but the spread of quality improvement systems described in this chapter contains one lesson that should not be ignored.

The adoption of quality improvement systems has depended on the preliminary development of the profession of general practice. Once that development has reached a certain level, in almost all countries the initial steps in quality improvement take place. This reflection leads to the conclusion that to make quality improvement systems truly effective, we need once again to examine the status of the profession. Restoration or reinvigoration of professionalism is likely to prove to be the key to the next stage of quality improvement in Europe. In some ways this is a surprising conclusion given the general assumption of a trend in which patients and planners gain power at the expense of professionals, yet if professionals have little authority over the quality of care, they will have very little authority to share with others, and they will have only limited power to improve the quality.

In some countries, planners have already instituted programmes to improve leadership in health care institutions. This is an important step in revitalising the profession, but other steps are also needed. National colleges and associations need to consider reforms to strengthen their ability to promote a culture, provide standards and create self-esteem that make steady quality improvement a routine part of the GP's working life. Planners must also address the many pressures on GPs caused by increased demands, lack of resources and in some countries inadequate numbers of doctors and nurses. If the fundamental impediment to transforming the quality of care is the flagging energy of the profession, substantial progress cannot be expected until reforms such as these have been implemented. However, gradual but limited progress will still occur. Such developments will include progress in those countries that have not yet firmly established quality improvement programmes. They will have to decide to commit to necessary resources, and introduce regulations or laws that make quality improvement an integral component of systems to manage clinical care. Future developments in all countries are likely to include growing interest in patient safety and the avoidance of error, and the use of techniques to facilitate effective teamwork.

References

Baker, R. (1996). Characteristics of practices, general practitioners and patients related to levels of patients' satisfaction with consultations, *British Journal of General Practice*, **46**: 601–605.

Baker, R. (1997). Will the future GP remain a personal doctor? *British Journal of General Practice*, **47**: 831–834.

Baker, R. (2001). Principles of quality improvement. Part one – defining quality, *Journal of Clinical Governance*, **9**: 89–91.

Baker, R. and Grol, R. (2002). Principles and models for quality improvement, in Jones, R. (ed.) *Oxford Textbook of Primary Medical Care*. Oxford: Oxford University Press.

Baker, R., Preston, C., Cheater, F. and Hearnshaw, H. (1999). Measuring patients' attitudes to care across the primary/secondary interface: the patient career diary, *Quality in Health Care*, **8**: 154–160.

Basak, O. and Saatci, E. (1998). The developments of general practice/family medicine in Turkey, *European Journal of General Practice*, **4**: 126–129.

Bero, L., Grill, R. and Grimshaw, J.M. (1998). Closing the gap between research and practice: an overview of systematic reviews of interventions to promote implementation of research findings by health care professionals, *British Medical Journal*, **317**: 465–468.

Boland, M. (1991). My brother's keeper, *British Journal of General Practice*, **41**: 295–300.

Boland, M. and O'Riordan, M. (1999). A report from Ireland, *European Journal of General Practice*, **5**: 81–82.

Bower, P., Mead, N. and Roland, M. (2002). What dimensions underlie patient responses to the General Practice Assessment Survey? A factor analytic study, *Family Practice*, **19**: 489–495.

Buntinx, F., Winkens, R., Grol, R. *et al.* (1993). Influencing diagnostic and preventive performance in ambulatory care by feedback and reminders. A review, *Family Practice*, **10**: 219–228.

Department of Health (2003). *Investing in General Practice: The New General Medical Services Contract*. London: Department of Health. (http://www.dh.gov.uk/assetRoot/04/07/19/67/04071967.pdf, accessed 28 October 2004).

Donabedian, A. (1980). *Explorations in Quality Assessment and Monitoring. Vol. I: The Definition of Quality and Approaches to its Assessment*. Ann Arbor: Health Administration Press.

Doumenc, M. and Lafont, M. (1997). Practice evaluation: what's new in France? *European Journal of General Practice*, **3**: 161.

Eliasson, G., Berg, L., Carlsson, P., Lindstrom, K. and Bengtsson, C. (1998). Facilitating quality improvement in primary health care by practice visiting, *Quality in Health Care*, **7**: 48–54.

Elwyn, G., Rhydderch, M., Edwards, A. *et al.* (2004). Assessing organisational development in primary medical care using a group based assessment: the Maturity Matrix, *Quality and Safety in Health Care*, **13**: 287–94.

Geboers, H., Van der Horst, M., Mokkink, H. *et al.* (1999). Setting up improvement projects in small scale primary care practices: feasibility of a model for continuous quality improvement, *Quality in Health Care*, **8**: 36–42.

Gerlach, F. and Beyer, M. (1998). New concept for continuous documentation of development of quality circles in ambulatory care: initial results from an information system in Germany, *Quality in Health Care*, **7**: 55–61.

Gerlach, F. and Szecsenyi, J. (1997). A report from Germany, *European Journal of General Practice*, **3**: 32.

Gerlach, F. and Szecsenyi, J. (1998). Communication section, *European Journal of General Practice*, **4**: 171–172.

Gerlach, F.M., Beyer, M. and Romer, A. (1999). Quality circles in ambulatory care: state of development and future perspective in Germany, *International Journal for Quality in Health Care*, **10**: 35–42.

Glehr, R. (1997). Events in Austria, *European Journal of General Practice*, **3**: 78.

Glehr, R. (1999). An update from Austria, *European Journal of General Practice*, **5**: 165–166.

Goranov, M.N. and Balaskova, M.I. (1998). General practice in Bulgaria, *European Journal of General Practice*, **4**: 37–38.

Grol, R. and Wensing, M. (2000). *Patients evaluate general/family practice. The Europep instrument*. WOK, University of Nijmegen and Wonca/EQuiP.

Grol, R., Baker, R., Roberts, R. and Booth, B. (1997). Systems for quality improvement in general practice: A survey in 26 countries, *European Journal of General Practice*, **3**: 65–68.

Grol, R., Baker, R., Wensing, M. and Jacobs, A. (1994). Quality assurance in general practice: the state of the art in Europe, *Family Practice*, **11**: 460–467.

Grol, R. (1994). Quality improvement by peer review in primary care: a practical guide, *Quality in Health Care*, **3**: 147–152.

Grol, R., Wensing, M., Mainz, J. *et al.* (1999). Patients' priorities with respect to general practice care: an international comparison, *Family Practice*, **16**: 4–11.

Gudmundsson, G.H. and Mixa, O. (1998). A report from Iceland, *European Journal of General Practice*, **4**: 171.

Hearnshaw, H., Baker, R. and Cooper, A. (1998a). A survey of audit activity in general practice, *British Journal of General Practice*, **48**: 979–981.

Hearnshaw, H., Reddish, S., Peddie, D., Baker, R. and Robertson, N. (1998b). Introducing a quality improvement programme to primary health care teams, *Quality in Health Care* **7**: 200–208.

Hulscher, M.E.J.L., Wensing, M., Grol., R. *et al.* (1999). Interventions to improve the delivery of preventive services in primary care, *American Journal of Public Health*, **89**: 737–746.

Jack, B., Nagy, Z. and Varga, Z. (1997). Health care reform in central and eastern Europe. Family medicine in Hungary, *European Journal of General Practice*, **3**: 152–8.

Jensen, P.B. (1996). Progress in quality improvement in Denmark, *European Journal of General Practice*, **2**: 89–90.

Jurgova, E. (1998). The transposition of Slovak health care system and its influence on primary care services, *European Journal of General Practice*, **4**: 34–36.

Kersnik, J. (1997). Quality improvement in general practice in Slovenia, *European Journal of General Practice*, **3**: 110–111.

Kuenzi, B. and Egli, N. (1996). Progress from Switzerland, *European Journal of General Practice*, **2**: 134.

Kvamme, O.J., Olesen, F. and Samuelson, M. (2001). Improving the interface between primary and secondary care: a statement from the European Working Party on Quality in Family Practice (EQuiP), *Quality in Health Care*, **10**: 33–39.

Lancaster, T., Silagy, C., Fowler, G. *et al.* (1998). Training health professionals in smoking cessation, *The Cochrane Library*, 4.

Lawrence, M. and Olesen, F. (1997). Indicators of quality in health care, *European Journal of General Practice*, **3**: 103–108.

Lember, M. (1996). Revaluation of general practice/family medicine in the Estonian health care system, *European Journal of General Practice*, **2**: 72–73.

Macfarlane, F., Greenhalgh, T., Schofield, T. and Desombre, T. (2004). RCGP Quality Team Development programme: an illuminative evaluation, *Quality and Safety in Health Care*, **13**: 356–362.

Makela, M. (1996). Quality assurance in Finnish health care, *European Journal of General Practice*, **2**: 90–91.

Melander, E., Bjorgell, A., Bjorgell, P., Ovhed, I. and Molstad, S. (1999). Medical audit changes physicians' prescribing of antibiotics for respiratory tract infections, *Scandinavian Journal of Primary Health Care*, **17**: 180–184.

Munck, A.P., Gahm-Hansen, B., Sogaard, P. and Sogaard, J. (1999). Long-lasting improvement in general practitioners' prescribing of antibiotics by means of medical audit, *Scandinavian Journal of Primary Health Care*, **17**: 185–190.

Munck, A.P., Hansen, D.G., Lindman, A., Ovhed, I., Forre, S. and Torsteinsson, J.B. (1998). A Nordic collaboration on medical audit, *Scandinavian Journal of Primary Health Care*, **16**: 2–6.

National Primary Care Development Team (2004). *National Primary Care Development Team*. Manchester: National Primary Care Development Team (http://www.npdt.org/, accessed 24 January 2005).

NICE (2002). *Principles for Best Practice in Clinical Audit*. National Institute for Clinical Excellence. Abingdon: Radcliffe Medical Press.

Olesen, F. and Jensen, P.B. (1999). A report from Denmark, *European Journal of General Practice*, **5**: 38.

Persson, L. (1995). Activities in Sweden, *European Journal of General Practice*, **1**: 129.

Persson, L. (1997). A update on quality development in Sweden, *European Journal of General Practice*, **3**: 77.

Pisco, L. (1997). A report from Portugal, *European Journal of General Practice*, **3**: 32.

Plsek, P. (2001). Redesigning health care with insights from the science of complex adaptive systems. Appendix B in Institute of Medicine, *Crossing the Quality Chasm*. Washington, DC: National Academy Press, 309–322.

Polluste, K., Kalda, R. and Lember, M. (2000). Primary health care system in transition: the patient's experience, *International Journal of Quality in Health Care*, **12**: 503–509.

Rubin, G., George, A., Chinn, D.J. and Richardson, C. (2003). Errors in general practice development of an error classification and pilot study of a method for detecting errors, *Quality and Safety in Health Care*, **12**: 443–447.

Samuelson, M. (1999). A report from France, *European Journal of General Practice*, **5**: 37–8.

Solomon, D.H., Hashimoto, H., Daltroy, L. *et al.* (1998). Techniques to improve physicians' use of diagnostic tests. A new conceptual framework, *Journal of the American Medical Association*, **280**: 2020–2027.

Spies, T.H. and Mokkink, H.G.A. (1999). *Toetsen aan standaarden. Het medisch handelen van huisartsen in de praktijk getoetst*. Nijmegen/Utrecht: WOK/NHG.

Thomson, M.A., Oxman, A.D., Davis, D.A. *et al.* (1998). Outreach visits to improve health professional practice and health care outcomes, *The Cochrane Library*, 3.

Tiljak, H. (1998a). Quality assurance in GP/FM in Croatia, *European Journal of General Practice*, **4**: 88–89.

Tiljak, H. (1998b). An update from Croatia, *European Journal of General Practice*, **4**: 130.

Timmermans, A.E. and In't Veld, C.J. (2001). The implementation of guidelines in the Netherlands, *Zeitschrift für Artzliche Fortbildung und Qualitatitsicherung*, **95**: 719–724.

UEMO (1997). UEMO Statement on Quality Assurance in general practice (UEMO 94/055), in UEMO. *European Union of General Practitioners Reference Book* 1996/97, 28–30. London: Kensington Publications Ltd.

Wensing, M., Van der Weijden, T. and Grol, R. (1998). Implementing guidelines and innovations in general practice: which interventions are effective? *British Journal of General Practice*, **48**: 991–997.

Wensing, M., Vedstedt, P., Kersnik, J. *et al.* (2002). Patient satisfaction with availability of general practice: an international comparison, *International Journal of Quality in Health Care*, **14**: 111–118.

Windak, A. (1998). The return of old family doctors in the new Europe, *European Journal of General Practice*, **4**: 168–170.

Windak, A., Tomasik, T. and Kryj-Radziszewska, E. (1998). The Polish experience of quality improvement in primary care, *Joint Commission Journal on Quality Improvement*, **24**: 232–239.

Wood, D., De Backer, G., Faergeman, O., Graham, I., Mancia, G. and Pyorala, K. (1999). Prevention of coronary heart disease in clinical practice, *European Journal of General Practice*, **5**: 154–161.

Worrall, G., Chaulk, P. and Freake, D. (1997). The effects of clinical practice guidelines on patient outcomes in primary care: a systematic review, *Canadian Medical Association*, **156**: 1705–1712.

chapter twelve

The role of new information and communication technologies in primary care

Mårten Kvist and Michael Kidd

Introduction

Rapid technological advances have been continuous in medicine over the past century. In primary care, the impact of new technologies has been variable as these have often been coopted and harnessed by hospital-based clinicians. Since the 1960s, however, one domain of technological development has had rapidly increasing effects on the organization and provision of primary care: the development and implementation of clinically oriented information and communication technologies.

This chapter explores the impact of these new information and communication technologies in primary care. It begins by discussing principles of use of information and communication technology (ICT) and the consequences of its use in the clinical arena, by distinguishing between the "hard technologies" of clinical systems, as against the "soft technologies" of clinical practice. Recent policy debates in the domain of e-health have hypothesized the development of a "future patient", who harnesses the developments of the information age and accesses health care knowledge and practices on a global scale. The truth is always more mundane, so we begin our analysis by relating the principal "technology" of clinical practice – the structured encounter between clinician and patient – with the potential range of technological agents that might be brought into play. The shift to information technologies in primary care runs in parallel with two wider social shifts in the organization of medicine: one, the shift towards patient-centred clinical practice, and two, the move towards shared decision-making. Additionally, coordination of care, over time and across levels of provision, can also be improved by easier exchange of information, and this offers new opportunities for continuity of care. This leads to a discussion of information management tools (a) *within* the doctor-patient interaction in the encounter; (b) in providing *external input* for the benefit of the consultation within an episode and (c) as a tool in facilitating the *coordination* of primary care services across providers/levels of care.

This chapter goes further by discussing the role of electronic records, guidelines and decision support. It analyses the need for hardware and quality of the telecom infrastructure such as computers, networks and telematics. Professionals (but also patients) need to be prepared for the utilization of ICT and the consequences for their roles. These subjects are discussed in the section about education and training. There also will be a need for new legislation to enable further development without damaging safety and confidentiality of information. This issue is dealt with at the end of the chapter. Finally, some ICT-technologies are listed, which can provide better patient care when dealt with appropriately.

ICT and quality and coordination of care

An Australian Government report examined the role of information technology in quality health care (AHMAC, 1996). This report included the recommendations that:

1. *Information is central to improving health care safety and quality*. Routine feedback systems are required in order to inform health care workers of the outcomes of their care and to provide information to health care policy-makers and consumers in order to drive necessary changes in the health system.

2. *There is a mismatch between the use of technology to deliver care to people, and the use of technology to ensure that the care delivered is safe*. Preventable adverse reactions continue to occur despite the best endeavours of clinicians, administrators and government. Computerized decision support systems offer the potential to revolutionize safety through the use of alerts and prompts. They can also improve continuity of care by improving information flows between health care providers.

3. *The use of technology has risks*. Not only risks of possible breaches of confidentiality and privacy but also risks of failing to use technology in increasingly complex health care systems and the risk of potentially preventable injuries and deaths continuing to occur in health care systems if solutions are not found.

A major area of quality improvement has been in the use of computerized prescription packages. It has been clearly demonstrated that these can be used to provide the general practitioner with information about individual medications, access to clinical guidelines and warnings about potential contra-indications, adverse reactions and allergies. Computer generated prescriptions are legible and accurate. Moreover, the systems allow audits of prescribing for individual patients and for the practitioner's patient population.

Quality of health care in general practice also can be improved through the use of electronic medical management, computerized clinical decision support systems and improved information flows between general practice and the rest of the health care system.

The breadth of clinical knowledge necessary for safe, competent and current primary health care delivery is constantly expanding. Most clinicians now accept that we cannot carry all the facts we need in our heads. A cultural shift is evident as clinicians seek current information based on the best available evidence, attempt to access current clinical guidelines and treatment protocols, and look for answers to clinical questions arising during the consultation.

It is no coincidence that the culture of evidence-based medicine has emerged at the same time as the information technology revolution and especially at a time when the world's information resources have become available to everybody through the Internet. Computers provide possible solutions to many of the challenges posed by the advocates of evidence-based medicine. They have the potential to assist in planning the management of patients, in coordination of their care, in provision of professional continuing education and in the process of accessing the findings of clinical research. Computer-based assistance also can help make clinicians more efficient and effective health care providers if used carefully in the consultation (Purves, 1996). Information technology thus has the potential to be the cornerstone of the delivery of modern evidence-based primary care.

The role of electronic records, guidelines and decision support

The electronic patient record is a necessary tool for providing patient-centred and continuing health care safely and efficiently in the modern health care information environment (Heard *et al.*, 2000). Appropriate utilization of information about patient contacts in primary health care requires the use of electronic patient records.

The way in which data are introduced into electronic medical records must be structured to allow later data retrieval. Different coding systems have been developed for primary care in different parts of the world. The Read codes are in use in the United Kingdom. Sweden has developed its own coding system. The International Classification of Diseases, 10th edition (ICD-10) is used in many countries even if it is not the most appropriate system for primary health care.

Based on the recognized weaknesses of the ICD system for use in primary health care, the Classification Committee of WONCA (The World Organization of Family Doctors) developed a three-dimensional coding system called International Classification of Primary Care (ICPC). The second edition of this coding system, ICPC-2, was published in 1998 and is appropriate for coding reasons for encounters (RFE) between doctors and patients. The RFE coding can also be linked to diagnostic procedures, medications, therapeutic procedures and diagnoses.

The Transhis project in Japan, the Netherlands and Poland has been able to demonstrate the superiority of this classification for use in primary medical care (Okkes *et al.*, 2002). ICPC has been accepted as a coding standard in a number of

European countries, including Belgium, Denmark, France, the Netherlands, Norway, Portugal, and some parts of Finland.

GPs and their patients often express concern about the possible impact of the use of electronic patient records on the patient-doctor relationship. Is it possible to maintain as close a relationship when the doctor is often communicating with a computer during each consultation instead of exclusively paying attention to each individual patient? In practice this should not cause any real problem if each patient is informed about how the information is entered, if the doctor ensures that adequate time is spent communicating directly with the patient, and if the patient is engaged as a partner in the process. The use of computerized records may even increase the trust patients feel in the way in which such information can be utilized to lead to improvements in their health care.

One of the key skills which will be required of primary care clinicians will be the ability to access, assess, select and apply suitable treatment guidelines, adapted for local circumstances, and to communicate and record variations in the treatment plan from the guidelines (Coiera, 1998). However, there is a problem in getting clinical research findings and evidence-based medicine recommendations into daily clinical practice. One reason for this is that many clinicians find it difficult to gain rapid and timely access to the systematic reviews, evidence-based summaries and original scientific reports that may be relevant to the care of the individual patient in front of them.

Timely computer-based access to relevant knowledge is becoming a reality. Connection to the Internet means that, as new research findings are made and guidelines are adapted by learned bodies, the knowledge available to the clinician through the desktop computer could be continuously updated. Unfortunately there is still a problem with the consolidation of information into databases of systematic reviews and the preparation of guidelines for delivery through CD-ROM or web sites (Langley *et al.*, 1998).

Computerized clinical decision support delivered through the computer on the GP's desk may however offer a practical solution. It is believed that electronic decision support tools will soon become an increasingly integral component of high quality general practice (Kidd and Mazza, 2000). In the future a clinical decision support system will be able to compare patient characteristics with a credible knowledge base and then guide a clinician by offering patient-specific and situation-specific advice. By incorporating evidence-based guidelines, it is believed that the clinical decision-making process can be enhanced, thereby improving the quality of care.

At present, rudimentary computerized clinical decision support for medication management and preventive care is a reality for many GPs. The most popular clinical use of computers in general practice in many countries is for generating prescriptions. Users of computerized prescribing software programs in some countries will be familiar with systems of prompts for overdue preventive health interventions, and computer-generated cautions about potential contra-indications, adverse events or allergic reactions in relation to prescribing decisions (Nolan *et al.*, 1999). In many cases these prompts are based on elements of clinical practice guidelines for therapeutic management and preventive care.

Another important area for development and adoption in this field could well be the use of clinical decision support related to the interpretation of pathology and radiology test results. In many countries general practices are already connected online to their pathology providers and receive pathology results electronically. Soon computerized assistance in the interpretation of diagnostic results in relation to details in an individual patient's electronic medical record could start to take place and advice could be generated through prompts generated from appropriate clinical guidelines.

Chronic disease management poses a greater challenge. The electronic medical record is currently seen as an essential element in triggering the delivery of guidelines in chronic and acute disease management. As mentioned earlier there are impediments to realizing the full potential of the electronic patient record. In the United Kingdom for example there has been a significant problem in getting doctors to use the full electronic medical record, although much of the currently available research relates to past software which often lacked functionality and speed (Watkins *et al.*, 1999; Ellis and Kidd, 2000).

Whatever happens, the individual style of consultation of many doctors may well have to change if these features are to be utilized. Many GPs have long been aware that the computer is becoming somewhat of an imposition in the doctor-patient relationship and that it is impeding the flow of communication (Purves *et al.*, 1998). This situation will be exacerbated as more time and attention during consultations is paid to information on the computer screen at the expense of direct communication between doctor and patient.

Another key problem is that most clinical guidelines have not been developed in a format that allows for easy incorporation into computerized clinical decision support systems. It is not a simple matter of transferring paper-based guidelines into a computerized format (Purves, 1996). The whole process of guideline development may have to change if we are to match the information provided by the guideline with the decision-making processes of individual clinicians.

The need for supporting technologies: computers, networks and telematics

With the rapid evolution of information technology, huge possibilities have been identified for handling large amounts of data about the health care needs of populations. An EU working group was established in 1993 to identify how the applications of telematics to general practice, in the framework of primary health care, could be further developed in order to improve the quality of health care in Europe (De Maeseneer and Beolchi, 1994). In the United Kingdom the government decided in 1989 to start collecting financial data from all practices, which gave impetus to a rapid increase in the computerization of primary care. Surveys of general practice computing suggest that over 95% of practices in the United Kingdom now have computers (Gilles, 2000). The use of those computers for specific clinical and administrative tasks is much more variable.

In other countries, the use of computers is usually dependent on how primary care is organized (group practices or solo practices, the existence of a list system of patients, a national health insurance system, etc.). Even if computers are used in most practices in a certain country, the extent to which primary care staff use computers in their everyday work varies.

It is difficult to quantify the current clinical usage of computers in consultations. While some clinicians in a number of countries have full electronic medical records and are moving towards embracing the concept of "The Paperless Practice" (Ellis, 2001), others use their computers for one or more of a variety of clinical purposes. These include, among others, word processing reports and referral letters, electronic prescribing and medication management, decision support in chronic disease management, recall and prompting about preventive care interventions, access to electronic information resources, electronic connectivity to pathology and other service providers, and data collection and reporting to meet government requirements or financial imperatives.

Rates of computer use in primary care consultations also vary significantly between countries. In the European Survey of the Task Profiles of GPs, it was found that there was a big variation between 30 European countries in the percentage (0–74%) of all GPs using computers for patient records (Boerma and Fleming, 1998). While GPs in countries such as the United Kingdom, the Netherlands and Scandinavia have been early adopters, many colleagues in other parts of the world, and especially the United States, are still to adopt clinical computerization in large numbers. In a European survey on computer use it was found that there was a correlation between a better structured primary care system, with patient lists, gatekeeping by the GP, organization in group practices and higher computer use rate among GPs (Strobbe *et al.*, 1995).

In a study aimed to test the feasibility of deriving comparative quality indicators in 18 practices within a primary care group in the United Kingdom, the researchers made a retrospective audit using practice computer systems (McColl *et al.*, 2000). They found that it was possible to derive eight out of 26 indicators in all practices. It was concluded that practices will need greater conformity and compatibility of computer systems, improved computer skills for their staff, and appropriate funding in order to derive indicators.

Connecting computers together in an internal network within a practice creates the opportunity for increased sharing of information about patients between health professionals. Patient data can be stored as securely as in a paper archive. Linking computer networks by modems or data transmission using the Internet further increases the possibilities for sharing patient data with other health professionals in different locations but of course raises security and privacy concerns. Even the use of e-mails may speed up and increase the efficiency of many of the GPs' daily activities. It should be stressed, however that a network only presents a medium, while the content is composed of the messages transferred within that network (e.g. electronic guidelines). Sometimes these concepts are mixed, which results in confusion, because related requirements and obstacles are so different.

Easy access to the Internet can provide the clinician with immediate access to treatment guidelines, which may, or may not, be kept continuously up to date. A network in a group practice can provide access to shared CD-ROMs containing medical information. This may include manuals, evidence-based guidelines, drug formularies, picture collections of dermatological conditions, etc. Easy access to such guidelines at the time when they are really needed may improve clinician compliance with treatment guidelines (Young and Beswick, 1995; Mäkelä and Kunnamo, 2001).

Efficient use of new communication tools requires a sufficient degree of computerization among other health care providers and organizations. An ideal system would have all health workers who need to enter patient information with easy access to a computer preferably located in their immediate working environment. This may be on the GP's desktop, or mobile technology to allow for visits to hospitals and homes. If access is made more troublesome then it is more likely that information will be handled in more traditional ways. This will result in computerized records which may lack essential information about individual patients.

Howcroft and Mitev made an empirical case study in 2000 of Internet usage and difficulties among medical practice management in the UK. They reported results from interviews with 37 GPs and as a conclusion they found that the majority of GPs wanted local electronic links, particularly as regards secondary care. Given the existing levels of computerization, a surprising number of GPs failed to use Internet technology and saw little benefit from its use. Some GPs enthused about technology, while others were positively "techno phobic". Non-fundholding general practices in socially deprived areas were far less willing to embrace information management and technology. One explanation suggested for this is based on priorities: when faced with the option of 'cruising' the information superhighway, as opposed to treating seriously ill patients living in socially deprived areas, the former may simply be relegated as less important.

Telemedicine is by definition a science focused on the transmission of health information in an electronic network, but practically it has been focused on problems with transmission of both still and live pictures. When cameras are connected to computers, digital images can easily be transferred over the existing network to other destinations and be retrieved with the same quality as they were recorded. X-ray pictures have been transferred between hospitals and radiologists for more than 35 years. The same technique can also be used in primary care settings which have X-ray facilities but no consultant radiologist on site. There are considerable investments required in the essential infrastructure, and needs should be carefully assessed before purchasing expensive technology.

Accumulated experience from those centres which have introduced telemedicine technology reveals that in more than 50% of cases telemedicine has been used for educational purposes (Wootton, 2001). Time and travel costs can be saved for health professionals but increased efforts are needed in preparing for educational events mediated as videoconferences. In some instances the transmission of live pictures can be slow and the pictures distorted. This problem can be eliminated by using rapid data transmission lines.

Since 1995, Queen's University, Northern Ireland, has organized real-time teledermatology consultations using videoconferencing for a number of primary health care institutions and the results have been impressive (Loane, 1999). This example has later been followed by others, for example in Nottingham (Lawton *et al.*, 2004).

All disciplines where images play an important role in the diagnostic process can use telemedicine. When the video-cable is moved from a camera to a microscope or to endoscopic equipment, live pictures can easily be transmitted from the general practice to a consultant located far away. Over the last decade there have been developments in teleradiology, teledermatology, telepathology, teleorthopaedics, telesurgery and teleophthalmology (Kvist, 1996; Lamminen and Nevalainen, 1999; Gonzales *et al.*, 2001). Telepsychiatry is a field with huge opportunities and good results have been demonstrated in many studies (Mielonen *et al.*, 1998; Gammon, 1999).

Studies on the interpretation differences between radiologists assessing real film pictures and screen pictures, scanned and transferred to remote sites and assessed on a computer screen, have shown good correlation (Krupinski *et al.*, 1996). Theoretically, if the pictures are taken initially with digitized X-ray equipment there should be no difference in quality as the identical information is available at the remote site. The trend is toward digitized X-ray equipment where no film is actually needed. However, the high cost of such equipment will still result in normal X-ray equipment as a required alternative for group practices of limited size.

In Finland the first demonstration of telegastroscopy was performed in 1995 with the consulting physician 900 kilometres away from the patient, providing immediate feedback about the status of the gastric mucosa and the best location for a possible biopsy (Kvist, 1995). In cases where gastroscopies are performed by clinicians with insufficient experience (less than 100–300 procedures), the addition of a telemedicine consultation with a more experienced clinician, or training with an endoscopic simulator, can make this a more reliable method of investigation (Bar-Meir, 2001).

All endoscopies are examples illustrating where telemedicine may add value to procedures performed in primary care. Experiments with distance ultrasound diagnostics of the upper abdomen have shown that it is possible to use it for these purposes too (Kormano, 1995). In a pilot study in northern Norway a GP was provided with the necessary equipment to carry out otorhinolaryngological consultations using telemedicine connections. This clinician's skills have increased and many patients have avoided the need to travel 700 km to the nearest university clinic (Pedersen *et al.*, 1999).

The cost-effectiveness of telemedicine services still needs to be fully evaluated. Taking into account the necessary investments in new technology it appears that for regular clinical use there may be little, if any, savings of health care resources. However, patients may benefit from significant savings in travel time to specialists or reduction in delays between the initial presentation of symptoms and the time when a correct diagnosis can be made and appropriate treatment initiated.

The Internet has arrived at the same time as health consumers are starting to seriously question the traditional doctor-patient relationship and to play a greater role in the management of their own health care (Jadad, 1999; Eysenback, 2000). If GPs are to continue to be the trusted cornerstone of health care delivery in each of our countries, they will need to start to adapt to the changing expectations of their patients and the use of the Internet by patients as a tool for health care.

Internet visionary Nicholas Negroponte wrote: 'On the Internet, no-one need know you're a dog' (Negroponte, 1995). Anyone can establish a web site on a health related topic and claim to be an expert. The Internet is littered with potentially dangerous sites, and patients need to be wary of all information gained through it. As do their GPs. It is up to each individual to make a judgement about the quality of a site. One needs to scrutinize the source of the information. 'Can I trust the information on this site? Can I trust the author? Do their qualifications and affiliations sound genuine? Is this information current?'

Many consumer groups and medical organizations and professional bodies offer links to sites which they have evaluated and believe will be of benefit to their members and other visitors to their own home pages. There may well be a place for the home page of each general practice to become the portal to useful and validated information on the Internet, specifically chosen for their patient population. One online survey showed that 50% of respondents would be interested in using a web site operated by their own doctor's office (Pyke, 1999).

One of the more recent challenges for GPs is the patient who presents with information gained from a search of the Internet. This seems to be particularly relevant for people with chronic health problems who may have a degree of dissatisfaction with some aspect of their current health care management. One approach is to try to determine what has motivated this person to bring in this information, and what concerns led to this fact-finding mission (Kidd, 2001).

It is also becoming apparent that many patients would like to communicate with their doctors online. Cyberconsultations, consulting with patients through e-mail or the Internet, represent a challenge to traditional methods of clinical care delivery. E-mail could be used by patients to request the results of pathology and radiology tests, to request repeat prescriptions or letters of referral, or to ask questions which arise after a consultation has ended.

E-mail communication does, however, carry some risks. Just as GPs have developed methods for handling telephone-based consultations with patients, they will also have to develop ways of handling requests for information received via the Internet. There are risks to the security of personalized health information sent by e-mail. There are risks if patients misinterpret information provided to them by e-mail. There are risks that doctors will end up with a large volume of unpaid extra computer work.

This poses additional challenges to the doctor-patient relationship. Each e-mail message to a patient becomes a legal document. It is possible that e-mail, through the creation of a "virtual relationship" which did not previously exist, could create a duty of care relationship where the doctor did not intend to create one. It is possible that doctors could find themselves with increased responsibility to respond to enquiries that they might otherwise have not been able to receive. Delays in response may bring added risks for patients (Kidd *et al.*, 2002).

However, these developments may also revolutionize health care delivery. In the place of discrete episodic visits to the doctor, contact and management advice may be able to be delivered in a continuous and ongoing manner. This could become a powerful clinical tool with the added ability for home monitoring and Internet-based transmission of vital signs and home pathology results. The role of the GP could become even more central in the management of many chronic health care problems. True continuity of care could become a reality as the GP's computer system allows the doctor to keep track of the care of individual patients on a daily basis.

For health care managers a new technology has recently been made available on Internet for managers of Primary Care Trusts. Web-based interactive maps of PCT star ratings are accessible for all managers, who want to compare the performance of their trust with the corresponding results of other trusts. By acting as an enhanced alternative or supplement to purely textual online interfaces, interactive web maps can further empower organizations and decision-makers (Boulos, 2004).

Education and training

Education and training of the clinical workforce are essential if new technologies are to be successfully incorporated in general practice and have an impact on clinical care. Many authors have addressed the need to include training about information technology in clinical education programmes and have outlined ways of educating health care workers and students on how to use information technology in their daily clinical practice (Hardy et al., 1996; Carlile and Sefton, 1998; Lawson et al., 1998; Kidd and McPhee, 1999). Unfortunately many health care professionals find that current education about the use of computers in health care can be dry and not very appealing, especially if the emphasis is on the technology, rather than its applications in clinical care. Working through clinical scenarios and identifying the information issues and their personal implications for learners can be far more effective education strategies (National Health Service, 1997). However, education solely about basic computer use is not sufficient for health care professionals. Clinicians also need to be equipped with advanced skills in information management if they are going to be able to meet the challenges of evidence-based medicine, provide truly coordinated care and tackle the problems associated with information overload.

It has been argued that education about information technology for health care workers requires a three-pronged approach (Koschmann, 1995). Clinicians need to learn about computers (i.e. their potential applications in health care). They need to learn through computers (i.e. how to use the technology to receive continuing education). Most powerfully, they need to learn with computers (i.e. through using this technology as part of their daily work, and through using its features to assist them to identify and meet their educational needs while working).

The National Health Service in the United Kingdom has produced recommendations for health informatics training in the education of their clinicians (National Health Service, 1999). These recommendations identify common elements across clinical practice relevant to all health care workers and provide advice on education strategies. The eight elements addressed are communication, knowledge management, data quality and management, confidentiality and security, secondary uses of clinical data and information, clinical and service audit, working clinical systems and telemedicine and telecare. The recommendations also provide a list of ten basic computing skills that are required by all health care professionals (Figure 12.1)

A more clinically targeted list of essential clinical informatics skills (Coiera,

Figure 12.1   Ten basic computing skills for health care professionals

1. Organize electronic information (e.g. naming documents, setting up directories, moving files, renaming files);
2. Use a word-processing package to generate simple documents;
3. Enter and manipulate data using a spreadsheet;
4. Search a simple database;
5. Undertake searches and access relevant sites on the World Wide Web and relevant health-related databases;
6. Retrieve/download electronic documents from various sources and transfer data from one application to another;
7. Explain the reasons for electronic networking and give examples of its use in health care;
8. Send, retrieve and acknowledge e-mails and attachments;
9. Identify examples of the use of information technology as an effective tool in the delivery and management of health care;
10. Evaluate the effective use of information systems in the National Health Service. Discuss why different examples should be paper-based or electronic.

Source: National Health Service (1999).

1998) has been recommended for health care professionals in Australia (Figure 12.2).

Together these recommendations can form the basis for an informatics education curriculum for GPs and other primary health care workers.

Legal aspects and data safety

The introduction of new technology can also face barriers when conflicts arise with existing legislation in individual countries. In some cases legislation has not foreseen or kept up to date with the developments taking place in clinical care. A transfer to completely paper-free records may not be legally possible without revision of existing legislation in some countries. The same rules apply to the storage of X-ray images. The data of these huge picture files may cause problems and necessitate new approaches to archiving. While technical solutions are often available, considerable investment may also often be required. A requirement of health authorities is that, from a legal point of view, it should be possible to audit all changes which have been made to original records both by date, content and provider. There are technical solutions to these problems.

New ways of interacting with patients using telemedicine or through the Internet can pose other legislative challenges. These new consultations can transcend traditional geographic boundaries and it is possible to consult with patients in other parts of the same country or across international borders. These innovations do not sit easily where legal and regulatory systems are often

Figure 12.2 Ten essential clinical informatics skills

1. Understand the dynamic and uncertain nature of medical knowledge, and be able to keep personal knowledge and skills up to date;
2. Know how to search for and assess knowledge according to the statistical basis of scientific evidence;
3. Understand some of the logical and statistical models of the diagnostic process;
4. Interpret uncertain clinical data and deal with artefact and error;
5. Structure and analyse clinical decisions in terms of risks and benefits;
6. Apply and adapt clinical knowledge to the individual circumstances of patients;
7. Access, assess, select and apply a treatment guideline, adapt it to local circumstances, and communicate and record variations in treatment plans and outcome;
8. Structure and record clinical data in a form appropriate for the immediate clinical task, for communication with colleagues, or for epidemiological purposes;
9. Select and operate the most appropriate communication method for a given task (e.g. face-to-face conversation, telephone, e-mail, video, voice-mail, letter);
10. Structure and communicate messages in a manner most suited to the recipient, task and chosen communication medium.

Source: Coiera (1998).

very 'jurisdiction-specific', and it is assumed that clinical service delivery has taken place in the 'traditional' face-to-face manner.

It is apparent that the introduction of ICT systems can 'raise the bar' of expectations, especially around privacy, security and confidentiality of personal health information. There are, as yet, few established legal principles, but the application of 'first principles' will give some preliminary guidance. These principles demonstrate that 'the bottom line' is whether or not a professional has exercised 'reasonable' care. The computer is likely to be regarded as a tool. Like all other tools, professionals who choose to use ICT will be expected to know how to use such tools safely.

GPs may find themselves legally exposed if they rely on an electronic clinical decision support tool that 'leads them astray'. It is possible that patient harm could be caused by the use of high technology tools. In such an event, users may complain that the technology was faulty, misleading or confusing. The manufacturer could respond that user error was to blame.

Conversely clinicians may – in the not too distant future – find themselves legally exposed if they fail to use appropriate electronic clinical decision support tools and computerized patient record systems. Community and legal expectations are likely to change as technology becomes more widespread and accepted as 'best' clinical practice. Clinicians may find themselves being criticized if they turn off decision support tools with drug-drug interaction information, or if they fail to access best practice guidelines known to be available on the Internet (Milstein and Togno, 2001).

The reorganization of the NHS in England into 303 Primary Care Trusts in 2002 increased expectations, that they could be powerful agents for change in a more devolved, clinically driven and locally responsive NHS. There is, however, a growing belief that these trusts have failed to fulfil these expectations, and that the organizations are perhaps ineffective. Further reorganization would reduce the number of primary care trusts to about 100–150 across England. Thus, the organizational restructuring seems to promote a change back towards the size of the original units, from which the trusts were originally created. The wave-like change of organizational structures has stressed the importance of well-functioning communication technology in public health networks, but there is no definitive evidence that structural reorganization of Primary Care Trusts would be of benefit to patients (Fahey *et al.*, 2003; Walshe *et al.*, 2004).

Conclusions

ICT offer good opportunities to further develop a coordinative role in primary health care. The use of new information and telecommunication technologies within the primary care consultation may extend its reach and make its boundaries more permeable. The widespread use of e-mail and the Internet by "information literate" patients may reshape doctor-patient interaction, but it brings in its wake problems of quality control relating to information, and of licensing and liability. If the boundaries of doctor-patient interaction are made permeable by the Internet and e-mail, they are also reshaped by new communications systems within health care organizations themselves, in particular telemedicine. These technologies do not simply change the procedures by which information moves through health care systems, but they also impact upon the professional identities of the clinicians that use them.

The proliferation and expansion of new technologies in primary health care draws into view not only a "future patient", but also a "future clinician". New technologies confront clinicians with new ethical questions about safety and liability, privacy and evidence, and the globalization of medical knowledge and clinical practice. We are moving toward an ICT-based practice with special conditions and requirements.

As clinical computer use in general practice becomes more widespread, evidence of the quality benefits is being accumulated. Systematic reviews of trials on the effects of computer-based clinical decision support systems on physician performance have been shown to improve antibiotic prescribing, drug dosing, preventive care and other aspects of primary medical care (Sullivan and Mitchell, 1995; Balas *et al.*, 1996; Pestonik *et al.*, 1996; Baker, 1997; Beilby and Silagy, 1997; Hunt *et al.*, 1998; Mitchell and Sullivan, 2001). Good knowledge of these opportunities offered by the ICT technology, are necessary if the future GP is going to be in the primary care driver's seat.

Conditions for an ICT-based primary care are:

- continuity of care/patient and doctor knowing each other;
- practice organization/scale of practice;
- financing/insurance system;
- cooperation between primary and secondary care;
- staff skills;
- compatible systems/software in own language/availability of coding and classification systems;
- legislation;
- infrastructure;
- well-developed professional infrastructure (CME, guideline production);
- informed patients.

References

AHMAC (Australian Health Ministers' Advisory Council) (1996) Taskforce on Quality in Australian Health Care of the Australian Health. Canberra: Department of Health and Aged Care, Australia.

Baker, R. (1997). Review: computerized reminders increase the rate of use of most preventive services, *ACP Journal Club* **126**(3): 80.

Balas, E.A., Austin, S.M., Mitchell, J.A., Ewigman, B.G., Bopp, K.D., Brown, G.D. (1996). The clinical value of computerized information services: a review of 98 randomized clinical trials, *Archives of Family Medicine* **5**(5): 271–278.

Bar-Meir, S. (2001). Training models – why and how, in *Poster Abstracts from the Falk Symposium on Medical Imaging in Gastroenterology and Hepatology*, in Hannover, Germany, 28–29.9, 19. www.falkfoundation.com/pdf/FS124-Internet.pdf.

Beilby, J.J. and Silagy, C.A. (1997). Trials of providing costing information to general practitioners: a systematic review, *Medical Journal of Australia* **167**(2): 89–92.

Boerma, W.G.W. and Fleming, D.M. (1998). *The Role of General Practice in Primary Health Care*. London: World Health Organization.

Boulos, K.M.N. (2004). Web GIS in practice: an interactive geographical interface to English Primary Care Trust performance ratings for 2003 and 2004, *International Journal of Health Geographics* **3**(1): 16.

Carlile, S. and Sefton, A.J. (1998). Healthcare and the information age: implications for medical education, *Medical Journal of Australia* **168**: 340–343.

Coiera, E. (1998). Medical informatics meets medical education, *Medical Journal of Australia* **168**: 319–320.

De Maeseneer, J. and Boelchi, L. (1994). Telematics in primary health care: a concerted action (AIM-PRIMACARE A 2015), *Computer Methods and Programs in Biomedicine* **45**: 145–147.

Ellis, N. (2001). *Going Paperless: A Guide to Computerisation in Primary Care*. Abingdon: Radcliffe Medical Press.

Ellis, N. and Kidd, M.R. (2000). What lessons can Australia learn from the computerisation of General Practice in the United Kingdom? *Medical Journal of Australia* **172**: 22–24.

Eysenback, G. (2000). Consumer health informatics, *British Medical Journal* **320**: 1713–1716.

Fahey, D.K., Carson, E.R., Cramp, D.G. and Muir Gray, J.A. (2003). User requirements and understanding of public health networks in England, *Journal of Epidemiology and Community Health* **57**(12): 938–944.

Gammon, D. (1999). Telepsychiatry in Norway, in Wootton, R. (ed.) *European Telemedicine 1998/1999*. London: Kensington Publications Ltd, 89–90.

Gilles, A. (2000). Information support for general practice in the new NHS, *Health Libraries Review* **17**: 91–96.

Gonzales, F., Iglesias, R., Suarez, A., Gomez-Ulla, F. and Perz, R. (2001). Teleophtalmology link between primary health care centre and a reference hospital, *Med Inform Internet Med* **26**(4): 251–263.

Hardy, J.L., Conrick, M., Foster, J., McGuiness, B. and Bostock, E. (1996). Computerised education for health professionals, in Hovenga, E., Kidd, M. and Cesnik, B. (eds), *Health Informatics: An Overview*. Melbourne: Churchill Livingstone.

Heard, S., Givel, T., Schloeffel, P. and Doust, J. (2000). The benefits and difficulties of introducing a national approach to electronic health records in Australia. Report to the electronic health records taskforce. Adelaide: Commonwealth Department of Health and Aged Care.

Howcroft, D. and Mitev, N. (2000). An empirical study of Internet usage and difficulties among medical practice management in the UK, *Internet Research: Electronic Networking Applications and Policy* **10**: 170–181.

Hunt, D.L., Haynes, R.B., Hanna, S.E. and Smith, K. (1998). Effects of computer-based clinical decision support systems on physician performance and patient outcomes – a systematic review, *Journal of the American Medical Association*, **280**(15): 1339–1346.

Jadad, A.R. (1999). Promoting partnerships: challenges for the internet age, *British Medical Journal*, **319**: 761–764.

Kidd, M.R. (2001). General practice and consumers on the Internet, *Australian Family Physician* **4** .

Kidd, M.R. and Mazza, D. (2000). Clinical practice guidelines and the computer on your desk, *Medical Journal of Australia* **173**: 373–375.

Kidd, M.R. and McPhee, W. (1999). The "Lost Generation": IT education for healthcare professionals, *Medical Journal of Australia* **171**: 510–511.

Kidd, M.R., Milstein, B. and Togno, J. (2002). The computer on your desk: new roles, new rules and new challenges for general practice, *New Zealand Family Physician* **29**(4): 226–228. (http://www.rnzcgp.org.nz/NZFP/Issues/Aug2002/Kidd-August-02.pdf, accessed 17 February 2004).

Kormano, M. (1995). Presentation at the National Conference in Telemedicine, Turku, Finland, 24–25 October.

Koschmann, T. (1995). Medical education and computer literacy: learning about, through, and with computers, *Academic Medicine*, **70**(9): 818–821.

Krupinski, E.A., Weinstein, R.S. and Rozek, L.S. (1996). Experience-related differences in diagnosis from medical images displayed on monitors, *Telemedicine Journal* **2**: 101–108.

Kvist, M. (1995). Telemedicine. Presentation at the Annual Medical Conference, Helsinki, Finland, 11 January.

Kvist, M. (1996). Telemedicine applications in Finland 1996. Helsinki: National Agency for Welfare and Health; FinOHTA publication No 2. (http://www.stakes.fi/finohta/e/reports/002/r002f.html, accessed 17 February 2004).

Lamminen, H. and Nevalainen, J. (1999). Telemedicine in orthopaedics, in Wootton, R. (ed.) *European Telemedicine 1998/1999*. London: Kensington Publications Ltd, 93–96.

Langley, C., Faulkner, A., Watkins, C., Gray, S., and Harvey, I. (1998). Use of guidelines in primary care – practitioners' perspectives, *Family Practice* **15**: 105–111.

Lawson, K., Armstrong, R. and Van der Weyden, M. (1998). A sea change in Australian medical education, *Medical Journal of Australia* **169**: 653–658.

Lawton, S., English, J., McWilliam, J., Wildgust, L. and Patel, R. (2004). Development of a district-wide teledermatology service, *Nursing Times* **100**(14): 38–41.

Loane, M. (1999). Real/time dermatology, in Wootton, R. (ed.) *European Telemedicine 1998/ 1999*. London: Kensington Publications Ltd, 76–78.

Mäkelä, M. and Kunnamo, I. (2001). Implementing evidence in Finnish primary care. Use of electronic guidelines in daily practice, *Scandinavian Journal of Primary Health Care* **19**(4): 214–217.

McColl, A., Roderick, P. and Smith, H. *et al.* (2000). Clinical governance in primary care groups: the feasibility of deriving evidence-based performance indicators, *Quality in Health Care* **9**: 90–97.

Mielonen, M-L., Ohinmaa, A., Moring, J. and Isohanni, M. (1998). The use of videoconferencing for telepsychiatry in Finland, *Journal of Telemedicine and Telecare* **4**: 125–131.

Milstein, B. and Togno, J. (2001). *Legal Issues in General Practice Computerisation*. Barton: General Practice Computing Group. (http://www.gpcg.org/publications/docs/ projects2001/GPCG_Project22_01.pdf, accessed 17 February 2004).

Mitchell, E., and Sullivan, F. (2001). A descriptive feast but an evaluative famine: systematic review of published articles on primary care computing during 1980–97, *British Medical Journal* **322**: 279–282.

National Health Service (1997). *Approaches for informatics in postgraduate medical and dental education: an account from four national pilot sites. National Health Service Education and Training Program in Information Management and Technology for Clinicians*. London: NHS.

National Health Service (1999). *Learning to Manage Health Information*. Bristol: National Health Service Executive.

Negroponte, N. (1995). *Being Digital*. New York: Knopf.

Nolan, A., Norquay, C., Dartnell, J., and Harvey, K. (1999). Electronic prescribing and computer-assisted decision support systems, *Medical Journal of Australia* **171**(10): 541–543.

Okkes, I.M., Polderman, G.O., Fryer, G.E. *et al.* (2002). The role of family practice in different health care systems: a comparison of reasons for encounter, diagnoses, and interventions in primary care populations in the Netherlands, Japan, Poland, and the United States, *The Journal of Family Practice* **51**: 72. (www.jfponline.com/content/ 2002/01/jfp_0102_00072.asp, accessed 17 February 2002).

Pedersen, S., Haga, D. and Arild, E. (1999). Tele-otorhinolaryngology (tele-ENT), in Wootton, R. (ed.) *European Telemedicine 1998/1999*. London: Kensington Publications Ltd.

Pestonik, S.L., Classen, D.C., Scott Evans, R. and Burke, J.P. (1996). Implementing antibiotic practice guidelines through computer-assisted decision support: clinical and financial outcomes, *Annals of Internal Medicine* **124**(10): 884–890.

Purves, I. (1996). Facing future challenges in general practice: a clinical method with computer support, *Family Practice* **13**(6): 536–543.

Purves, I., Nestor, G. and Williams, K. (1998). Testing of PRODIGY continues, *British Medical Journal* **316**: 776.

Pyke, B. (1999). The rise of the Internet health consumer: impacts of the Internet on the doctor-patient relationship. (http://www.cyberdialogue.com/pdfs/wp/wp-cch-1999-doctors.pdf, accessed 19 February 2004).

Strobbe, J., De Maeseneer, J. and Ceenaeme, R. (1995). A picture of primary health care in Europe, in de Maeseneer, J. and Beolchi, L. (eds) *Telematics in Primary Care in Europe*. Amsterdam: IOS Press.

Sullivan, F. and Mitchell, E. (1995). Has general practitioner computing made a difference to patient care? A systematic review of published reports, *General Practice* **311**: 848–852.

Walshe, K., Smith, J., Dixon, J. *et al.* (2004). Primary care trusts. Premature reorganisation, with mergers, may be harmful, *British Medical Journal*, **329**: 871–872.

Watkins, C., Harvey, I., Langley, C., Gray, S. and Faulkner, A. (1999). General practitioners' use of guidelines in the consultation and their attitudes to them, *British Journal of General Practice* **49**: 11–15.

Wootton, R. (2001). Recent advances: telemedicine, *British Medical Journal* **323**: 557–560.

Young, A. and Beswick, K. (1995). Protocols used by UK general practitioners, what is expected of them and what solutions are provided, *Computer Methods and Programs in Biomedicine* **48**: 85–90.

Key references for further reading

1. www.globalfamilydoctor.com (web site of WONCA, The World Organization of Family Doctors, featuring links to many useful resources for primary medical care providers).
2. www.gpcg.org (web site of the General Practice Computing Group, the peak national organization for primary medical care computing in Australia, featuring resources targeted to the needs of general practitioners involved in the computerization of the consultation).
3. www.imia.org (web site of the International Medical Informatics Association with links to resources which promote informatics in health care and biomedical research).
4. www.phcsg.org.uk (web site of The Primary Health Care Specialist Group of the British Computer Society with a link to *The Journal of Primary Care Informatics*).
5. www.amia.org (web site of the American Medical Informatics Association with links to *The Journal of the American Medical Informatics Association*, a peer-reviewed journal published bimonthly containing articles about all aspects of medical informatics).
6. www.fimnet.fi/telemedicine/index2.html (web site of the Finnish Society of Telemedicine with useful links to telemedicine web sites).
7. www.americantelemed.org (web site of the American Telemedicine Association).

Acknowledgements

This chapter draws on the following previous publications of the authors:

Kidd, M.R. (2001). General practice and consumers on the Internet, *Australian Family Physician* 4.

Kidd, M.R., Milstein, B. and Togno, J. (2002). The computer on your desk: new roles, new rules and new challenges for general practice. *New Zealand Family Physician* 29(4): 226–228 (http://www.rnzcgp.org.nz/NZFP/Issues/Aug2002/Kidd-August-02.pdf, accessed 17 February 2004).

Kidd, M.R. and Mazza, D. (2000). Clinical practice guidelines and the computer on your desk, *Medical Journal of Australia* 173: 373–375.

Kidd, M.R. and McPhee, W. (1999). The "Lost Generation": IT education for healthcare professionals, *Medical Journal of Australia* 171: 510–511.

Kvist, M. (1991). Telephone contacts in Finnish urban general practice [Dissertation]. Turku University Publication, series D, No. 71, Turku.

Kvist, M. (1996). Telemedicine applications in Finland 1996. Helsinki: National Agency for Welfare and Health, 1996; FinOHTA publication No. 2 (http://www.stakes.fi/finohta/e/reports/002/r002f.html, accessed 15 March 2004).

Index

Page numbers in *italics* refer to tables; in chapter 2 the location of figures is indicated by cross references in the relevant text.

Related books from Open University Press

Purchase from www.openup.co.uk or order through your local bookseller

SOCIAL HEALTH INSURANCE SYSTEMS IN WESTERN EUROPE

Richard B. Saltman, Reinhard Busse and Josep Figueras (eds)

- What are the characteristics that define a Social Health Insurance system?
- How is success measured in SHI systems?
- How are SHI systems developing in response to external pressures?

Using the seven Social Health Insurance countries in western Europe – Austria, Belgium, France, Germany, Luxembourg, the Netherlands and Switzerland – as well as Israel, this important book reviews core structural and organizational dimensions, as well as recent reforms and innovations.

Covering a wide range of policy issues, the book:

- Explores the pressures these health systems confront to be more efficient, more effective, and more responsive
- Reviews their success in addressing these pressures
- Examines the implications of change on the structure of SHI's as they are currently defined
- Draws out policy lessons about past experience and likely future developments in SHI systems in a manner useful to policymakers in Europe and elsewhere

Social Health Insurance Systems in Western Europe will be of interest to students of health policy and management as well as health managers and policy-makers.

Contributors
Helmut Brand, Jan Bultman, Reinhard Busse, Laurent Chambaud, David Chinitz, Diana M.J. Delnoij, André P. den Exter, Aad A. de Roo, Anna Dixon, Isabelle Durand-Zaleski, Hans F.W. Dubois, Josep Figueras, Bernhard Gibis, Stefan Greß, Bernhard J. Güntert, Jean Hermesse, Maria M. Hofmarcher, Martin McKee, Pedro W. Koch-Wulkan, Claude Le Pen, Kieke G.H. Okma, Martin Pfaff, Richard B. Saltman, Wendy G.M. van der Kraan, Jürgen Wasem, Manfred Wildner, Matthias Wismar.

Contents
*List of contributors – Introduction – Foreword – Acknowledgements – **Part One – Social health insurance in perspective: the challenge of sustaining stability** – The historical and social base of social health insurance systems – Organization and financing of social health insurance systems: current status and recent policy developments – Patterns and performance in social health insurance systems – Assessing social health insurance systems: present and future policy issues – **Part Two – The challenge to solidarity** – Governance and (self-)regulation in social health insurance systems – Solidarity and competition in social health insurance countries – Key organizational issues – Shifting Criteria for benefit decisions in social health insurance systems – Contracting and paying providers in social health insurance systems – The role of private health insurance in social health insurance countries – The changing role of the individual in social health insurance systems – Beyond acute care – Prevention and public health in social health insurance systems – Long-term care in social health insurance systems – Index.*

328pp   0 335 21363 4 (Paperback)   0 335 21364 2 (Hardback)

HEALTH POLICY AND EUROPEAN UNION ENLARGEMENT

Martin McKee, Laura MacLehose and Ellen Nolte (eds)

European national policy makers broadly agree on the core objectives that their health care system should pursue. The list is straightforward: universal access for all citizens, effective care for better health outcomes, efficient use of resources, and high quality services responsive to patients' concerns. It is a formula that resonates across the political spectrum and which, in various, sometimes inventive configurations, has played a role in most recent European national election campaigns.

While there may be consensus on the broader issues, expectations differ between EU countries, and, with the enlargement of 2004, matters become more complex. This book seeks to assess the impact of the enlargement process and to analyse the challenges that lie ahead in the field of health and health policy. Written by leading health policy analysts, the book investigates a host of areas including:

- health care investment
- international recruitment of nurses and doctors
- health and safety
- communicable disease control
- European pharmaceutical policy

Health Policy and European Union Enlargement will be of interest to students of health policy, economics, public policy and management, as well as health managers and policy makers.

Contents
Health and enlargement – The process of enlargement – Health status and trends in candidate countries – Health and health care in the candidate countries to the European Union: Common challenges, different circumstances, diverse policies – Investing in health for accession – Integration of East Germany into the EU: Investment and health outcomes – The challenges of the free movement of health professionals – Free movement of health professionals: The Polish experience – The market for physicians – Not from our own backyard? The United Kingdom, Europe and international recruitment of nurses – Free movement of patients – Closing the gap: Health and safety – Communicable disease control: Detecting and managing communicable disease outbreaks across borders – Free Trade versus the protection of health: The examples of alcohol and tobacco – Opportunities for inter-sectoral health improvement in new Member States – the case for health impact assessment – European pharmaceutical policy and implications for current Member States and candidate countries – Lessons from Spain: Accession, pharmaceuticals and intellectual property rights – Looking beyond the new borders: Stability Pact countries of south-east Europe and accession and health – Index

312pp   0 335 21353 7 (paperback)   0 335 21354 5 (hardback)

HUMAN RESOURCES FOR HEALTH IN EUROPE

Carl-Ardy Dubois, Martin McKee, and Ellen Nolte

Health service human resources are key determinants of health service performance. The human resource is the largest and most expensive input into healthcare, yet it can be the most challenging to develop. This book examines some of the major challenges facing health care professions in Europe and the potential responses to these challenges.

The book analyses how the current regulatory processes and practices related to key aspects of the management of the health professions may facilitate or inhibit the development of effective responses to future challenges facing health care systems in Europe. The authors document how health care systems in Europe are confronting existing challenges in relation to the health workforce and identify the strategies that are likely to be most effective in optimizing the management of health professionals in the future.

Human Resources for Health in Europe is key reading for health policy-makers and postgraduates taking courses in health services management, health policy and health economics. It is also of interest to human resource professionals.

Contributors
Carl Afford, Rita Baeten, James Buchan, Anna Dixon, Carl-Ardy Dubois, Sigrún Gunnarsdóttir, Yves Jorens, Elizabeth Kachur, Karl Krajic, Suzy Lessof, Ann Mahon, Alan Maynard, Martin McKee, Ellen Nolte, Anne Marie Rafferty, Charles Shaw, Bonnie Sibbald, Ruth Young.

Contents
Foreword – Human resources for health in Europe – Analysing trends, opportunities and challenges – Migration of health workers in Europe: policy problem or policy solution? – Changing professional boundaries – Structures and trends in health profession education in Europe – Managing the performance of health professionals – Health care managers as a critical component of the health care workforce – Incentives in health care: the shift in emphasis from the implicit to the explicit – Enhancing working conditions – Reshaping the regulation of the workforce in European health care systems – The challenges of transition in CEE and the NIS of the former USSR – The impact of EU law and policy – Moving forward: building a strategic framework for the development of the health care workforce – Index.

288pp   0 335 21855 5 (Paperback)   0 335 21856 3 (Hardback)

PURCHASING TO IMPROVE HEALTH SYSTEMS PERFORMANCE

Edited by Josep Figueras, Ray Robinson and Elke Jakubowski

Purchasing is championed as key to improving health systems performance. However, despite the central role the purchasing function plays in many health system reforms, there is very little evidence about its development or its real impact on societal object-ives. This book addresses this gap and provides:

- A comprehensive account of the theory and practice of purchasing for health services across Europe
- An up-to-date analysis of the evidence on different approaches to purchasing
- Support for policy-makers and practitioners as they formulate purchasing strategies so that they can increase effectiveness and improve performance in their own national context
- An assessment of the intersecting roles of citizens, the government and the providers

Written by leading health policy analysts, this book is essential reading for health policy makers, planners and managers as well as researchers and students in the field of health studies.

Contributors
Toni Ashton, Philip Berman, Michael Borowitz, Helmut Brand, Reinhard Busse, Andrea Donatini, Martin Dlouhy, Antonio Duran, Tamás Evetovits, André P. van den Exter, Josep Figueras, Nick Freemantle, Julian Forder, Péter Gaál, Chris Ham, Brian Hardy, Petr Hava, David Hunter, Danguole Jankauskiene, Maris Jesse, Ninel Kadyrova, Joe Kutzin, John Langenbrunner, Donald W. Light, Hans Maarse, Nicholas Mays, Martin McKee, Eva Orosz, John Øvretveit, Dominique Polton, Alexander S. Preker, Thomas A. Rathwell, Sabine Richard, Ray Robinson, Andrei Rys, Constantino Sakellarides, Sergey Shishkin, Peter C. Smith, Markus Schneider, Francesco Taroni, Marcial Velasco-Garrido, Miriam Wiley.

Contents
List of tables – List of boxes – List of figures – List of contributors – Series Editors' intro-duction – Foreword – Acknowledgements – **Part One** *– Introduction – Organization of purchasing in Europe – Purchasing to improve health systems –* **Part Two** *– Theories of purchasing – Role of markets and competition – Purchasers as the public's agent – Purchas-ing to promote population health – Steering the purchaser: Stewardship and government – Purchasers, providers and contracts – Purchasing for quality of care – Purchasing and paying providers – Responding to purchasing: Provider perspectives – Index.*

320pp   0 335 21367 7 (Paperback)   0 335 21368 5 (Hardback)

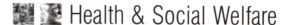
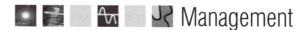
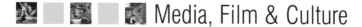
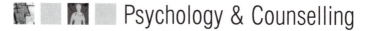
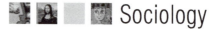
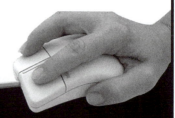